# New Approaches for the Discovery of Pharmacologically-Active Natural Compounds

# New Approaches for the Discovery of Pharmacologically-Active Natural Compounds

Special Issue Editor

**José L. Medina-Franco**

MDPI • Basel • Beijing • Wuhan • Barcelona • Belgrade

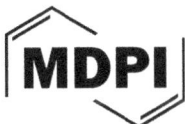

**MDPI**

*Special Issue Editor*
José L. Medina-Franco
National Autonomous University of
Mexico (UNAM)
Mexico


*Editorial Office*
MDPI
St. Alban-Anlage 66
4052 Basel, Switzerland

This is a reprint of articles from the Special Issue published online in the open access journal *Education Sciences* (ISSN 2227-7102) from 2018 to 2019 (available at: https://www.mdpi.com/journal/education/special_issues/Visible_Learning)

For citation purposes, cite each article independently as indicated on the article page online and as indicated below:

LastName, A.A.; LastName, B.B.; LastName, C.C. Article Title. *Journal Name* **Year**, *Article Number*, Page Range.

ISBN 978-3-03921-104-3 (Pbk)
ISBN 978-3-03921-105-0 (PDF)

# About the Special Issue Editor

**José L. Medina-Franco** holds a BSc (1998) and an MSc and Ph.D. degree (2005) in Chemistry. In 2005, Dr. Medina- Franco joined the University of Arizona as a postdoctoral fellow and was named Assistant Member at the Torrey Pines Institute for Molecular Studies in Florida in August 2007. In 2013, he conducted research at the Mayo Clinic, and in 2014, he joined UNAM as Principal Investigator and Full Time Research Professor. He currently leads the DIFACQUIM research group at UNAM.

Since 2007, Dr. Medina-Franco has been a member of the National Researcher System, National Council of Science and Technology in Mexico at the highest level (III). In 2016, he was appointed as Research Collaborator of the Mayo Clinic and in 2017, he was named Fellow of the Royal Society of Chemistry (UK).

Dr. Medina-Franco has published more than 200 peer-reviewed papers, 20 chapters in books, and has issued one international patent. He has edited the books Epi-Informatics and Food Informatics. He serves as an Associate Editor for the journals RSC Advances and Molecular Diversity.

Since 2007, he has been the principal investigator in several research grants funded by government institutions and pharmaceutical companies.

# Contents

*biomolecules*

MDPI

*Editorial*

# New Approaches for the Discovery of Pharmacologically-Active Natural Compounds

José L. Medina-Franco

Department of Pharmacy, National Autonomous University of Mexico, Mexico City 04510, Mexico;
medinajl@unam.com.mx; Tel.: +5255-5622-3899

Received: 21 March 2019; Accepted: 22 March 2019; Published: 23 March 2019

Natural products continue to be a major source of active compounds. Natural products from different sources have provided a large number of molecules approved for clinical use or that have been used as the starting points of optimization programs [1,2]. Similarly, natural products have inspired the synthesis and development of biologically active molecules [3,4]. However, identifying pharmacologically active natural products in an efficient and systematic manner is not an easy task. To this end, a broad range of experimental and computational approaches have emerged and evolved in recent years, boosted by the progress in the technological advances of screening strategies. In many cases, both experimental and theoretical methods are used in synergy [5,6].

This special issue includes nine papers including eight full articles and one review paper from more than 45 scientists from around the world. The papers illustrate the development and/or application of a broad range of computational and experimental techniques applied to natural product research. As described below, several papers also integrate either the creation or the mining of compound databases and web-based resources open to the scientific community interested in research into natural products.

The issue begins with the article by Prieto-Martínez et al. describing the computational and experimental characterization of the flavonoid amentoflavone as a novel inhibitor of bromodomain 4 [7]. The computational studies were performed with docking using four algorithms. This work is an example of a successful synergistic combination of informatic methods with natural products and experimental validation. The work of González et al. discussed the biological activity of a diterpenoid previously extracted from the octocoral *Pseudopterogorgia acerosa* [8]. The marine natural product inhibited the proteasomal chymotrypsin-like activity of murine macrophages in the presence of lipopolysaccharide, but not in its absence. The authors also conducted docking simulations that provided a hypothesis regarding the inhibitory activity of the chymotrypsin-like activity. Loza-Mejía et al. reported on an in silico study of secondary metabolites isolated from plants of the *Calceolaria* genus as bioinsecticides [9]. The compounds were docked with three molecular targets, namely; acetylcholinesterase, prophenoloxidase, and the ecdysone receptor. The findings of the informatics studies were in good agreement with previously published experimental results. In the same work, the authors concluded that verbascoside is a promising candidate for the development of a multitarget insecticide. Soo Moon et al. presented the results of the synthesis of new derivatives of ginsenosides that are distinctive triterpenoidal saponins considered to be responsible for most of the pharmacological activities of *Panax ginseng* (Korean ginseng). One of the newly synthesized compounds, α-glycosylated ginsenoside F1 had increased solubility, lower cytotoxicity toward human dermal fibroblast cells, and higher tyrosinase activity and ultraviolet A (UVA)-induced inhibitory activity against matrix metalloproteinase-1 than the parent ginsenoside F1. The authors concluded that the new compound has potential interest in cosmetic applications [10]. In their research article, Lu et al. reported the identification of squalene in five alpine grasslands soils from the Tibetan Plateau, which is characterized by high altitude, strong solar radiation, drought, low temperatures, and thin air. To this end, the research team used the pyrolysis gas chromatography–mass spectrometry technique and concluded that the harsh environmental conditions of the Tibetan Plateau seemed to stimulate the biosynthesis of squalene. One of the significances of this work is that squalene is a natural product broadly used in the food, cosmetics, and medical industries because of its antioxidant, antistatic, and anti-carcinogenic properties [11]. Pilón-Jiménez et al. described the construction, curation, and informatic analysis of BIOFACQUIM, a compound database of natural products isolated and characterized in Mexico. The compound database is annotated with the name of the compound, source, and link to the original peer-reviewed paper that describes the characterization and potential biological evaluation. The authors mention that the compound database described in their paper is freely accessible online and will be updated [12]. Chen et al. presented the development of a novel machine learning methodology that enabled the identification of natural products in large compound databases. The algorithm can be further employed to measure the product-likeness of small-molecules and visualize atoms that are part of small molecules that are characteristic of natural products or synthetic molecules. The authors of that work have made the best performing models freely accessible [13]. Sánchez-Salgado et al. discussed a systematic literature search of flavonoids as compounds for the treatment of cholestatic liver disease and reported the results of naringenin as a representative flavonoid in an obstructive cholestasis model. The multidisciplinary team found that naringenin had beneficial effects by improving specific metabolic and liver damage biomarkers [14]. The issue ends with the review by Del Prado-Audelo et al., who reviewed the analysis of the chemical composition and the main mechanisms for brain applications of curcumin. The review paper also covered the application of nanoparticles with curcumin and their extensive health benefit applications [15].

In all, the papers in this special issue illustrate examples of the recent progress on the technological advances and applications of different approaches to identify pharmacologically active natural products. Our aim is that the research presented here contributes to advance the field and further encourages multidisciplinary teams and young scientists and students to further advance the discovery of pharmacologically-active natural compounds.

## References

1. Newman, D.J. From natural products to drugs. *Phys. Sci. Rev.* **2018**. [CrossRef]
2. Rodrigues, T.; Reker, D.; Schneider, P.; Schneider, G. Counting on natural products for drug design. *Nat. Chem.* **2016**, *8*, 531. [CrossRef] [PubMed]
3. Thomford, N.; Senthebane, D.; Rowe, A.; Munro, D.; Seele, P.; Maroyi, A.; Dzobo, K. Natural products for drug discovery in the 21st century: Innovations for novel drug discovery. *Int. J. Mol. Sci.* **2018**, *19*, 1578. [CrossRef] [PubMed]
4. Yao, H.; Liu, J.; Xu, S.; Zhu, Z.; Xu, J. The structural modification of natural products for novel drug discovery. *Expert Opin. Drug Discov.* **2017**, *12*, 121–140. [CrossRef] [PubMed]
5. Chen, Y.; de Bruyn Kops, C.; Kirchmair, J. Data resources for the computer-guided discovery of bioactive natural products. *J. Chem. Inf. Model.* **2017**, *57*, 2099–2111. [CrossRef] [PubMed]
6. Saldívar-González, F.I.; Gómez-García, A.; Chávez-Ponce de León, D.E.; Sánchez-Cruz, N.; Ruiz-Rios, J.; Pilón-Jiménez, B.A.; Medina-Franco, J.L. Inhibitors of DNA methyltransferases from natural sources: A computational perspective. *Front. Pharmacol.* **2018**, *9*, 1144. [CrossRef] [PubMed]
7. Prieto-Martínez, F.D.; Medina-Franco, J.L. Flavonoids as putative epi-modulators: Insight into their binding mode with BRD4 bromodomains using molecular docking and dynamics. *Biomolecules* **2018**, *8*, 61. [CrossRef] [PubMed]
8. González, Y.; Doens, D.; Cruz, H.; Santamaria, R.; Gutiérrez, M.; Llanes, A.; Fernández, P.L. A marine diterpenoid modulates the proteasome activity in murine macrophages stimulated with lps. *Biomolecules* **2018**, *8*, 109. [CrossRef] [PubMed]
9. Loza-Mejía, M.A.; Salazar, J.R.; Sánchez-Tejeda, J.F. In silico studies on compounds derived from calceolaria: Phenylethanoid glycosides as potential multitarget inhibitors for the development of pesticides. *Biomolecules* **2018**, *8*, 121. [CrossRef] [PubMed]

10. Moon, S.S.; Lee, H.J.; Mathiyalagan, R.; Kim, Y.J.; Yang, D.U.; Lee, D.Y.; Min, J.W.; Jimenez, Z.; Yang, D.C. Synthesis of a novel alpha-glucosyl ginsenoside f1 by cyclodextrin glucanotransferase and its in vitro cosmetic applications. *Biomolecules* **2018**, *8*, 142. [CrossRef] [PubMed]

11. Lu, X.; Ma, S.; Chen, Y.; Yangzom, D.; Jiang, H. Squalene found in alpine grassland soils under a harsh environment in the Tibetan plateau, China. *Biomolecules* **2018**, *8*, 154. [CrossRef] [PubMed]

12. Pilón-Jiménez, B.A.; Saldívar-González, F.I.; Díaz-Eufracio, B.I.; Medina-Franco, J.L. BIOFACQUIM: A Mexican compound database of natural products. *Biomolecules* **2019**, *9*, 31. [CrossRef] [PubMed]

13. Chen, Y.; Stork, C.; Hirte, S.; Kirchmair, J. NP-scout: Machine learning approach for the quantification and visualization of the natural product-likeness of small molecules. *Biomolecules* **2019**, *9*, 43. [CrossRef] [PubMed]

14. Sánchez-Salgado, J.C.; Estrada-Soto, S.; García-Jimenez, S.; Montes, S.; Gómez-Zamudio, J.; Villalobos-Molina, R. Analysis of flavonoids bioactivity for cholestatic liver disease: Systematic literature search and experimental approaches. *Biomolecules* **2019**, *9*, 102. [CrossRef] [PubMed]

15. Del Prado-Audelo, M.L.; Caballero-Floran, I.H.; Meza-Toledo, J.A.; Mendoza-Munoz, N.; González-Torres, M.; Floran, B.; Cortés, H.; Leyva-Gómez, G. Formulations of curcumin nanoparticles for brain diseases. *Biomolecules* **2019**, *9*, 56. [CrossRef] [PubMed]

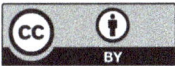

*biomolecules*

MDPI

*Review*

# Formulations of Curcumin Nanoparticles for Brain Diseases

María L. Del Prado-Audelo [1], Isaac H. Caballero-Florán [2,3], Jorge A. Meza-Toledo [3,4], Néstor Mendoza-Muñoz [5], Maykel González-Torres [6,7], Benjamín Florán [2], Hernán Cortés [8,*] and Gerardo Leyva-Gómez [3,*]

[1] Laboratorio de Posgrado en Tecnología Farmacéutica, FES-Cuautitlán, Universidad Nacional Autónoma de México, Cuautitlán Izcalli 54740, Mexico; ml.delprado@iim.unam.mx

[2] Departamento de Fisiología, Biofísica & Neurociencias, Centro de Investigación y de Estudios Avanzados del Instituto Politécnico Nacional, Ciudad de México 07360, Mexico; hiram.qfohead@gmail.com (I.H.C.-F.); bfloran@fisio.cinvestav.mx (B.F.)

[3] Departamento de Farmacia, Facultad de Química, Universidad Nacional Autónoma de México, Ciudad Universitaria, Circuito Exterior S/N, Del. Coyoacán, C.P. Ciudad de México 04510, Mexico; jamtoledo90@outlook.com

[4] Escuela de Ciencias de la Salud, Universidad del Valle de México, Campus Coyoacán, Ciudad de México, 04910, Mexico

[5] Facultad de Ciencias Químicas, Universidad de Colima, C.P. Colima 28400, México; nmendoza0@ucol.cmx

[6] CONACyT-Laboratorio de Biotecnología, Instituto Nacional de Rehabilitación Luis Guillermo Ibarra Ibarra, Ciudad de México 14389, Mexico; mikegcu@gmail.com

[7] Instituto Tecnológico y de Estudios Superiores de Monterrey, Campus Ciudad de México 14380, Mexico

[8] Laboratorio de Medicina Genómica, Departamento de Genética, Instituto Nacional de Rehabilitación Luis Guillermo Ibarra Ibarra, Ciudad de México 14389, Mexico

* Correspondence: hcortes@inr.gob.mx or hcortes_c@hotmail.com (H.C.); gerardoleyva@hotmail.com (G.L.-G.); Tel.: +52-55-59991000 (ext. 14710) (H.C.); +52-55-56223899 (ext. 44408) (G.L.-G.)

Received: 14 December 2018; Accepted: 1 February 2019; Published: 8 February 2019

**Abstract:** Curcumin is a polyphenol that is obtained from *Curcuma longa* and used in various areas, such as food and textiles. Curcumin has important anti-inflammatory and antioxidant properties that allow it to be applied as treatment for several emerging pathologies. Remarkably, there are an elevated number of publications deriving from the terms "curcumin" and "curcumin brain diseases", which highlights the increasing impact of this polyphenol and the high number of study groups investigating their therapeutic actions. However, its lack of solubility in aqueous media, as well as its poor bioavailability in biological systems, represent limiting factors for its successful application. In this review article, the analysis of its chemical composition and the pivotal mechanisms for brain applications are addressed in a global manner. Furthermore, we emphasize the use of nanoparticles with curcumin and the benefits that have been reached as an example of the extensive advances in this area of health.

**Keywords:** curcumin; nanoparticles; inflammation; protein aggregation; brain diseases; Alzheimer's disease; Parkinson's disease

## 1. Introduction

Curcumin is an active natural polyphenol component of *Curcuma longa*. Due to its chemical structure, this molecule could be applied in several different fields, such as food, textile, and the pharmaceutical industry. It has been shown that curcumin possess anti-inflammatory and antioxidant properties [1,2]. It also presents a spread spectrum of molecular targets such as transcription factors and their receptors, growth factors, cytokines, genes, and adhesion molecules. For example, curcumin could inhibit the cell signaling pathway of nuclear factor kappa B (NF-κB), which is an important cellular target of cancer cells [3–5]. Additionally, the blockade of NF-κB triggers the reduction in the expression of different NF-κB-regulated products, such as tumor necrosis factor alpha (TNF-α), interleukin 8 (IL-8), and cyclooxygenase 2 (COX-2), which play key roles in the inflammation process [6]. Furthermore, it has been recently demonstrated that curcumin may inhibit protein aggregation, such as amyloid-β (Aβ) protein, which is related to several neurological pathologies, such as Alzheimer's disease (AD) [7].

For these reasons, in recent years, there has been an increasing interest in curcumin-based treatments as managements for many disorders, such as brain diseases. However, its poor bioavailability, low solubility in aqueous media, instability in body fluids, and elevated degradation rate have limited the therapeutic applications of this drug. Different strategies, such as the use of nanotechnology, have emerged to tackle these problems. In general, nanoparticles-based drug delivery systems present important advantages, such as a long lifetime circulation, ability to improve the drug's aqueous solubility as well the bioavailability, and the capacity to overcome physiological barriers [8–10].

Many authors have demonstrated that curcumin-loaded nanoparticles comprise a very effective and attractive treatment for several diseases. Therefore, the main objective of this work is to present an extensive review of the properties of curcumin, the nanotechnology-based curcumin delivery systems, and its potential application for the treatment of brain diseases, particularly AD, Parkinson's disease (PD), and cancer.

## 2. Curcumin Chemical Information

Chemically, curcumin is a naturally polyphenol denominated (1E,6E)-1,7-bis(4-hydroxy-3-methoxyphenyl)-1,6-heptadiene-3,5-dione) (Figure 1), which is isolated from the rhizomes of *C. longa*. From a structural point of view, there are three chemical entities in the molecule: two aromatic ring systems containing *o*-methoxy phenolic groups linked by a seven-carbon spacer consisting of an α,β-unsaturated β-diketone moiety [11]. Therefore, the diketo group exhibits keto–enol tautomerism, meaning that curcumin can exist in equilibrium between the keto and the enol tautomer. However, nuclear magnetic resonance (NMR) studies carried out on a variety of solvents concluded that the enol form of curcumin is essentially the only form of this molecule in solution [12]. The relevance of the tautomerism was explored by Yanagizawa et al. [13]; these authors suggested that curcumin and its analogues exist predominantly in the enol form during binding to Aβ fibrils/aggregates, in turn suggesting that the enolization of curcumin derivatives is crucial for binding to Aβ aggregates in the treatment of AD. In this respect, some physicochemical properties are described below.

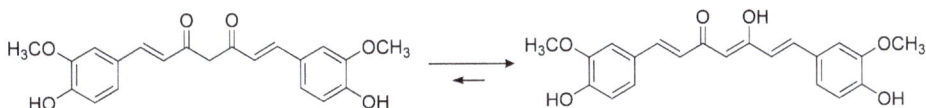

**Figure 1.** Chemical structure of curcumin and keto–enol tautomerism.

### 2.1. Thermal Analysis of Curcumin

Thermogravimetric analysis is a common complementary tool to describe this molecule. Therefore, we performed an evaluation of the thermal degradation of curcumin at a heating rate of 10 °C/min and under a nitrogen atmosphere. As can be observed in Figure 2a, the initial temperature of the mass loss is approximately 193 °C. This behavior results in the decomposition of the turmeric powder; below this temperature, weight loss in the curcumin follows a gradual decrease related to the loss of moisture. In a complementary way, a differential scanning calorimetry thermogram (Figure 2b) showed a melting temperature for curcumin of 174.05 °C, which is in agreement with data reported previously [14].

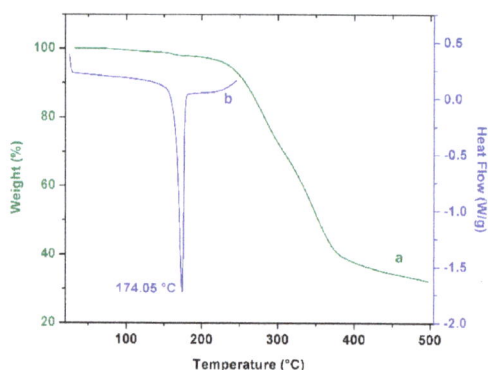

**Figure 2.** Thermal analysis of curcumin. Thermogravimetric analysis ((a), green line) and differential scanning calorimetry ((b), blue line). Melting point of curcumin is indicated at 174.05 °C.

## 2.2. Ultraviolet-Visible Spectrophotometric Analysis of Curcumin

The chemical reactivity and solubility of curcumin depends on the medium pH in which it is dissolved; that is, under acidic conditions, curcumin exhibits moderate solubility, and the solution maintains a yellow color (Figure 3A), whereas at a neutral pH, curcumin is not fully soluble, as can be observed in Figure 3B. On the other hand, within the basic pH range, curcumin is more water-soluble than in the neutral form, and the color of the solution changes to red (Figure 3C). The color change under alkaline conditions could be an effect deriving from the deprotonation. It is known that the photophysical and photochemical properties of curcumin are related to the solvents polarity because of the keto–enol structure of curcumin that involves intramolecular proton transfer [15]. Kharat M. et al. [16] mentioned the formation of condensation yellow products (such as feruloymethane) as a potential reason for this color increment under an alkaline environment.

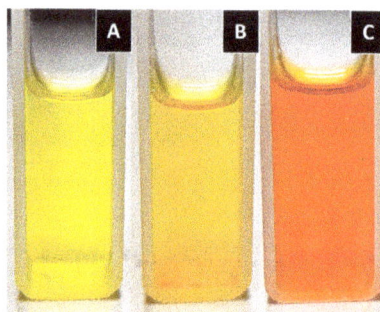

**Figure 3.** Curcumin dissolved in different mediums. (**A**) Curcumin in an acidic solution (pH 3.5); and (**B**) curcumin in a neutral solution (pH 7.4); both with the addition of 1% Tween 80 in order to increase solubility. (**C**) Curcumin in a basic solution (pH 12).

In order to corroborate the solubility of curcumin, we tested the drug incorporated in solvents with different pH levels (maintaining a concentration of eight mg/mL), through ultraviolet (UV)-vis spectrophotometry. Figure 4 depicts that at a neutral pH (lines a and b), the maximum absorption peak of curcumin was found at 420 nm, which is in agreement with the literature [17], while the maximum absorption in alkaline pH was found at 470 nm (Figure 4, line c). This result is in agreement with the reported by Priyadarsini [11], who reported that the maximum absorption peak of the fully deprotonated curcumin is found at 467 nm under alkaline conditions (>pH 10).

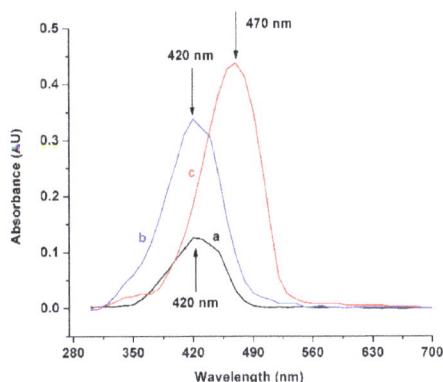

**Figure 4.** Ultraviolet-Visible spectrophotometric scanning of curcumin. (a) Absorption in methanol, maximum peak of absorption found at 420 nm; (b) Absorption in neutral medium, maximum peak of absorption found at 420 nm; and (c) Absorption in basic medium, maximum peak of absorption found at 470 nm.

### 2.3. Fourier Transform Infrared Spectroscopy of Curcumin

Infrared spectroscopy is commonly employed to study the molecules' chemical structure; a curcumin spectrum is shown in Figure 5. As depicted, the characteristic band of the O—H bond stretching appears at 3506 cm$^{-1}$. The infrared (IR) band at 2915 cm$^{-1}$ and its doublet at 2847 cm$^{-1}$ are due to the asymmetric and symmetric stretching vibrations of the C–H$_2$ group. For C–C stretching, a peak at 1624 cm$^{-1}$ is found. The C=O stretching vibration of the carboxylic groups (methyl esters and triglycerides) can be attributed to the strong band at 1510 cm$^{-1}$ [18]. In plane C–OH bending vibration can be assigned to the IR bands at 1375 cm$^{-1}$. Curcumin shows a peak at around 1270 cm$^{-1}$, which corresponds to the C—O stretching frequency of the ether group in curcumin. The peaks at 729 cm$^{-1}$, 806 cm$^{-1}$, and 955 cm$^{-1}$ indicate the bending vibrations of the —CH bond of the alkene group [19].

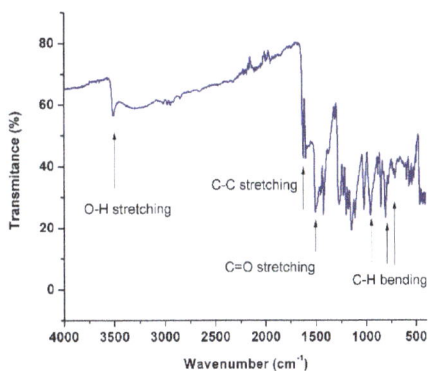

**Figure 5.** Fourier transform infrared spectroscopy of curcumin. Characteristic bands of the molecule are indicated with arrows.

## 2.4. Solubility

Curcumin has poor solubility in water (an estimated of 3.21 mg/L at 25 °C); however, it is soluble in ethanol, dimethyl sulfoxide (DMSO), methanol, acetonitrile, chloroform, and ethyl acetate [11,20]. The theoretical Hansen solubility parameters (HSP), which were calculated on the basis of the group contribution method, are $\delta_d = 17.46$, $\delta_p = 3.66$, $\delta_h = 13.84$, and $\delta_{total} = 22.46$ for the enol form of curcumin [21]. The first $pKa_1 = 7.5–8.5$ corresponds to the deprotonation of the enolic proton group, while $pKa_2 = 8.5–10.4$ and $pKa_3 = 9.5–10.7$ are for the phenolic protons, indistinctly [11]. The log octanol–water partition coefficient (log Kow) is 3.29 (estimated), conferring hydrophobic characteristics on the molecule [20].

Curcumin is unstable in aqueous and alcoholic solution, and it is more stable in acidic pH (1.2–6) than in alkaline pH (Figure 3); the degradation products found under hydrolytic conditions are: trans-6-(4'-hydroxy-3'-methoxyphenyl)-2,4-dioxo-5-hexenal, ferulic acid, ferulic aldehyde, feruloylmethane, and vanillin [22,23]. However, new evidence suggests that the major degradation product is bicyclopentadione, which is the result of the autoxidation of curcumin [24], and is formed by the oxygenation and double cyclization of the heptadienedione chain connecting the two methoxyphenol rings of curcumin [25]. Curcumin is also sensitive to light. It has been shown to decompose when it is exposed to UV/visible light, both in solution and in the solid state [26].

## 3. Biological Activity

Curcumin has a broad spectrum of biological activities. For example, it has been reported as possessing antioxidant, anti-AD, anticarcinogenic, antimutagenic, and anti-inflammatory properties (Figure 6).

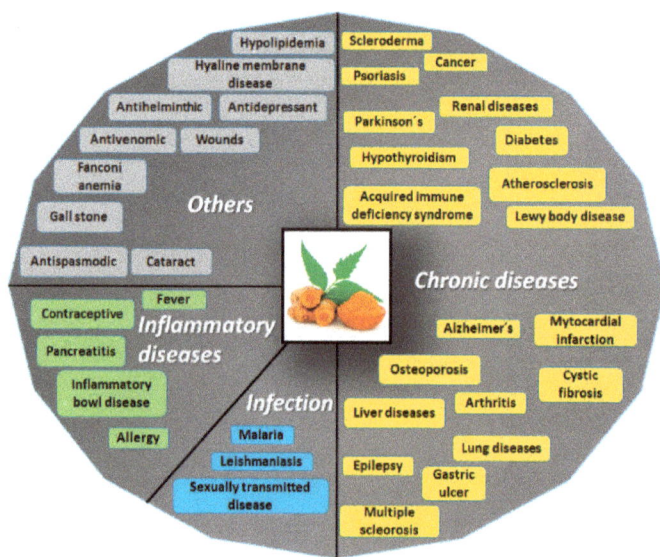

**Figure 6.** Potential applications of curcumin. Due to the structure of curcumin, this molecule could be applied as treatment for a wide range of disorders, such as chronic diseases, inflammatory disorders, infections of diverse etiology, and other conditions. Adapted with permission from [26]. 2007, Springer Nature.

With respect to antioxidant activity, evidence has shown that curcumin can directly scavenge several free radicals as the result of its two phenolic sites. Likewise, curcumin has been effective against the generation of reactive oxygen species (ROS) and reactive nitrogen species (RNS) in the cellular environment. Curcumin also reduces low-density lipoprotein (LDL), and inhibits the oxidation of proteins and DNA. At the enzymatic level, curcumin inhibits lipoxygenase/cyclooxygenase and xanthine dehydrogenase/oxidase, which are two enzymes related to the generation of ROS, and upregulates superoxide dismutase and glutathione peroxidase, which are two first-line enzymes of defense against oxygen-free radicals [22].

In AD, curcumin protects against Aβ-induced oxidative stress, prevents the formation and extension of Aβ fibrils, destabilizes Aβ fibrils, inhibits acetylcholinesterase, decreases neuroinflammation, and sequesters transition metals [22]. A variety of structure–activity studies have proven that the three moieties in the chemical structure of curcumin play different roles in its interaction with the Aβ peptide: one of the hydroxyl substitutions in the aromatic end group is necessary for inhibition, while the other one of the hydroxyl substitutions is required for activity. Finally, the diketo chain contributes to the flexibility and correct length between aromatic rings [27]. Curcumin has been extensively evaluated and possesses potential antioxidant and anti-inflammatory activity in AD. The most important mechanism of the anti-inflammatory action of curcumin is based on the inhibition of NF-kB, which leads to the decreased formation of cytochemokines and Aβ fibrils. Other molecular targets inhibited by curcumin are inducible nitric oxide synthase (iNOs), c-Jun N-terminal kinase (JNK) activation, and activating protein-1 (AP-1) [28].

In anticancer therapy, curcumin inhibits oxidative stress, reduces lipid peroxidation and DNA single-strand breakage, inhibits the COX-1 and COX-2 enzymes, suppresses NF-kB activation, and possesses antiproliferative effects. Moreover, it induces apoptosis by targeting mitochondria, and affects tumor protein p53 (p53)-related signaling [22]. The specific molecular targets for curcumin that are therapeutically important in cancer-signaling pathways include cyclin-dependent kinases (CDKs), p53, Ras, phosphoinositide 3-kinase (PI3K), Protein kinase B (Akt), Wnt/β-catenin, and mammalian target of rapamycin (mTOR) [29]. During angiogenesis, curcumin can inhibit and/or downregulate the expression of various pro-angiogenic growth factors such as the vascular endothelial growth factor (VEGF), fibroblast growth factor (FGF), and the endothelial growth factor (EGF) [30]. An overview of the molecular targets of curcumin is represented in Figure 7.

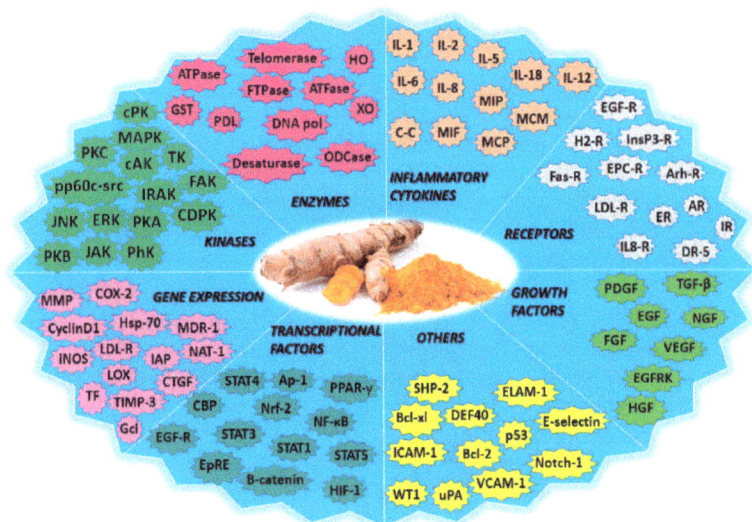

**Figure 7.** Curcumin is a pleiotropic agent with multiple molecular targets. This molecule could modify the expression of genes, inflammatory cytokines, transcriptional and growth factors, enzymes, and receptors, among others. Adapted with permission from [26]. 2007, Springer Nature.

### 3.1. Effect of Curcumin on Aggregation Protein

Protein aggregation is the process by which misfolded proteins assume a conformation that cause their polymerization into aggregates and organized fibrils. The adequate aggregation of protein is a precise progression that requires extensive guidance from an excellent control network, which comprises approximately 800 proteins in humans. Many neurodegenerative diseases are associated with inappropriate protein aggregation [31]. These neuronal diseases include disorders in which the aggregates may accumulate in the nucleus, such as for example in polyglutamine expansion diseases (such as spinocerebellar ataxias and Huntington's disease (HD)), which are pathologies that are characterized by inclusions in cytoplasm (for example, α-synuclein in PD), disorders in which the aggregates are found outside of the cell (prion diseases), or both intracellularly and extracellularly (such as Aβ in AD) [31].

The effect of curcumin on prion disease has been studied by several authors. Hafner-Bratkovič et al. [32] reported that the binding of curcumin to the α-intermediate could block conformational change into the β-structure, and that the binding of curcumin to prion fibrils could prevent further growth, thus, the formation of new seeds. Similarly, Caughey et al. [33] concluded in their work that curcumin inhibits prion protein resistance (PrP-Res) accumulation in neuroblastoma cells infected with the scrapie agent. In addition, these authors reported the partial inhibition of the conversion of PrP into PrP-res.

Additionally, Pandey et al. [34] analyzed the curcumin effect both in vitro and in cell culture models of α-synuclein aggregation. The authors concluded that curcumin induces the inhibition of α-synuclein aggregation in a dose-dependent manner. Also, their results suggested that curcumin increased α-synuclein solubility in cells containing aggregates.

The oligomerization of α-synuclein aggregates is structurally similar to the Aβ-protein aggregates of AD. Therefore, curcumin has been investigated as a potential AD treatment. Brahmkhatri et al. [35] reported that curcumin-loaded gold nanoparticles inhibited Aβ aggregation, and that these were capable of dissolving aggregates. Likewise, Mithu et al. [36] reported that curcumin disorganizes Aβ fibrils; the disruption of Aβ-fibrils was achieved by means of structural changes in the salt bridge region and near the C terminus. A more detailed report on the inhibition of Aβ aggregation revealed that, besides curcumin inhibiting fibril formation in vitro, it also inhibited the formation of Aβ oligomers and their toxicity in vivo [37].

It has been reported that amyloid formation could be limited by mechanisms such as metal chelation [38], and reducing the induction of the β-secretase enzyme (BACE1) by proinflammatory cytokines [39]. It has been suggested that BACE1 has a main role in the initiation of the formation of Aβ [40]; therefore, it is an attractive drug target for AD. The sequential proteolytic cleavage of the Aβ precursor protein (APP), which is a type I transmembrane protein, produced the formation of Aβ.

Zhang et al. [7] studied the interaction between curcumin and Aβ. These authors proposed the modulation of APP levels in the secretory pathway as the cellular mechanism by which curcumin reduces Aβ levels. In addition, they reported that the use of curcumin considerably increased the retention of immature APP in the endoplasmic reticulum. Furthermore, the authors suggested that APP endocytosis could be attenuated by treatment with curcumin.

In order to identify the chemical features that are most important for preventing Aβ accumulation, Reinke et al. [27] examined the effect of three features on the inhibition of amyloid aggregation: the presence of aromatic groups at both extremes of the molecule, the substitution pattern of these aromatics, and the distance and flexibility of the linker section. They demonstrated that the presence of just one single aromatic group did not decrease the protein aggregation; thus, the curcumin efficiency as an aggregation inhibitor could be related to its two phenyl groups. Also, their results suggested that the substitution of these aromatics groups is important for activity, since these are capable of taking part in hydrogen bonding. In addition, the authors reported the approximate distance between the docking sites, which are found between eight and 16 Å from each other; this is similar to the distance between the terminal aromatic regions of curcumin.

## 3.2. Effect of Curcumin in Neuroinflammation

In recent years, interest in the identification and application of natural compounds that limit neuroinflammation has been growing. The term neuroinflammation has been used to describe several different pathological events, from modifications in the morphology of glial cells to fully fledged tissue invasion and destruction by leukocytes. Neuroinflammation plays a key role in the progression of neurodegenerative diseases and in the invasion of central nervous system (CNS) parenchyma by leukocytes, it is one of its main characteristics, as well as a severe loss of the blood–brain barrier (BBB) integrity [6].

Due to the latter, lymphocytes and myeloid cells express cytokines in the tissue, increasing the inflammatory cascade. Interleukins such as IL-1β, IL-6, and IL-23, and cytokines such as TNF, interferon gamma (IFNγ), and granulocyte/macrophage colony-stimulating factor (GM-CSF), chemokines (such as CCL2, CCL5, and CXCL1), secondary messengers (nitric oxide and prostaglandins), and ROS are also mediators for the neuroinflammatory response [41]. The excessive production of these inflammatory mediators could cause neuronal damage and death. It has been demonstrated that curcumin reduces the expression of several inflammatory cytokines, including IL-1α, IL-1β, IL-6, TNF, IFNγ, and many others (Figure 8) [42,43].

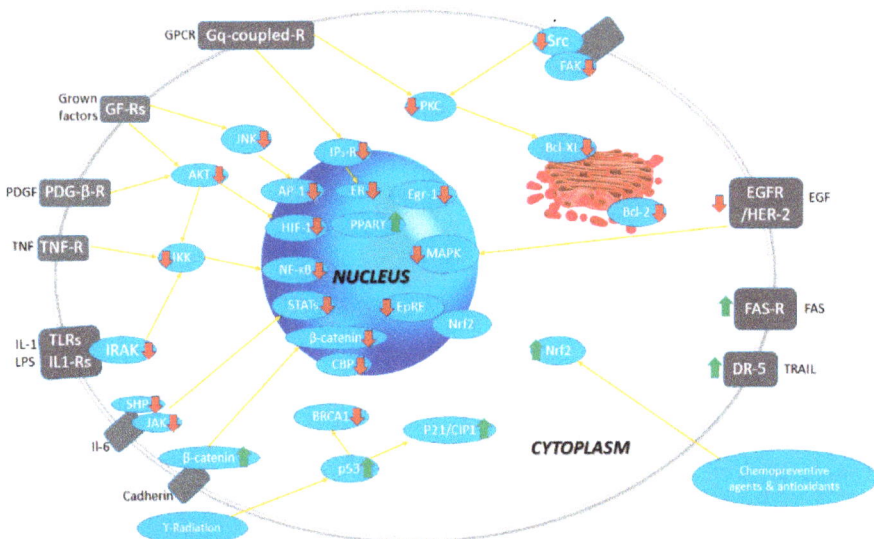

**Figure 8.** Signaling pathways modulated by curcumin. Up and green arrows indicate the intermediaries upregulated by curcumin; meanwhile, down and red arrows indicate the intermediaries downregulated by curcumin. Adapted with permission from [26]. 2007, Springer Nature.

Some authors have reported that curcumin suppresses the expression of IL-1β [44,45]. This mechanism suggests that curcumin inhibits the activation of the Nod-like receptor protein 3 (NLRP3) inflammasome, which is the most characterized inflammasome, and an important innate immune sensor. The NLRP3 inflammasome is activated by an extensive variety of signals of pathogenic, endogenous, and environmental origin. Some authors found that curcumin suppressed inflammation via a strong inhibition of NLRP3-dependent caspase-1 activation and IL-1 β secretion [44].

In the same manner, Devi et al. [46] reported that curcumin could exert a direct effect on constitutive signal transducer and activator of transcription 3 (STAT3) phosphorylation. These authors also mentioned that curcumin is a potent inhibitor of IL-6 expression in stromal cells. They suggested that this inhibition was related to the IκB kinase (IKK)/NF-κB pathway. Likewise, NF-κB is a ubiquitous transcription factor; its activation is linked with the promotion or inhibition of apoptosis, depending on the cell type and condition. Likewise, the inflammatory response induced by TNF-α is strongly linked to the activation of NF-kB.

On the other hand, TNF-α is a very important inflammatory mediator; thus, its reduction is a therapeutic target in several inflammatory diseases [47]. For the interaction of the TNF-α and curcumin, Wang et al. [4] found inhibition in the expression of this factor through downregulating the expression of NF-κB. These authors reported that curcumin reduced the transcription and secretion of TNF-α, and also IL-6, which is induced by palmitate, and induces the nuclear translocation of NF-κB in a concentration-dependent manner [48,49].

Similarly, the suppression of CCL2 function may decrease the attraction of cells of the immune system to the sites of inflammation, which could result in a slowdown of the advancement of inflammation [50]. Zhang et al. [51] investigated the inhibitory effect of curcumin on lipopolysaccharide (LPS)-induced chemokine CCL production. First, these authors induced the upregulation of CCL2 mRNA and protein in C6 cells, utilizing one μg/mL of LPS. After this, they probed three doses of curcumin as treatments (2.5 μM, 10 μM, and 25 μM), and found that the expression of CCL2 mRNA decreased with these concentrations in a dose-dependent manner. Moreover, their results suggested that in astrocytoma cells, curcumin induces the downregulation of CCL2 expression through the JNK pathway. However, it appears that CCL2 could be inhibited by curcumin through other pathways besides the JNK pathway. Herman et al. [52] suggested that curcumin downregulates CCL2 activity via the inhibition of protein kinase C (PKC) and matrix metalloproteinases.

On the other hand, IFN-γ exerts important effects on epithelial integrity, promotes barrier dysfunction, and increases epithelial permeability through numerous mechanisms. The loss of integrity in BBB is involved in neuronal diseases. For example, Midura-Kiela et al. [53] studied the interaction of IFN-γ and curcumin in epithelial cells. They concluded that curcumin induces the inhibition of the signaling of IFN-γ. Furthermore, curcumin also inhibits the COX-2 pathway. COX-2 is overexpressed in malignant tissues. Accordingly, its inhibition could be a key to cancer and tumor treatments.

*3.3. Effect of Curcumin on Oxidative Stress*

Although oxygen plays an important role in energy production processes in cells (ATP), this molecule could be transformed into very toxic forms in the cells, which are denominated ROS [54]. Antioxidant systems are complex and act in concert to decrease the ROS load. A process known as oxidative stress occurs if an imbalance between ROS and antioxidant systems takes place in favor of oxidants. Oxidative stress has been related to mechanisms leading to neuronal cell injury in various neuronal diseases.

Antioxidants are compounds that can prevent biomolecules from undergoing oxidative damage through free radical-mediated reactions [55]. The majority of the antioxidants present a phenolic group or a β-diketone group in their structure [56].

To explain the protective properties of phenolic groups in antioxidants, two different mechanisms have been proposed. In the first mechanism (Equation (1)), the free radical becomes a radical by hydrogen atom transfer from the antioxidant (ArOH). This antioxidant activity is related to phenolic O–H bond dissociation enthalpy (BDE); thus, if the O–H bond attraction is weak, free radical inactivation will be easier.

In the second mechanism, the free radical receives an electron from the antioxidant. The free radical becomes a radical cation, which could be reacting with another antioxidant molecule (Equations (2) and (3)). In terms of this mechanism, the important parameter to analyze for antioxidant activity is the ionization potential (IP). With a low IP, electron abstraction will be easier. In addition to BDE and IP, proton dissociation enthalpy, proton affinity (PA), and electron transfer enthalpy are important factors for evaluating antioxidant activity [55,57].

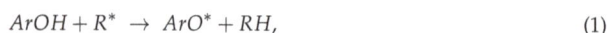

$$ArOH + R^* \rightarrow ArO^* + RH, \tag{1}$$

$$ArOH + R^* \rightarrow ArOH^* + R^-, \tag{2}$$

$$ArOH + R^- \rightarrow ArO^* + RH. \tag{3}$$

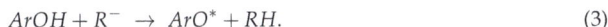

As previously mentioned, curcumin possesses a wide range of biological functions, including antioxidant activity. Curcumin contains a variety of functional groups, including phenolic rings that act as electron traps to prevent $H_2O_2$ production and scavenge superoxide radicals, the β-diketo group that is involved in metal–ligand complexation, and carbon–carbon double bonds (Figure 9) [56,58]; together, these provide the molecule with unique antioxidant properties.

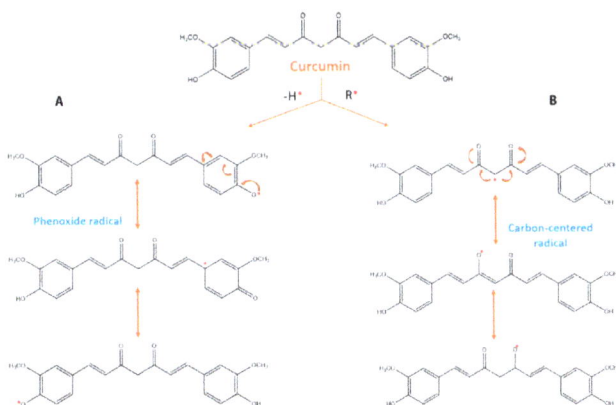

**Figure 9.** Antioxidant mechanism of curcumin. There are two mechanisms to form phenoxyl radicals. The first mechanism (**A**) begins by initial electron transfer to the free radical; thus, a radical cation is formed, which produces a phenoxyl radical by a proton loss. The second mechanism (**B**) is related to direct hydrogen abstraction. Based on the bond dissociation energies, many authors suggest that the most susceptible target for free radicals in curcumin is phenolic OH.

Under acidic to neutral conditions (pH = 3−7), the keto conformation is the major form. On the other hand, under basic conditions (pH > 8), the enol conformation is predominant, which presents powerful free radical-scavenger properties [59].

Using erythrocyte sedimentation rate (ESR), the reduction of ferric iron in aqueous medium, and intracellular ROS/toxicity assays, Barzegar et al. [60] analyzed the antioxidant properties of curcumin. Their results demonstrated that curcumin confers protection on the cells against the mortal effects of cumene hydroperoxide.

In addition, Zbarsky et al. [58] applied, in the unilateral 6-hydroxydopamine (6-OHDA) rat model of PD, natural compounds, with phenolic groups in their structure to evaluate the neuroprotection level. These authors reported that, with the sub-chronic administration of curcumin, the loss of dopaminergic neurons in the *substantia nigra pars compacta* was reduced significantly.

The antioxidant protective effect of curcumin was also evaluated against hemin-induced neuronal death. In 2013, González-Reyes et al. [61] evaluated the neuroprotection of curcumin in the primary cultures of the cerebellar granule neurons of rats. They concluded that the use of curcumin as a pretreatment induces antioxidant protection against hemin-induced neuronal death.

The antioxidant effect of curcumin has been evaluated in other applications in addition to neuronal pathologies. For example, Haryuna et al. [62] investigated the antioxidant action of curcumin against oxidative stress caused by diabetes mellitus. These authors worked with cochlear fibroblasts in rat models of diabetes mellitus, and reported that curcumin confers antioxidant protection via the increased expression of superoxide dismutase. These results showed that curcumin presents a wide range of applications.

## 4. Limitation of Chemical Properties and New Proposals

There are two main limitations when curcumin is formulated for therapeutic purposes: limited solubility in water and low permeability [63]. In addition, the low permeability is related to chemical degradation, a high rate of biotransformation, especially glucuronidation and sulfation [22], and rapid systemic elimination, resulting in low curcumin absorption and poor bioavailability. Therefore, curcumin can be classified as a BCS Class IV molecule. In fact, the majority of oral curcumin is excreted in the feces—about 90%—and the rest in urine (6%) after 72 hours in rats [64]. Consequently, high doses of curcumin are necessary to produce detectable plasma concentrations. For example, in a human clinical trial, 3.6 g of curcumin via the oral route was found to produce a plasma curcumin level of 11.1 nmol/L after one hour of dosing on days one, two, eight, and 29 of the administration [65]. Due to these limitations, novel drug delivery systems have been proposed to increase the bioavailability of curcumin.

## 5. New Formulations of Curcumin

As previously mentioned, one of the reasons that curcumin has poor bioavailability is due to its limited solubility in water; therefore, one of the directions in the development of new formulations for this molecule (as for other lipophilic compounds) is to increase solubility, following strategies such as modification of the solid state, reduction of particle size, the creation of supersaturated solutions, or the encapsulation into nanoparticles. Some new formulations are briefly described later.

Amorphous solid dispersions (ASD) are an interesting strategy of modification of the solid state to improve the rate of dissolution of drugs, and thus their bioavailability. Solid dispersion involves the incorporation of water-insoluble compounds into a hydrophilic carrier matrix. In a study performed by Gangurde et al. [66], the authors demonstrated that curcumin formulated in an Eudragit E (Evonik Nutrition & Care GmbH, Essen, Germany) polymeric matrix dissolved more rapidly (20–45% release after 60 min) than curcumin alone (2–5% release after 120 min) at pH 1.2. Solubility also was increased: with curcumin alone, solubility was 0.02%, whereas curcumin containing Eudragit E (Evonik Nutrition & Care GmbH) exhibited solubility of 40.29% and 18.78% by the spray-drying and rotoevaporation techniques, respectively. In other studies, curcumin revealed an increase of >1000 times when it was formulated as ASD in hydroxypropyl methylcellulose matrixes [67].

Nanosuspension is a carrier-free nanoparticle system containing only pure drug crystals, and is sometimes accompanied by a stabilizer. Nanosuspension can greatly increase the saturation solubility as well as the dissolution velocity (by increasing the superficial area). Curcumin has been formulated as a nanosuspension with good results. For example, Wang et al. [68] found an increase in the oral bioavailability of curcumin of about three to four times after the administration of curcumin in nanosuspensions in rats. Similarly, Li et al. [69] found an increase in bioavailability after the intravenous administration of a nanosuspension of about 4.2-fold compared to a curcumin solution.

Self-microemulsifying drug delivery systems (SMEDDS) are isotropic mixtures of oil, hydrophilic surfactant, and co-solvents that rapidly form oil-in-water (o/w) microemulsion upon gentle agitation followed by dilution in an aqueous medium [70]. This class of supersaturated systems has been effective in increasing the solubility of drugs at the absorption site. Formulated curcumin in SMEDDS has been proposed by Wu et al. [71]. The formulation, which is composed of 20% ethanol, 60% Cremophor RH40 (BASF Personal Care and Nutrition GmbH, Monhein, Germany) and 20% isopropyl myristate, improved the relative oral bioavailability of SMEDDS compared with the curcumin suspension by about 1213%. Similar studies conducted by other researches can be found in the references [72–74].

In addition, the encapsulation of curcumin into nanoparticles not only enhances its bioavailability and solubility (Figure 10), it also increases its stability by protecting it from the influence of the outside environment.

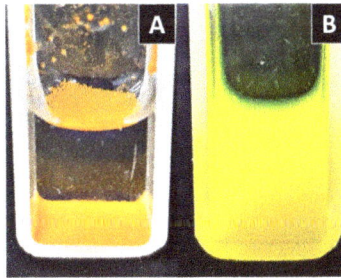

**Figure 10.** Curcumin solubility: (**A**) Curcumin showed poor solubility in aqueous medium; (**B**) the use of the nanoplatforms increased the drug solubility. Curcumin was entrapped in poly-ε-caprolactone nanoparticles stabilized by Pluronic F68 (Thermofisher, Whaltam, USA), with size of 170 nm and zeta potential of −7 mV.

Novel curcumin-nanoparticulated delivery approaches, including liposomes, polymeric nanoparticles, solid lipid nanoparticles, polymeric micelles, and others, are emerging as suitable and promising systems. This is because they can be designed and adapted to the desired size, chemical composition, surface charge, and surface functionalization, rendering them potent tools for the treatment of specific diseases such as neurodegenerative disorders and cancer [75,76]. In this review, a more detailed description on the development of formulations based on nanoparticles, specifically for neurodegenerative disorders are discussed in the following sections.

## 6. Formulations of Curcumin in Nanoparticles

Nanoparticles for medical purposes comprise a variety of drug transport systems; they traditionally have dimensions of fewer than 200 nm for brain applications, and are expandable up to 1000 nm, in concept. The small aggregation size confers a high degree of tissue penetration. Nanoparticles for medical and brain purposes are considered non-invasive systems. Although they are designed to flank and cross various tissues, their small size and composition guarantee, in the majority of cases, minimal invasion without risk. The main security provided comprises the chemical composition and the mechanisms of elimination and/or biodegradation. However, several research groups that have delved into this topic have always highlighted the need for a broad assessment in the area of nanotoxicology, because some materials, only by the change of size of aggregation from bulk to nanoparticles can increase their toxicity; contrariwise, other materials exhibit new and better properties.

Conventionally, nanoparticles for medical purposes arise from the combination of two master ideas: from Paul Ehrlich with the concept of magical bullets [77], and Richard Feynman with the notion of miniaturization [78]. However, the materialization of the investigation of new carriers for the transport of drugs to the brain with the use of nanoparticles dates from the first conceptions of Peter Speiser in 1969 [79]. Subsequently, J. Kreuter et al. [80] began the initial assessments on the coating of nanoparticles with polysorbate 80 to facilitate their passage into the CNS. These pioneering works set the standard for the development of polymeric nanoparticles. In parallel, R.H. Müller et al. [81] worked on the development of lipid nanoparticles that would later allow for wide applications in the same area.

The subsequent epochs were accompanied by pharmacokinetic and mechanistic studies at the cellular level with the intention of achieving greater degrees of vectorization. Therefore, some of the examples cited in the application of nanoparticles for the transport of curcumin to the CNS have employed as a strategy the coupling of ligands that permit targeting to the brain. Drug vectorization has advanced substantially, even to the achievement of reaching intranuclear levels in neurons. Some of the most commonly used systems for administering curcumin for the purpose of brain impairment are described below.

*6.1. Polymeric Nanoparticles*

Polymeric materials were the first to have been used to transport drugs to the brain, and a significant number of curcumin-carrying applications can be found in the literature. Some examples of traditional polymers include poly (butyl cyanoacrylate) (PBCA), poly (lactic-co-glycolic acid) (PLGA), and chitosan. In particular, the synthetic polymers PBCA and PLGA allow adequate control of the particle size, which results in highly reproducible production batches (Figure 11).

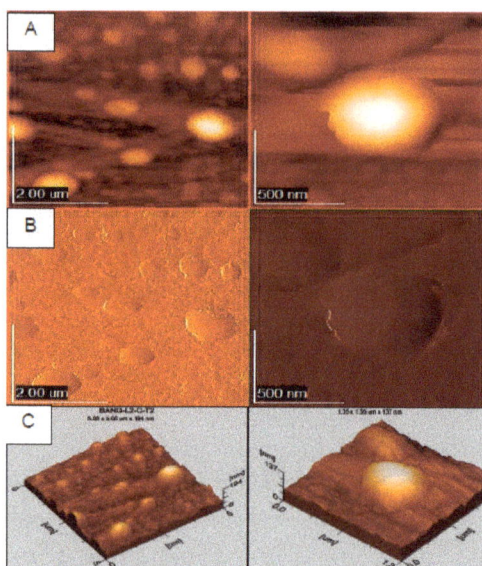

**Figure 11.** Atomic force microscopy (AFM) microscopy of curcumin poly-ε-caprolactone nanoparticles in two magnifications, left and right. Images in AFM (**A**), 2D (**B**) and 3D (**C**) mode.

Subsequent steps have been directed toward the synthesis of new polymers to couple different ligands that can permit adequate vectorization. Usually, these systems allow suitable stability with a zeta potential of at least –15 mV with polyvinyl alcohol (PVA), while with systems prepared with chitosan, although they appear very promising by the simple and rapid methods of ionic gelation, one of the disadvantages is usually the control of molecular weight. In general, PLGA polymer nanoparticles have shown adequate biocompatibility at the cellular level, and in studies in more complex biological models, even at high amounts up to one mg/mL at a cell density of $1 \times 10^4$. However, other studies have indicated that the degradation of PLGA could induce cellular damage by the generated acidic medium, although this is restricted to the amount of polymer that was administered [82].

*6.2. Lipid Nanoparticles*

Even when a broad demonstration of the biocompatibility of polymeric systems is available, doubt remains concerning their possible effects in prolonged administrations, due to the possible interactions within the nanometric range with biological systems or accumulation in some tissues. One of the main alternatives to the possible effects deriving from polymers are lipid nanoparticles. This term includes solid lipid nanoparticles and nanostructured lipid carriers. One of the great advantages of these systems is the use of lipids with high biocompatibility and biodegradation. The majority of lipid matrices are constituted of glyceride derivatives that are easily assimilated by our metabolism. We can imagine that several of these are also present in foods, and that they follow the same route of biotransformation. Therefore, this aspect is crucial in the choice of the type of nanoparticle matrix for the transport of curcumin, and it is reflected in a considerable percentage of the published information for brain diseases. The majority of production methods employ temperatures above the melting point of the lipids used. One aspect to be considered is the possible stability of lipid nanoparticles in aqueous dispersion and the exchange between polymorphic structures that can promote the expulsion of the drug. Interestingly, some lipids exhibit biological properties in addition to the nutritional aspect, and their applications are enhanced when handled in the nanometer state. Some of these demonstrate novel biological properties due to an increase in interaction with the biological environment, and to the high degree of distribution and penetration in tissues. If this were the case, the new properties that were exhibited can be complemented with the drugs encapsulated in the same system.

*6.3. Liposomes*

Liposomes are spherical vesicles with one or several layers of phospholipids with an internal aqueous compartment. They usually have a size of less than 100 nm. Due to the high percentage of phospholipids, they are also recognized as highly biocompatible and biodegradable systems. The difference with the previous systems, besides the composition, is the type of architecture. Lipid nanoparticles derive from a solid and compact matrix, and the liposomes do not; even there are some variants that confer flexibility to the structure. The development and evaluation of liposomes is evidenced by a long history in pharmaceutical technology. In fact, the first drug approved by the Food and Drug Administration (FDA) in the nano order was with liposomes, i.e., Doxil (Janssen, Titusville, FL, USA) for the treatment of certain types of cancer [83]. The long trajectory in liposome research also confers the establishment of well-implemented industrial processes that facilitate the subsequent development of similar formulations. This is somewhat different from the polymeric and lipid systems, in which there remain critical systems to be reinforced, especially when they involve high agitation speeds.

*6.4. Cyclodextrins*

Cyclodextrins are glucopyranose structures in the form of a glass with a hydrophobic interior and a hydrophilic exterior by the exposure of hydroxyl units [84]. Cyclodextrins can be used to transport drugs to different organs, and can also be derivatized to increase their vectorization. They have shown high biocompatibility for deriving from the starch. Unlike previous systems, cyclodextrins are prefabricated carriers for the direct incorporation of the cargo. In theory, competition is mentioned between the liquid medium inside the vessel and the new molecule that one wishes to enter. Therefore, it is necessary to know the constants of affinity and dissociation. As with a traditional glass, when transported to the table, the interior can spill. In the case of drugs, the cargo may also get in the way. The hydrophobic characteristic allows some lipid extraction at the BBB level, which could also facilitate passage into the brain region. Even in other pathologies, effects can be found with empty cyclodextrins due to the effect generated in lipophilic components.

*6.5. Tools for Drug Targeting of Curcumin*

The BBB is a highly sophisticated barrier that is designed to maintain the integrity and homeostasis of the brain. From a technological point of view, it is a great challenge to direct different carriers toward the brain region under the concept of "non-invasive". Some strategies that have been employed include the surface coupling of the nanoparticles of ligands to specific receptors, the coupling of transporter substrates overexpressed in the BBB, and transport by adsorption through the interaction of opposite electrical charges (negative of the endothelial cell membrane and positive of the carrier). In other situations, various pathologies related with neuroinflammation produce a relative opening of the narrow junctions, therefore increasing the probability of the passage of carriers into the nanoparticle architecture. Intentional opening has not comprised a viable option because of the risk involved. Other strategies include furtive aggressive participation. The use of peptides, some of these from virus fragments or modified versions to ensure efficacy without toxicity, is a highly effective option. The transactivating-transduction peptide (TAT) has been a classic example of this type of mechanism.

It is noteworthy that the presence of surface agents substantially modifies the targeting capacity of the curcumin nanoparticles toward the CNS. However, a study in the literature mentions the formulation of PLGA nanoparticles with curcumin obtained by flash nanoprecipitation without a stabilizing agent. These authors demonstrated a 20-fold reduction in the administered dose compared with bulk curcumin (see Table 1). It is even more important to point out that the majority of the studies mentioned in Table 1, some of these that have been widely extended in biological elucidation mechanisms do not involve the application of highly sophisticated systems. In other brain pathologies, it has become a challenge to possess the most sophisticated. On the other hand, some formulations of curcumin in nanoparticles even include the combination of two active molecules, such as puerarin and dexanabinol. In addition, in the search for multifunctional systems, or theranostics, curcumin has been conjugated in magnetic nanoparticles for the detection of Aβ plaques in AD and in combination with gold–iron oxide nanocomposite systems for brain-cancer theranostics (see Table 1 for details).

**Table 1.** Examples of nanoparticle formulation for transport of curcumin to the brain.

| Carrier | Composition | Ligand/Stabilizer | Size, PI and Ψ (mV) | % of EE and DL | Model of Evaluation | Reference |
|---|---|---|---|---|---|---|
| Solid lipid nanoparticles | Polyoxyethylene stearate, stearic acid | Lecithin | 60, Ψ = −21.7 | DL = 21.61 | Major depression (in vitro and in vivo models) | [85] |
| | Compritol 888 ATO (Gattefossé, Saint-Priest, France) | Tween 80, soya lecithin | 136 | 81.9, 92.3 | Cerebral ischemic injury (in vivo model) | [86] |
| | Stearic acid | Lecithin, taurocholate | 148 | EE = 93.2 | Huntington's disease (in vivo model) | [87] |
| | Glyceryl monooleate | Pluronic F-68, vitamin E TPGS | 93, Ψ = −30.9 | EE = 65 | Rotenone-induced mouse model of Parkinson's disease (in vitro and in vivo models) | [88] |
| | Palmitic acid, cholesterol | N-trimethyl Chitosan vitamin E TPGS | 412, 0.26, Ψ = 35.7 | 93, 4 | Biodistribution (in vitro and in vivo models) | [89] |
| | Compritol 888 ATO | Tween 80, soya lecithin | 136 | 81.9, 92.3 | Aluminum-induced behavioral (in vivo model) | [90] |
| Solid lipid nanoparticles (SLNs) and nanostructured lipid carriers (NLCs) | Cetyl palmitate (SLN), cetyl palmitate + oleic acid (NLC) | Tween 80 | 204.7, 0.194 and 117.36, 0.188 | SLN = 83.98, 4.54 NLC = 82.60, 4.67 | Pharmacokinetic (in vivo model) | [91] |
| Nanostructured lipid carriers | Precirol, capmul MCM | Tween 80, soya lecithin | 146, 0.18, Ψ = −21.4 | EE = 90.86 | Astrocytoma-glioblastoma (in vitro and in vivo models) | [92] |
| | Glyceryl monostearate, soy lecithin, medium chain triglycerides | Poloxamer 188 | 129, 0.25 Ψ = −27.8 | 95.9, 4.21 | Pharmacokinetic and biodistribution (in vivo model) | [93] |
| | Phosphatidyl choline, cholesterol oleate, glycerol trioleate | Lactoferrin | 103.8, PI = 0.15, Ψ = −5.80 | 96.51, 2.60 | Alzheimer's disease (in vitro and in vivo models) | [94] |
| | PC, cholesterol oleate, glycerol trioleate | Polysorbate 80 | 90.5, 0.14, Ψ = −20.3 | EE = 94.39, DL = 3.29 | Biodistribution (in vitro and in vivo models) | [95] |
| Polymeric nanoparticles | PLGA | Lipid monolayer | 193.4, PI=0.115, Ψ = −43.8 | 13.23, 2.31 | Inflammation model (in vitro model) | [96] |
| | Poly(butyl) cyanoacrylate | Apolipoprotein E3 | 197, 0.18, Ψ = −22.44 | - | Beta amyloid induced cytotoxicity in neuroblastoma cells (in vitro model) | [97] |
| | Poly(butyl) cyanoacrylate | Apolipoprotein E3 | 197, 0.18, Ψ = −22.44 | EE = 77.85 | Anticancer activity in neuroblastoma cells (in vitro model) | [98] |
| | PLGA | - | 100 | 94.7, 47.3 | Bioavailability in the CNS (in vivo model) | [99] |
| | PLGA | PVA | 163, 0.053, Ψ = −12.5 | EE = 46.9 | Pharmacokinetic (in vivo model) | [100] |
| | PLGA | - | - | - | Opioid tolerance and dependence (in vivo model) | [101] |
| | Chitosan | Tween 80 | 10, Ψ = −16.8 | - | Arsenic toxicity (in vivo model) | [102] |
| | Chitosan-alginate | - | 50 | - | Epilepsy (in vivo model) | [103] |
| | Chitosan | Bovine serum albumin | 143.5, 0.021, Ψ = −10.8 | EE = 95.4 | Phagocytosis of the Aβ peptide (in vitro model) | [104] |
| | PLGA | PVA | 200, Ψ = −19 | EE = 77 | Neurogenesis (in vitro and in vivo models) | [105] |

**Table 1.** *Cont.*

| Carrier | Composition | Ligand/Stabilizer | Size, PI and Ψ (mV) | % of EE and DL | Model of Evaluation | Reference |
|---|---|---|---|---|---|---|
| | PLGA | PVA | 153, 0.15 | 90, 9.5 | Pain (*in vivo* model) | [106] |
| | PLGA | Tet-1 | 150-200, Ψ = −30 to −20 | - | Amyloid aggregates (*in vitro* model) | [107] |
| | PLGA | PEG-B6 peptide | 150, Ψ = 3.8 | DL = 15.6 | Alzheimer transgenic mice (*in vitro* and *in vivo* models) | [108] |
| | PLGA | PEG, cyclic hexapeptide | 97.3, 0.16 | EE = 80.5 | Glioma tumor cells (*in vitro* and *in vivo* models) | [109] |
| | PLGA | PEG, transferrin receptor-binding peptide T7 | 130, Ψ = −15.9 | EE = 18 | Brain tumor (*in vitro* and *in vivo* models) | [110] |
| | PLGA | 1,2-distearoyl-glycerol-3-phospho-ethanolamine-N-[methoxy (polyethylene glycol)-2000 | 169, 0.22 | EE = 35 | Glioblastoma (*in vitro* and *in vivo* models) | [111] |
| | PLGA | PVA | 220, Ψ = −20.6 | 81.7, 16.3 | Subarachnoid hemorrhage-induced BBB disruption (*in vivo* model) | [112] |
| | PLA–PEG | PVP | 55, 0.09, Ψ = −0.29 | EE = 99 | Alzheimer's Disease Tg2576 Mice (*in vitro* and *in vivo* models) | [113] |
| | Hyaluronic acid/chitosan | - | 207, Ψ = 25.3 | 89.9, 6.5 | Glioma cells (*in vitro* model) | [114] |
| Polymeric micelle | Oleoyl chloride, polyethylene glycol 400 | - | 142, 0.4, Ψ = −7 | EE = 87 | Glioblastoma cells (*in vitro* model) | [115] |
| | Labrafac Lipophile WL 1349, Solutol HS 15, Transcutol HP | Tween 80, Tween 20 | 67, 0.137, Ψ = −37 | - | Malignant glioma cells (*in vitro* model) | [116] |
| Nanoemulsion | Labrafac Lipophile | Cremophor RH40 | 114, 0.25, Ψ = −21.8 | - | Biodistribution (*ex vivo* and *in vivo* models) | [117] |
| | Castor oil | Soybean lecithin, PEG 660-stereate | 20.7, 0.19, Ψ = −9.7 | EE ≥ 99 | Permeation in Franz cells (*ex vivo* model) | [118] |
| Metallic nanoparticles | Au | PEG | - | - | Lipopolysaccharide-induced inflammation (*in vitro* and *in vivo* models) | [119] |
| | Iron (II) sulfate heptahydrate | PEG-PLA | 94, 0.14, Ψ = −0.01 | EE = 99 | Detection of amyloid plaques in Alzheimer's (*in vitro* and *in vivo* models) | [120] |
| | Gold-iron oxide | Glutathione | 40, 0.185, Ψ = −16 | EE = 70, 0.7 | Brain cancer (*in vitro* model) | [121] |
| Magnetic nanoparticles | Fe3O4 | - | 185, Ψ = −37.5, | EE = 75 | Schizophrenic rats (*in vivo* model) | [122] |
| | Iron oxide. SPIO nanoparticles, 10,12-pentacosadiynoic acid | PVA, Lactoferrin | 100 | EE = 90.3 | Orthotopic Brain Tumor-Bearing Rat (*in vitro* and *in vivo* models) | [123] |
| Liposomes | 1,2-dipalmitoyl-sn-glycerol-3-phosphatidylcholine, cholesterol | - | 207, 0.25, Ψ = −10.5 | - | Amyloid peptide plaques (*in vivo* model) | [124] |
| β-cyclodextrin (BCD), nanoliposome (NL) | β-cyclodextrin, phosphatidylcholine: cholesterol (5:1) | Tween 80 for liposome | 133.49, −31.76 and 121.81, −7.91 | BCD = 76.6, 19.73 NL = 88.2, 4.13 | Dimethylhydrazine induced poison (*in vivo* model) | [125] |

PVA: polyvinyl alcohol, PLGA: poly (lactic-co-glycolic acid), PVP: polyvinylpyrrolidone, PI: polidispersity index, PEG: polyethylene glycol, EE: entrapment efficiency, DL: drug load, D-α-tocopheryl polyethylene glycol 1000 Succinate: vitamin E TPGS, CNS: central nervous system, BBB: blood–brain barrier.

## 7. Applications of Curcumin in Nanoparticles

### 7.1. Alzheimer's Disease

Alzheimer's disease is the most frequent neurodegenerative disorder worldwide; it is characterized by extracellular Aβ aggregation, intracellular neurofibrillary tangles, tau hyperphosphorylation, and progressive neuron loss. Its main clinical features are memory loss, behavioral changes, and cognitive impairment [126,127]. At present, the limited efficacy of the available therapies has encouraged the search for new treatments. In this regard, recent investigations undertaken in diverse experimental models have suggested that curcumin could be helpful for AD treatment. However, limitations in the bioavailability of curcumin have hindered its use and promoted the search for suitable vehicles to improve its pharmacological activity, such as nanoparticle formulations.

In recent years, the development of nanocarriers to transport curcumin to the brain in AD models has increased considerably; however, the efficacy, safety, and suitability of these formulations is still a main concern. Thus, in addition to the cellular uptake, the evaluation of cell viability has become pivotal to demonstrate the biocompatibility of these formulations.

It has been suggested that aluminum is involved in the etiology of AD; thus, in an early study, the neuroprotective effect of solid lipid nanoparticles loaded with curcumin (SLN-Cur) was proved in an AD mouse model induced by 100 mg/kg of aluminum chloride [91]. The results showed that treatment with SLN-Cur (50 mg/kg) produced a 73% recovery in acetylcholinesterase and a 97.46% recovery in membrane lipids with respect to the group treated with aluminum chloride alone. In addition, mice treated with SLN-Cur underwent less learning impairment and cognition loss, as measured by the Morris water maze test, which suggests the potential of SLN-Cur as an alternative therapeutic for AD.

Similarly, evidence for a reduction of neurogenesis in AD has been shown, which suggests that the induction of this neuronal process mediated by endogenous neuronal stem cells (NSC) would be a probable therapeutic target. In this regard, Tiwari et al. [105] explored the effect of PLGA nanoparticles loaded with curcumin (PLGA–NP–Cur) on neuronal differentiation and NSC proliferation. Through transmission electron microscopy (TEM) analysis, these authors showed that PLGA-NP-Cur had the ability to internalize into NSC derived from the hippocampus. Moreover, Alamar blue reduction and MTT assays suggested that PLGA-NP-Cur (0.001–50 μM) increased NSC proliferation and cell viability, with the highest effect at 0.5 μM. It is noteworthy that bulk curcumin enhanced NSC proliferation only at 0.5 μM, whereas PLGA-NP-Cur significantly increased NSC proliferation at much lower doses (0.001 μM, 0.01 μM, 0.1 μM, and 0.2 μM). Likewise, the results demonstrated that PLGA-NP-Cur reversed deficits in hippocampal neurogenesis and in learning and memory dysfunction in an AD rat model induced by the brain injection of Aß. Interestingly, a more pronounced effect was exhibited by PLGA-NP-Cur when compared with bulk curcumin. Collectively, the results suggested that PLGA-NP-Cur could offer an alternative for the treatment of AD and regenerative medicine.

On the other hand, diverse evidences suggest that oxidative stress participates in the pathophysiology of AD; thus, Djiokeng Paka et al. [128] evaluated the antioxidant and anti-inflammatory activities of curcumin-loaded PLGA nanoparticles (Cur–PLGA–NP) in SK-N-SH cells, which are human neuroblastoma-derived cells. Through assays of radical scavenging activity, the authors found that Cur-PLGA-NP exhibited 1.5-fold and 2.2-fold greater antioxidant activity against peroxyl radical than curcumin alone and empty NP, respectively. They also showed that Cur-PLGA-NP prevented Tau phosphorylation and Akt activity, which have been shown as altered in AD brains. Therefore, the authors suggested that Cur-PLGA-NP could be potentially useful for treating AD.

In another study, Meng et al. [94] developed a low-density lipoprotein-mimic nanocarrier attached to lactoferrin encapsulated in curcumin (Lf–mNLC–Cur) and evaluated its effect on the progression of disease in a rat model of AD. The rat model was generated by means of an intraperitoneal injection of D-gal (0.3 mL/100 g/d for six weeks) and a bilateral injection of $A\beta_{1-42}$ in the dorsal hippocampus (one mg/mL; 5 μL). Through fluorescence images, it was shown that Lf-mNLC-Cur had the ability to cross the BBB, to penetrate into the brain, and to release curcumin. In order to evaluate the therapeutic effect of the formulation, histological preparations to examine the state of the nerve cells in the hippocampal region after the administration of Lf-mNLC-Cur and measurements of malondialdehyde (MDA) in blood were performed. Hematoxylin–eosin staining revealed a lower damage in the treatment with Lf-mNLC-Cur, and the content of MDA was reduced with respect to the control, which suggested that the formulation was effective for decreasing the oxidative stress associated with the progression of AD [94].

Similarly, Barbara et al. [129] designed and engineered a curcumin-encapsulated PLGA nanoparticle bound to peptide g7 (Cur-NP-g7) to promote BBB crossing. The authors demonstrated that Cur-NP-g7 can internalize hippocampal neurons, and that concentrations to around 200 μM were not toxic. Furthermore, the authors determined the effect of Cur-NP-g7 on Aβ aggregation, employing an in vitro AD model generated in the primary hippocampal culture derived from the rat brain. The results revealed an important decrease of Aβ; thus, they concluded that their formulation represent a promising tool for the treatment of AD.

On the other hand, a recent study demonstrated the anti-inflammatory effects of curcumin-loaded spherical polymeric nanoparticles (Cur-SPN). In that study, it was demonstrated that Cur-SPN (10 μM) reduced cytokines IL-1ß, IL-6, and TNF-α expression in macrophages stimulated by Aβ fibrils (2 μM). Likewise, cell viability assays revealed that Cur-SPN did not induce apoptosis, and no evidence of toxicity was detected. Based on their findings, the authors claimed that this approach could be helpful for the amelioration of inflammation observed in AD [94].

In a study undertaken by Huang et al. [130], PLGA nanoparticles were designed conjugated with the S1 peptide (an inhibitor of Aβ generation), brain-targeting calreticulin (CRT) (a peptide that binds to the transferrin receptor), and curcumin (as a therapeutic substance to tackle the disorder). The results revealed that the nanocarrier (S1-CRT-NP+Cur) was taken up into a cellular model of the BBB (brain microvascular bEnd.3 cells), suggesting that it can permeate across the BBB. In support of this hypothesis, S1-CRT-NP+Cur was distributed in mouse brain after intravenous administration, as demonstrated by in vivo bioluminescence imaging system and post-mortem studies. The therapeutic effect of S1-CRT-NP+Cur was explored by means of a Y-maze and a new object recognition test, the determination of astrogliosis and microgliosis, and the measurement of cytokines, superoxide dismutase (SOD), and ROS levels in a transgenic AD mouse model (APP/PS1dE9). Interestingly, S1-CRT-NP+Cur attenuated cognitive deficits, reduced astrogliosis and microgliosis, increased the number of synapses, decreased inflammatory cytokines, enhanced SOD levels, and reduced ROS levels. These findings highlight S1-CRT-NP+Cur as a promising approach for future use in AD treatment.

Finally, in a recent report, PLGA–PEG nanoparticles attached to the B6 peptide with curcumin encapsulated (PLGA/PEG-B6-Cur) were designed [108]. PLGA–PEG was employed to enhance the bioavailability, and the B6 peptide was employed to permit BBB crossing. In order to explore their potential usefulness in AD treatment, PLGA/PEG-B6-Cur were proven in HT22 cells and an AD rodent model (APP/PS1 transgenic mice). Cytotoxicity studies in HT22 cells demonstrated that PLGA/PEG-B6-Cur did not affect cell viability up to 500 μg/mL. To evaluate the effect of PLGA/PEG-B6-Cur on memory capability and spatial learning, the Morris water maze test was performed in animals intraperitoneally injected with the nanocarrier. The experimental results revealed that PLGA/PEG-B6-Cur significantly improved cognitive performance, which correlated with a decrease in tau phosphorylation and Aβ production in the hippocampus. Altogether, these findings suggest that PLGA/PEG-B6-Cur may represent a promising alternative for treating AD.

*7.2. Parkinson's Disease*

Parkinson's disease is the second most frequent neurodegenerative disorder and is characterized by abnormalities in the control of voluntary movements. The pathological hallmarks of PD include neuronal cell death, oxidative stress, mitochondrial dysfunction, and the accumulation of α-synuclein. The gold standard for the treatment of PD is L-Dopa; however, its chronic employment leads to a severe collateral problem known as dyskinesia. Therefore, the lack of a permanent cure has triggered the search for novel treatments. In this respect, curcumin has shown good effects in different experimental models; thus, it could be a key molecule for developing new strategies to reach a definitive treatment.

In this regard, in a first approach, alginate–curcumin nanoparticles (Alg-NP-Cur) were developed, and their probable therapeutic actions were evaluated in a PD Drosophila model. Alg-NP-Cur exhibited antioxidant power by the reduction of the lipid peroxidation in the PD Drosophila brain after a diet supplemented with the nanocarrier for 24 days. The effective prevention of the progression of the Parkinsonian symptoms in the PD flies was evidenced by the inhibition of the loss of climbing ability in flies with respect to PD flies without exposure to Alg-NP-Cur. Therefore, this report provided a rationale for employing curcumin-encapsulated nanoparticles in preclinical and clinical studies [131].

In this respect, in another study, Kundu et al. [88] designed glyceryl monooleate nanoparticles loaded with piperine and curcumin (GMO-NP-Pip/Cur). The anti-aggregate and anti-fibrillar effects of GMO-NP-Pip/Cur on α-synuclein oligomers were evaluated employing atomic force microscopy (AFM). The results showed that GMO-NP-Pip/Cur produced a pronounced inhibition of α-synuclein aggregation. Similarly, GMO-NP-Pip/Cur were able to ameliorate motor dysfunction when co-administered with rotenone in a PD mouse model. Interestingly, GMO-NP-Pip/Cur exhibited anti-apoptotic and antioxidant activities with no evidence of cytotoxicity. Therefore, GMO-NP-Pip/Cur could be an interesting approach for the treatment of PD.

In another study, Bollimpelli et al. [132] elaborated lactoferrin nanoparticles by sol-oil chemistry, which were loaded with curcumin (Lf-NP-Cur). The potential neuroprotective usefulness of this formulation was evaluated against toxicity induced by rotenone in SK-N-SH cells, employing microscopy, a lactate dehydrogenase (LDH) release assay, and an MTT assay. The findings suggested that Lf-NP-Cur protect the cells from the toxicity of rotenone, more than curcumin alone; thus, these may be a suitable drug-delivery strategy against PD.

Finally, nanoparticles with Polysorbate 80 are widely used to improve the BBB permeability of the nanoparticles; thus, Zhang et al. [133] developed curcumin-loaded polysorbate 80-modified cerasomes (PS80-NP-Cur). The formulation was able to modify the release time of curcumin monitored in C57BL/6 mice, producing a prolonged circulation time in the blood. Furthermore, PS80-NP-Cur produced a remarkable reduction of PD symptoms in a PD mouse model induced by 1-methyl-4-phenyl-1,2,3,6-tetrahydropyridine (MPTP), when these were administered concomitantly with ultrasound-targeted microbubble destruction (UTMD). Despite these promising results, the utilization of techniques such as UTMD should be evaluated to a greater extent, because its employment for prolonged times could lead to severe undesirable effects.

### 7.3. Huntington's Disease

Huntington's disease is a genetic neurodegenerative disorder whose clinical manifestations include involuntary movements and anxiety. To date, there is no specific medication to treat the disease; however, since mitochondrial impairment appears to contribute to neuronal death in HD, approaches to decrease mitochondrial dysfunction could represent a therapeutic alternative. In this regard, it has been reported that dietary curcumin possesses beneficial effects in HD. Therefore, Sandhir et al. [87] fabricated solid lipid nanoparticles loaded with curcumin (SLNP-Cur) and explored their neuroprotective effectiveness in a HD rat model induced by 3-nitropropionic acid (3-NP). The administration of SLNP-Cur was able to restore SOD activity and glutathione levels. Furthermore, SLNP-Cur decreased ROS, protein carbonyls, and lipid peroxidation. In addition, the formulation reduced the motor impairment induced by the treatment with 3-NP. Therefore, these results indicate that SLNP-Cur could be helpful for the treatment of HD.

### 8. Conclusions

Curcumin is an example of an ancestral phytochemical whose health benefits have been confirmed and new applications have been discovered with a high impact for incurable diseases. The study of curcumin is one of the few cases of broad applications demonstrated under methodological principles and in a reproducible manner. Recently, the greatest impacts of this molecule are due to the novel technological proposals for its biological administration. In particular, the use of nanoparticles has made it possible to demonstrate benefits at the brain level, which can even revolutionize medicine. However, as with any chemical substance, it is convenient to emphasize toxicity issues in order to ensure the safety of all clinical trials. In addition to the clear results in brain models, the increase in benefits can be addressed with an improvement in the functioning of nanotechnological carriers.

**Author Contributions:** Conceptualization, G.L.-G. and H.C.; Methodology, M.L.D.P.-A.; Software, J.A.M.-T.; Validation, B.F., M.G.-T. and I.H.C.-F.; Formal Analysis, M.L.D.P.-A.; Investigation, I.H.C.-F., N.M.-M.;

*Biomolecules* **2019**, *9*, 56

Writing—Original Draft Preparation, N.M.-M., M.L.D.P.-A., G.L.-G., H.C.; Writing–Review and Editing, M.L.D.P.-A., G.L.-G., H.C.; Visualization, G.L.-G.; Supervision, G.L.-G. and H.C.

**Funding:** This research was funded by Dirección General de Asuntos del Personal Académico, Universidad Nacional Autónoma de México (Becas Posdoctorales, PAPIIT TA 200318), Consejo Nacional de Ciencia y Tecnología, 526864.

**Acknowledgments:** The authors would like to thank Carlos Flores-Morales for his assistance with AFM assessment, Miguel Ángel Canseco-Martínez for the help providing FTIR analysis, Karla Eriseth Reyes-Morales for her technical assistance with thermal tests.

**Conflicts of Interest:** The authors declare no conflict of interest. The funders had no role in the design of the study; in the collection, analyses, or interpretation of data; in the writing of the manuscript, or in the decision to publish the results.

## Abbreviations

| | |
|---|---|
| AD | Alzheimer disease |
| AP-1 | activating protein-1 |
| APP | amyloid-β precursor protein |
| AR | androgen receptor |
| Arh-R | aryl hydrocarbon receptor |
| AS | α-synuclein |
| ASD | Amorphous solid dispersions |
| Aβ | amyloid-β |
| BACE1 | β-secretase enzyme |
| BBB | blood–brain barrier |
| BCS | Biopharmaceutics Classification System |
| cAK | autophosphorylation-activated protein kinase |
| CBP | CREB-binding protein |
| CDPK | $Ca^{2+}$-dependent protein kinase cellular src kinase |
| CNS | central nervous system |
| COX-2 | cyclooxygenase-2 |
| cPK | protamine kinase |
| CTGF | connective tissue growth factor |
| DFF40 | DNA fragmentation factor; 40-kd subunit |
| DL | drug loading |
| DR-5 | death receptor-5 |
| EE | entrapment efficiency |
| EGF | epidermal growth Factor |
| EGF-R | EGF receptor |
| EGFRK | EGF receptor-kinase |
| Egr-1 | early growth response gene-1 |
| ELAM-1 | endothelial leukocyte adhesion molecule-1; Bcl-2, B-cell lymphoma protein 2 |
| EPC-R | endothelial protein C-receptor |
| EpRE | electrophile |
| ERK | extracellular receptor kinase |
| ER-α | estrogen receptor-α |
| FAK | focal adhesion kinase |
| Fas-R | Fas receptor |
| FDA | Food and Drug Administration |
| FGF | fibroblast growth factor |
| FPTase | farnesyl protein transferase |
| Gcl | Glutamate–cysteine ligase |
| GM-CSF | granulocyte-macrophage colony-stimulating factor |
| GST | glutathione-S-transferase |
| H2-R | histamine (2)-receptor |

| | |
|---|---|
| HGF | hepatocyte growth factor |
| HO | heme oxygenase |
| HSP-70 | heat shock protein 70 |
| IAP | inhibitory apoptosis protein |
| IARK | IL-1 receptor-associated kinase |
| ICAM-1 | intracellular adhesion molecule-1 |
| IFNγ | interferon gamma |
| IKK | IκB kinase |
| IL | interleukin |
| IL-8-R | interleukin-8-receptor |
| iNOS | inducible nitric oxide synthase |
| Inos | matrix inducible nitric oxide synthase |
| InsP3-R | inositol 1,4,5-triphosphate receptor |
| IR | Fourier transform infrared spectroscopy |
| IR | integrin receptor |
| JAK | janus kinase |
| JNK | c-jun N-terminal kinase |
| LDL-R | low-density lipoprotein-receptor |
| LOX | lipoxygenase |
| LPS | lipopolysaccharide |
| MAPK | mitogen-activated protein kinase |
| MCP | monocyte chemoattractant protein |
| MDR | multidrug resistance |
| MIF | migration inhibition protein |
| MIP | macrophage inflammatory protein |
| MMP | matrix metalloproteinase |
| Mv | Millivolts |
| NAT | arylamine N-acetyltransferases |
| NF-κB | nuclear factor-κB |
| NGF | nerve growth factor |
| NMR | nuclear magnetic resonance |
| Nrf-2 | nuclear factor erythroid 2-related factor |
| PBCA | poly (butyl cyanoacrylate) |
| PDGF | platelet-derived growth factor |
| PhK | phosphorylase kinase |
| PKA | protein kinase A |
| PKB | protein kinase B |
| PKC | protein kinase C |
| PLGA | poly lactic-co-glycolic acid |
| pp60c-src | non-receptor protein tyrosine kinase c-Src |
| PPARγ | peroxisome proliferator-activated receptor-γ |
| PrP | prion protein |
| PrP-Res | prion protein resistance |
| PVA | polyvinyl alcohol |
| SHP-2 | Src homology 2 domain containing tyrosine phosphatase 2 |
| SMEDDS | Self-microemulsifying drug delivery systems |
| STAT | signal transducers and activators of transcription |
| TAT | transactivating–transduction peptide |
| TGF-β1 | transforming growth factor-β1 |
| TIMP | tissue inhibitor of metalloproteinase-3 |
| TK | protein tyrosine kinase |
| TNF | tumoral necrosis factor |
| TNF-α | tumor necrosis factor-α |
| uPA | urokinase-type plasminogen activator |

*Biomolecules* **2019**, *9*, 56

| VCAM-1 | vascular cell adhesion molecule-1 |
|--------|----------------------------------|
| VEGF | vascular endothelial growth factor |
| Ψ | zeta potential |

## References

1. Aggarwal, B.B.; Harikumar, K.B. Potential therapeutic effects of curcumin, the anti-inflammatory agent, against neurodegenerative, cardiovascular, pulmonary, metabolic, autoimmune and neoplastic diseases. *Int. J. Biochem. Cell Biol.* **2009**, *41*, 40–59. [CrossRef] [PubMed]
2. Alsamydai, A.; Jaber, N. Pharmacological aspects of curcumin: Review article. *Int. J. Pharmacogn.* **2018**, *5*, 313–326.
3. Bengmark, S. Curcumin, an atoxic antioxidant and natural NFκB, cyclooxygenase-2, lipooxygenase, and inducible nitric oxide synthase inhibitor: A shield against acute and chronic diseases. *J. Parenter. Enter. Nutr.* **2006**, *30*, 45–51. [CrossRef]
4. Wang, S.L.; Ying, L.; Ying, W.; Chen, Y.F.; Na, L.X.; Li, S.T.; Sun, C.H. Curcumin, a potential inhibitor of Up-regulation of TNF-alpha and IL-6 induced by palmitate in 3T3-L1 adipocytes through NF-κB and JNK pathway. *Biomed. Environ. Sci.* **2009**, *22*, 32–39. [CrossRef]
5. Guo, Y.Z.; He, P.; Feng, A.M. Effect of curcumin on expressions of NF-κBp65, TNF-α and IL-8 in placental tissue of premature birth of infected mice. *Asian Pac. J. Trop. Med.* **2017**, *10*, 175–178. [CrossRef] [PubMed]
6. Becher, B.; Spath, S.; Goverman, J. Cytokine networks in neuroinflammation. *Nat. Rev. Immunol.* **2017**, *17*, 49–59. [CrossRef] [PubMed]
7. Zhang, C.; Browne, A.; Child, D.; Tanzi, R.E. Curcumin decreases amyloid-β peptide levels by attenuating the maturation of amyloid-β precursor protein. *J. Biol. Chem.* **2010**, *285*, 28472–28480. [CrossRef]
8. Fonseca-Santos, B.; Gremião, M.P.; Chorilli, M. Nanotechnology-based drug delivery systems for the treatment of Alzheimer's disease. *Int. J. Nanomed.* **2015**, *10*, 4981–5003. [CrossRef]
9. Li, J.; Sabliov, C. PLA/PLGA nanoparticles for delivery of drugs across the blood-brain barrier. *Nanotechnol. Rev.* **2013**, *2*, 241–257. [CrossRef]
10. Bhatia, S. Nanoparticles types, classification, characterization, fabrication methods and drug delivery applications. In *Natural Polymer Drug Delivery Systems*; Nanoparticles, Plants, and Algae; Springer International Publishing: Cham, Switzerland, 2016; pp. 33–85.
11. Priyadarsini, K. The Chemistry of Curcumin: From Extraction to Therapeutic Agent. *Molecules* **2014**, *19*, 20091–20112. [CrossRef]
12. Payton, F.; Sandusky, P.; Alworth, W.L. NMR study of the solution structure of curcumin. *J. Nat. Prod.* **2007**, *70*, 143–146. [CrossRef] [PubMed]
13. Yanagisawa, D.; Shirai, N.; Amatsubo, T.; Taguchi, H.; Hirao, K.; Urushitani, M.; Morikawa, S.; Inubushi, T.; Kato, M.; Kato, F.; et al. Relationship between the tautomeric structures of curcumin derivatives and their Aβ-binding activities in the context of therapies for Alzheimer's disease. *Biomaterials* **2010**, *31*, 4179–4185. [CrossRef] [PubMed]
14. Chen, Y.; Wu, Q.; Zhang, Z.; Yuan, L.; Liu, X.; Zhou, L. Preparation of curcumin-loaded liposomes and evaluation of their skin permeation and pharmacodynamics. *Molecules* **2012**, *17*, 5972–5987. [CrossRef] [PubMed]
15. Subramani, P.A.; Panati, K.; Lebaka, V.R.; Redd, D.D.; Narala, V.R. Nanostructures for curcumin delivery: Posibilities and challenges. In *Nano and -Micro Drug Delivery Systems*; Andrew, W., Ed.; Elsevier Science Ltd Desing and Fabrication: Amsterdam, The Netherlands, 2017; pp. 393–418.
16. Kharat, M.; Du, Z.; Zhang, G.; Mcclements, D.J. Physical and Chemical Stability of Curcumin in Aqueous Solutions and Emulsions: Impact of pH, Temperature, and Molecular Environment. *J. Agric. Food Chem.* **2017**, *65*, 1525–1532. [CrossRef] [PubMed]
17. Sharma, K.; Agrawal, S.S.; Gupta, M. Development and validation of UV spectrophotometric method for the estimation of curcumin in bulk drug and pharmaceutical dosage forms. *Int. J. Drug Dev. Res.* **2012**, *4*, 375–380.
18. Benassi, R.; Ferrari, E.; Lazzari, S.; Spagnolo, F.; Saladini, M. Theoretical study on Curcumin: A comparison of calculated spectroscopic properties with NMR, UV-vis and IR experimental data. *J. Mol. Struct.* **2008**, *892*, 168–176. [CrossRef]

19. Athira, G.K.; Jyothi, A.N. Preparation and characterization of curcumin loaded cassava starch nanoparticles with improved cellular absorption. *Int. J. Pharm. Pharm. Sci.* **2014**, *6*, 171–176.
20. O'Neil, M.J. (Ed.) *The Merck Index, An Encyclopedia of Chemicals, Drugs, and Biologicals*, 15th ed.; Royal Society of Chemistry: Cambridge, UK, 2013.
21. Doktorovova, S.; Souto, E.B.; Silva, A.M. Hansen solubility parameters (HSP) for prescreening formulation of solid lipid nanoparticles (SLN): In Vitro testing of curcumin-loaded SLN in MCF-7 and BT-474 cell lines. *Pharm. Dev. Technol.* **2018**, *23*, 96–105. [CrossRef]
22. Shen, L.; Ji, H.F. The pharmacology of curcumin: Is it the degradation products? *Trends Mol. Med.* **2012**, *18*, 138–144. [CrossRef]
23. Wang, Y.-J.; Pan, M.-H.; Cheng, A.-L.; Lin, L.-I.; Ho, Y.-S.; Hsieh, C.-Y.; Lin, J.-K. Stability of curcumin in buffer solutions and characterization of its degradation products. *J. Pharm. Biomed. Anal.* **1997**, *15*, 1867–1876. [CrossRef]
24. Schneider, C.; Gordon, O.N.; Edwards, R.L.; Luis, P.B. Degradation of Curcumin: From Mechanism to Biological Implications. *J. Agric. Food Chem.* **2015**, *63*, 7606–7614. [CrossRef] [PubMed]
25. Griesser, M.; Pistis, V.; Suzuki, T.; Tejera, N.; Pratt, D.A.; Schneider, C. Autoxidative and cyclooxygenase-2 catalyzed transformation of the dietary chemopreventive agent curcumin. *J. Biol. Chem.* **2011**, *286*, 1114–1124. [CrossRef] [PubMed]
26. Aggarwal, B.B.; Sundaram, C.; Malani, N.; Haruyo, I. Curcumin: The Indian solid gold. In *The Molecular Targets and Therapeutics Uses of Curcumin in Health and Disease*; Aggarwal, B.B., Surh, Y.-J., Shishodia, S., Eds.; Springer Science: Boston MA, USA, 2007; Volume 595, pp. 1–75.
27. Reinke, A.A.; Gestwicki, J.E. Structure-activity relationships of amyloid beta-aggregation inhibitors based on curcumin: Influence of linker length and flexibility. *Chem. Biol. Drug Des.* **2007**, *70*, 206–215. [CrossRef] [PubMed]
28. Ray, B.; Lahiri, D.K. Neuroinflammation in Alzheimer's disease: Different molecular targets and potential therapeutic agents including curcumin. *Curr. Opin. Pharmacol.* **2009**, *9*, 434–444. [CrossRef] [PubMed]
29. Kasi, P.D.; Tamilselvam, R.; Skalicka-Woźniak, K.; Nabavi, S.F.; Daglia, M.; Bishayee, A.; Pazoki-Toroudi, H.; Nabavi, S.M. Molecular targets of curcumin for cancer therapy: An updated review. *Tumor Biol.* **2016**, *37*, 13017–13028. [CrossRef] [PubMed]
30. Zhou, H.; Beevers, C.S.; Huang, S. The targets of curcumin. *Curr. Drug Targets* **2011**, *12*, 332–347. [CrossRef]
31. Aguzzi, A.; O'Connor, T. Protein aggregation diseases: Pathogenicity and therapeutic perspectives. *Nat. Rev. Drug Discov.* **2010**, *9*, 237–248. [CrossRef]
32. Hafner-Bratkovič, I.; Gašperšič, J.; Šmid, L.M.; Bresjanac, M.; Jerala, R. Curcumin binds to the α-helical intermediate and to the amyloid form of prion protein -A new mechanism for the inhibition of PrPSc accumulation. *J. Neurochem.* **2008**, *104*, 1553–1564. [CrossRef]
33. Caughey, B.; Raymond, L.D.; Raymond, G.J.; Maxson, L.; Silveira, J.; Baron, G.S. Inhibition of protease-resistant prion protein accumulation in vitro by curcumin. *J. Virol.* **2003**, *77*, 5499–5502. [CrossRef]
34. Pandey, N.; Strider, J.; Nolan, W.C.; Yan, S.X.; Galvin, J.E. Curcumin inhibits aggregation of α-synuclein. *Acta Neuropathol.* **2008**, *115*, 479–489. [CrossRef]
35. Brahmkhatri, V.; Sharma, N.; Punnepalli, S.; D'Souza, A.; Raghothama, S.; Atreya, H.S. Curcumin nanoconjugate Inhibits aggregation of N-terminal region (Aβ-16) of an amyloid beta peptide. *New J. Chem.* **2018**, *42*, 19881–19892. [CrossRef]
36. Mithu, V.S.; Sarkar, B.; Bhowmik, D.; Das, A.K.; Chandrakesan, M. Curcumin Alters the Salt Bridge-containing Turn Region in amyloid β(1-42) aggregates. *J. Biol. Chem.* **2014**, *289*, 11122–11131. [CrossRef] [PubMed]
37. Yang, F.; Lim, G.P.; Begum, A.N.; Ubeda, O.J.; Simmons, M.R.; Ambegaokar, S.S.; Chen, P.; Kayed, R.; Glabe, C.G.; Frautschy, S.A.; et al. Curcumin Inhibits Formation of Amyloid β Oligomers and Fibrils, Binds Plaques, and Reduces Amyloid in vivo. *J. Biol. Chem.* **2005**, *280*, 5892–5901. [CrossRef] [PubMed]
38. Huang, X.; Atwood, Æ.C.S.; Moir, Æ.R.D.; Hartshorn, M.A.; Tanzi, Æ.R.E.; Bush, A.I. Trace metal contamination initiates the apparent auto-aggregation, amyloidosis, and oligomerization of Alzheimer's Aβ peptides. *J. Biol. Inorg. Chem.* **2004**, *9*, 954–960. [CrossRef] [PubMed]
39. Cole, G.M.; Teter, B.; Frautschy, S.A. Neuropretective effects of curcumin. In *The Molecular Targets and Therapeutic Uses of Curcumin in Health and Disease*; Aggarwal, B.B., Surh, Y.J., Shishodia, S., Eds.; Springer: Boston, MA, USA, 2007; Volume 595, pp. 197–212.

40. Vassar, R. Bace 1 The β-secretase enzyme in alzheimer's disease. *J. Mol. Neurosci.* **2004**, *23*, 105–113. [CrossRef]

41. DiSabato, D.J.; Quan, N.; Godbout, J.P. Neuroinflammation: The Devil is in the Details. *J. Neurochem.* **2016**, *139*, 136–153. [CrossRef] [PubMed]

42. Karlstetter, M.; Lippe, E.; Walczak, Y.; Moehle, C.; Aslanidis, A.; Mirza, M.; Langmann, T. Curcumin is a potent modulator of microglial gene expression and migration. *J. Neuroinflammation* **2011**, *8*, 1–12. [CrossRef]

43. Tizabi, Y.; Hurley, L.L.; Qualls, Z.; Akinfiresoye, L. Relevance of the anti-inflammatory properties of curcumin in neurodegenerative diseases and depression. *Molecules* **2014**, *19*, 20864–20879. [CrossRef]

44. Yin, H.; Guo, Q.; Li, X.; Tang, T.; Li, C.; Wang, H.; Sun, Y.; Feng, Q.; Ma, C.; Gao, C.; et al. Curcumin Suppresses IL-1β Secretion and Prevents Inflammation through Inhibition of the NLRP3 Inflammasome. *J. Immunol.* **2018**, *200*, 2835–2846. [CrossRef]

45. Jurrmann, N.; Brigelius-Flohe, R.; Bol, G.F. Curcumin blocks interleukin-1 (IL-1) signaling by inhibiting the recruitment of the IL-1 receptor-associated kinase IRAK in murine thymoma EL-4 cells. *J. Nutr.* **2005**, *135*, 1859–1864. [CrossRef]

46. Devi, Y.S.; DeVine, M.; DeKuiper, J.; Ferguson, S.; Fazleabas, A.T. Inhibition of IL-6 signaling pathway by curcumin in uterine decidual cells. *PLoS ONE* **2015**, *10*, e0125627. [CrossRef] [PubMed]

47. Sahebkar, A.; Cicero, A.F.G.; Simental-Mendía, L.E.; Aggarwal, B.B.; Gupta, S.C. Curcumin downregulates human tumor necrosis factor-α levels: A systematic review and meta-analysis of randomized controlled trials. *Pharmacol. Res.* **2016**, *107*, 234–242. [CrossRef] [PubMed]

48. Singh, S.; Aggarwal, B.B. Activation of transcription factor NF-κ B is suppressed by curcumin (diferuloylmethane). *J. Biol. Chem.* **1995**, *270*, 24995–25000. [CrossRef] [PubMed]

49. Aggarwal, B.B.; Gupta, S.C.; Sung, B. Curcumin: An orally bioavailable blocker of TNF and other pro-inflammatory biomarkers. *Br. J. Pharmacol.* **2013**, *169*, 1672–1692. [PubMed]

50. Howe, C.L.; LaFrance-Corey, R.G.; Goddery, E.N.; Johnson, R.K.; Mirchia, K. Neuronal CCL2 expression drives inflammatory monocyte infiltration into the brain during acute virus infection. *J. Neuroinflamm.* **2017**, *14*, 1–14. [CrossRef] [PubMed]

51. Zhang, Z.-J.; Zhao, L.-X.; Cao, D.-L.; Zhang, X.; Gao, Y.-J.; Xia, C. Curcumin Inhibits LPS-Induced CCL2 Expression via JNK Pathway in C6 Rat Astrocytoma Cells. *Cell. Mol. Neurobiol.* **2012**, *32*, 1003–1010. [CrossRef] [PubMed]

52. Herman, J.G.; Stadelman, H.L.; Roselli, C.E. Curcumin blocks CCL2-induced adhesion, motility and invasion, in part, through down-regulation of CCL2 expression and proteolytic activity. *Int. J. Oncol.* **2009**, *34*, 1319–1327. [PubMed]

53. Midura-Kiela, M.T.; Radhakrishnan, V.; Kiela, P. Curcumin inhibits interferon-γ signaling in colonic epithelial cells. *Am. J. Physiol. Liver Phisiol.* **2012**, *302*, G86–G96. [CrossRef] [PubMed]

54. Ogadimma, I.; Uzairu, A.; Eyije, S.; Ola, S. Evaluation of the antioxidant properties of curcumin derivatives by genetic function algorithm. *J. Adv. Res.* **2018**, *12*, 47–54.

55. Bendary, E.; Francis, R.R.; Ali, H.M.G.; Sarwat, M.I.; Hady, S. El Antioxidant and structure—Activity relationships (SARs) of some phenolic and anilines compounds. *Ann. Agric. Sci.* **2013**, *58*, 173–181.

56. Menon, V.P.; Sudheer, A.R. Antioxidant and anti-inflamatory properties of curcumin. In *The Molecular Targets and Therapeutic Uses of Curcumin in Health and Disease*; Aggarwal, B.B., Surh, Y.-J., Shishodia, S., Eds.; Springer International Publishing: Cham, Switzerland, 2007; pp. 105–126.

57. Chen, Y.; Xiao, H.; Zheng, J.; Liang, G. Structure-Thermodynamics-Antioxidant Activity Relationships of Selected Natural Phenolic Acids and Derivatives: An Experimental and Theoretical Evaluation. *PLoS ONE* **2015**, *10*, e0121276. [CrossRef] [PubMed]

58. Zbarsky, V.; Datla, K.P.; Parkar, S.; Rai, D.K.; Okezie, I.; Dexter, D.T. Neuroprotective properties of the natural phenolic antioxidants curcumin and naringenin but not quercetin and fisetin in a 6-OHDA model of Parkinson's disease. *Free Radic. Res.* **2009**, *39*, 1119–1125. [CrossRef]

59. Maiti, P.; Dunbar, G.L. Use of curcumin, a natural polyphenol for targeting molecular pathways in treating age-related neurodegenerative diseases. *Int. J. Mol. Sci.* **2018**, *19*, 1637. [CrossRef]

60. Barzegar, A.; Moosavi-movahedi, A.A. Intracellular ROS Protection Efficiency and Free Radical- Scavenging Activity of Curcumin. *PLoS ONE* **2011**, *6*, e26012. [CrossRef]

61. González-Reyes, S.; Guzmán-Beltrán, S.; Medina-Campos, O.N.; Pedraza-Chaverri, J. Curcumin Pretreatment Induces Nrf2 and an Antioxidant Response and Prevents Hemin-Induced Toxicity in Primary Cultures of Cerebellar Granule Neurons of Rats. *Oxid. Med. Cell. Longev.* **2013**, *2013*, 1–14. [CrossRef] [PubMed]
62. Haryuna, T.; Munir, D.; Maria, A.; Bashiruddin, J. The Antioxidant Effect of Curcumin on Cochlear Fibroblasts in Rat Models of Diabetes Mellitus. *Iran J. Otorhinolaryngol.* **2017**, *29*, 197–202. [PubMed]
63. Wahlang, B.; Pawar, Y.B.; Bansal, A.K. Identification of permeability-related hurdles in oral delivery of curcumin using the Caco-2 cell model. *Eur. J. Pharm. Biopharm.* **2011**, *77*, 275–282. [CrossRef]
64. Holder, G.M.; Plummer, J.L.; Ryan, A.J. The metabolism and excretion of curcumin (1,7-bis-(4-hydroxy-3-methoxyphenyl)-1,6-heptadiene-3,5-dione) in the rat. *Xenobiotica* **1978**, *8*, 761–768. [CrossRef]
65. Sharma, R.A. Phase I Clinical Trial of Oral Curcumin: Biomarkers of Systemic Activity and Compliance. *Clin. Cancer Res.* **2004**, *10*, 6847–6854. [CrossRef]
66. Gangurde, A.B.; Kundaikar, H.S.; Javeer, S.D.; Jaiswar, D.R.; Degani, M.S.; Amin, P.D. Enhanced solubility and dissolution of curcumin by a hydrophilic polymer solid dispersion and its in silico molecular modeling studies. *J. Drug Deliv. Sci. Technol.* **2015**, *29*, 226–237. [CrossRef]
67. Chuah, A.M.; Jacob, B.; Jie, Z.; Ramesh, S.; Mandal, S.; Puthan, J.K.; Deshpande, P.; Vaidyanathan, V.V.; Gelling, R.W.; Patel, G.; et al. Enhanced bioavailability and bioefficacy of an amorphous solid dispersion of curcumin. *Food Chem.* **2014**, *156*, 227–233. [CrossRef] [PubMed]
68. Wang, Y.; Wang, C.; Zhao, J.; Ding, Y.; Li, L. Journal of Colloid and Interface Science A cost-effective method to prepare curcumin nanosuspensions with enhanced oral bioavailability. *J. Colloid Interface Sci.* **2017**, *485*, 91–98. [CrossRef] [PubMed]
69. Li, X.; Yuan, H.; Zhang, C.; Chen, W.; Cheng, W.; Chen, X.; Ye, X. Preparation and in-vitro/in-vivo evaluation of curcumin nanosuspension with solubility enhancement. *J. Pharm. Pharmacol.* **2016**, *68*, 980–988. [CrossRef] [PubMed]
70. Dokania, S.; Joshi, A.K. Self-microemulsifying drug delivery system (SMEDDS)—Challenges and road ahead. *Drug Deliv.* **2015**, *22*, 675–690. [CrossRef] [PubMed]
71. Wu, X.; Xu, J.; Huang, X.; Wen, C. Self-microemulsifying drug delivery system improves curcumin dissolution and bioavailability. *Drug Dev. Ind. Pharm.* **2011**, *37*, 15–23. [CrossRef] [PubMed]
72. Jaisamut, P.; Wiwattanawongsa, K.; Graidist, P.; Sangsen, Y.; Wiwattanapatapee, R. Enhanced Oral Bioavailability of Curcumin Using a Supersaturatable Self-Microemulsifying System Incorporating a Hydrophilic Polymer; In Vitro and In Vivo Investigations. *AAPS PharmSciTech* **2018**, *19*, 730–740. [CrossRef]
73. Bele, M.H.; Shaikh, A.A.; Paralkar, S.G. To enhance the solubility of curcumin by solid self-microemulsifying drug delivery system (SMEDDS). *Indo Am. J. Pharm. Res.* **2017**, *7*, 8587–8607.
74. Cui, J.; Yu, B.; Zhao, Y.; Zhu, W.; Li, H.; Lou, H.; Zhai, G. Enhancement of oral absorption of curcumin by self-microemulsifying drug delivery systems. *Int. J. Pharm.* **2009**, *371*, 148–155. [CrossRef]
75. Yallapu, M.M.; Jaggi, M.; Chauhan, S.C. Curcumin nanoformulations: A future nanomedicine for cancer. *Drug Discov. Today* **2012**, *17*, 71–80. [CrossRef]
76. Sun, M.; Su, X.; Ding, B.; He, X.; Liu, X.; Yu, A.; Lou, H.; Zhai, G. Advances in nanotechnology-based delivery systems for curcumin. *Nanomedicine* **2012**, *7*, 1085–1100. [CrossRef]
77. Kreuter, J. Nanoparticles-a historical perspective. *Int. J. Pharm.* **2007**, *331*, 1–10. [CrossRef] [PubMed]
78. Leson, A. There is plenty of room at the bottom. *Vak. Forsch. und Prax.* **2005**, *17*, 123. [CrossRef]
79. Khanna, S.C.; Soliva, M.; Speiser, P. Epoxy resin beads as a pharmaceutical dosage form II: Dissolution studies of epoxy-amine beads and release of drug. *J. Pharm. Sci.* **1969**, *58*, 1385–1388. [CrossRef] [PubMed]
80. Kreuter, J.; Alyautdin, R.N.; Kharkevich, D.A.; Ivanov, A.A. Passage of peptides through the blood-brain barrier with colloidal polymer particles (nanoparticles). *Brain Res.* **1995**, *674*, 171–174. [CrossRef]
81. Müller, R.H.; Maaßen, S.; Weyhers, H.; Mehnert, W. Phagocytic uptake and cytotoxicity of solid lipid nanoparticles (SLN) sterically stabilized with poloxamine 908 and poloxamer 407. *J. Drug Target.* **1996**, *4*, 161–170. [CrossRef] [PubMed]
82. Xu, Y.; Kim, C.S.; Saylor, D.M.; Koo, D. Polymer degradation and drug delivery in PLGA-based drug–polymer applications: A review of experiments and theories. *J. Biomed. Mater. Res. Part B Appl. Biomater.* **2017**, *105*, 1692–1716. [CrossRef] [PubMed]
83. Barenholz, Y. Doxil—The first FDA-approved nano-drug: Lessons learned. *J. Control. Release* **2012**, *160*, 117–134. [CrossRef]

84. Jansook, P.; Ogawa, N.; Loftsson, T. Cyclodextrins: Structure, physicochemical properties and pharmaceutical applications. *Int. J. Pharm.* **2018**, *535*, 272–284. [CrossRef]

85. He, X.; Zhu, Y.; Wang, M.; Jing, G.; Zhu, R.; Wang, S. Antidepressant effects of curcumin and HU-211 coencapsulated solid lipid nanoparticles against corticosterone-induced cellular and animal models of major depression. *Int. J. Nanomed.* **2016**, *11*, 4975–4990. [CrossRef]

86. Kakkar, V.; Muppu, S.K.; Chopra, K.; Kaur, I.P. Curcumin loaded solid lipid nanoparticles: An efficient formulation approach for cerebral ischemic reperfusion injury in rats. *Eur. J. Pharm. Biopharm.* **2013**, *85*, 339–345. [CrossRef]

87. Sandhir, R.; Yadav, A.; Mehrotra, A.; Sunkaria, A.; Singh, A.; Sharma, S. Curcumin nanoparticles attenuate neurochemical and neurobehavioral deficits in experimental model of Huntington's disease. *Neuromol. Med.* **2014**, *16*, 106–118. [CrossRef] [PubMed]

88. Kundu, P.; Das, M.; Tripathy, K.; Sahoo, S.K. Delivery of Dual Drug Loaded Lipid Based Nanoparticles across the Blood-Brain Barrier Impart Enhanced Neuroprotection in a Rotenone Induced Mouse Model of Parkinson's Disease. *ACS Chem. Neurosci.* **2016**, *7*, 1658–1670. [CrossRef] [PubMed]

89. Ramalingam, P.; Ko, Y.T. Enhanced oral delivery of curcumin from N-trimethyl chitosan surface-modified solid lipid nanoparticles: Pharmacokinetic and brain distribution evaluations. *Pharm. Res.* **2015**, *32*, 389–402. [CrossRef] [PubMed]

90. Kakkar, V.; Kaur, I.P. Evaluating potential of curcumin loaded solid lipid nanoparticles in aluminium induced behavioural, biochemical and histopathological alterations in mice brain. *Food Chem. Toxicol.* **2011**, *49*, 2906–2913. [CrossRef] [PubMed]

91. Sadegh, M.S.; Azadi, A.; Izadi, Z.; Kurd, M.; Dara, T.; Dibaei, M.; Sharif Zadeh, M.; Akbari Javar, H.; Hamidi, M. Brain Delivery of Curcumin Using Solid Lipid Nanoparticles and Nanostructured Lipid Carriers: Preparation, Optimization, and Pharmacokinetic Evaluation. *ACS Chem. Neurosci.* **2018**, *10*, 728–739. [CrossRef] [PubMed]

92. Madane, R.G.; Mahajan, H.S. Curcumin-loaded nanostructured lipid carriers (NLCs) for nasal administration: Design, characterization, and in vivo study. *Drug Deliv.* **2016**, *23*, 1326–1334. [PubMed]

93. Fang, M.; Jin, Y.; Bao, W.; Gao, H.; Xu, M.; Wang, D.; Wang, X.; Yao, P.; Liu, L. In vitro characterization and in vivo evaluation of nanostructured lipid curcumin carriers for intragastric administration. *Int. J. Nanomed.* **2012**, *7*, 5395–5404. [CrossRef]

94. Meng, F.; Asghar, S.; Gao, S.; Su, Z.; Song, J.; Huo, M.; Meng, W.; Ping, Q.; Xiao, Y. A novel LDL-mimic nanocarrier for the targeted delivery of curcumin into the brain to treat Alzheimer's disease. *Colloids Surfaces B Biointerfaces* **2015**, *134*, 88–97. [CrossRef]

95. Meng, F.; Asghar, S.; Xu, Y.; Wang, J.; Jin, X.; Wang, Z.; Wang, J.; Ping, Q.; Zhou, J.; Xiao, Y. Design and evaluation of lipoprotein resembling curcumin-encapsulated protein-free nanostructured lipid carrier for brain targeting. *Int. J. Pharm.* **2016**, *506*, 46–56. [CrossRef]

96. Ameruoso, A.; Palomba, R.; Palange, A.L.; Cervadoro, A.; Lee, A.; Di Mascolo, D.; Decuzzi, P. Ameliorating amyloid-β fibrils triggered inflammation via curcumin-loaded polymeric nanoconstructs. *Front. Immunol.* **2017**, *8*, 1411. [CrossRef]

97. Mulik, R.S.; Mönkkönen, J.; Juvonen, R.O.; Mahadik, K.R.; Paradkar, A.R. ApoE3 Mediated Poly(butyl) Cyanoacrylate Nanoparticles Containing Curcumin: Study of Enhanced Activity of Curcumin against Beta Amyloid Induced Cytotoxicity Using In Vitro Cell Culture Model. *Mol. Pharm.* **2010**, *7*, 815–825. [CrossRef] [PubMed]

98. Mulik, R.S.; Mönkkönen, J.; Juvonen, R.O.; Mahadik, K.R.; Paradkar, A.R. ApoE3 mediated polymeric nanoparticles containing curcumin: Apoptosis induced in vitro anticancer activity against neuroblastoma cells. *Int. J. Pharm.* **2012**, *437*, 29–41. [CrossRef]

99. Szymusiak, M.; Hu, X.; Leon Plata, P.A.; Ciupinski, P.; Wang, Z.J.; Liu, Y. Bioavailability of curcumin and curcumin glucuronide in the central nervous system of mice after oral delivery of nano-curcumin. *Int. J. Pharm.* **2016**, *511*, 415–423. [CrossRef]

100. Tsai, Y.M.; Chien, C.F.; Lin, L.C.; Tsai, T.H. Curcumin and its nano-formulation: The kinetics of tissue distribution and blood-brain barrier penetration. *Int. J. Pharm.* **2011**, *416*, 331–338. [CrossRef] [PubMed]

101. Hu, X.; Huang, F.; Szymusiak, M.; Liu, Y.; Wang, Z.J. Curcumin Attenuates Opioid Tolerance and Dependence by Inhibiting $Ca^{2+}$/Calmodulin-Dependent Protein Kinase II $\alpha$ Activity. *J. Pharmacol. Exp. Ther.* **2015**, *352*, 420–428. [CrossRef] [PubMed]

102. Yadav, A.; Lomash, V.; Samim, M.; Flora, S.J.S. Curcumin encapsulated in chitosan nanoparticles: A novel strategy for the treatment of arsenic toxicity. *Chem. Biol. Interact.* **2012**, *199*, 49–61. [CrossRef] [PubMed]

103. Hashemian, M.; Anisian, D.; Ghasemi-Kasman, M.; Akbari, A.; Khalili-Fomeshi, M.; Ghasemi, S.; Ahmadi, F.; Moghadamnia, A.A.; Ebrahimpour, A. Curcumin-loaded chitosan-alginate-STPP nanoparticles ameliorate memory deficits and reduce glial activation in pentylenetetrazol-induced kindling model of epilepsy. *Prog. Neuro-Psychopharmacol. Biol. Psychiatry* **2017**, *79*, 462–471. [CrossRef]

104. Yang, R.; Zheng, Y.; Wang, Q.; Zhao, L. Curcumin-loaded chitosan–bovine serum albumin nanoparticles potentially enhanced Aβ 42 phagocytosis and modulated macrophage polarization in Alzheimer's disease. *Nanoscale Res. Lett.* **2018**, *13*, 1–9. [CrossRef]

105. Tiwari, S.K.; Agarwal, S.; Seth, B.; Yadav, A.; Nair, S.; Bhatnagar, P.; Karmakar, M.; Kumari, M.; Chauhan, L.K.S.; Patel, D.K.; et al. Curcumin-loaded nanoparticles potently induce adult neurogenesis and reverse cognitive deficits in Alzheimer's disease model via canonical Wnt/β-catenin pathway. *ACS Nano* **2014**, *8*, 76–103. [CrossRef]

106. Pieretti, S.; Ranjan, A.P.; Di Giannuario, A.; Mukerjee, A.; Marzoli, F.; Di Giovannandrea, R.; Vishwanatha, J.K. Curcumin-loaded Poly (D, L-lactide-co-glycolide) nanovesicles induce antinociceptive effects and reduce pronociceptive cytokine and BDNF release in spinal cord after acute administration in mice. *Colloids Surf. B Biointerfaces* **2017**, *158*, 379–386. [CrossRef]

107. Mathew, A.; Fukuda, T.; Nagaoka, Y.; Hasumura, T.; Morimoto, H.; Yoshida, Y.; Maekawa, T.; Venugopal, K.; Kumar, D.S. Curcumin loaded-PLGA nanoparticles conjugated with Tet-1 peptide for potential use in Alzheimer's disease. *PLoS ONE* **2012**, *7*, e32616. [CrossRef] [PubMed]

108. Fan, S.; Zheng, Y.; Liu, X.; Fang, W.; Chen, X.; Liao, W.; Jing, X.; Lei, M.; Tao, E.; Ma, Q.; et al. Curcumin-loaded PLGA-PEG nanoparticles conjugated with B6 peptide for potential use in Alzheimer's disease. *Drug Deliv.* **2018**, *25*, 1091–1102. [CrossRef] [PubMed]

109. Zhang, X.; Li, X.; Hua, H.; Wang, A.; Liu, W.; Li, Y.; Fu, F.; Shi, Y.; Sun, K. Cyclic hexapeptide-conjugated nanoparticles enhance curcumin delivery to glioma tumor cells and tissue. *Int. J. Nanomed.* **2017**, *12*, 5717–5732. [CrossRef] [PubMed]

110. Cui, Y.; Zhang, M.; Zeng, F.; Jin, H.; Xu, Q.; Huang, Y. Dual-Targeting Magnetic PLGA Nanoparticles for Codelivery of Paclitaxel and Curcumin for Brain Tumor Therapy. *ACS Appl. Mater. Interfaces* **2016**, *8*, 32159–32169. [CrossRef] [PubMed]

111. Orunoğlu, M.; Kaffashi, A.; Pehlivan, S.B.; Şahin, S.; Söylemezoğlu, F.; Karlı-Oğuz, K.; Mut, M. Effects of curcumin-loaded PLGA nanoparticles on the RG2 rat glioma model. *Mater. Sci. Eng. C* **2017**, *78*, 32–38. [CrossRef] [PubMed]

112. Zhang, Z.Y.; Jiang, M.; Fang, J.; Yang, M.F.; Zhang, S.; Yin, Y.X.; Li, D.W.; Mao, L.L.; Fu, X.Y.; Hou, Y.; et al. Enhanced Therapeutic Potential of Nano-Curcumin Against Subarachnoid Hemorrhage-Induced Blood–Brain Barrier Disruption Through Inhibition of Inflammatory Response and Oxidative Stress. *Mol. Neurobiol.* **2017**, *54*, 1–14. [CrossRef] [PubMed]

113. Cheng, K.K.; Yeung, C.F.; Ho, S.W.; Chow, S.F.; Chow, A.H.L.; Baum, L. Highly Stabilized Curcumin Nanoparticles Tested in an In Vitro Blood–Brain Barrier Model and in Alzheimer's Disease Tg2576 Mice. *AAPS J.* **2013**, *15*, 324–336. [CrossRef]

114. Yang, L.; Gao, S.; Asghar, S.; Liu, G.; Song, J.; Wang, X.; Ping, Q.; Zhang, C.; Xiao, Y. Hyaluronic acid/chitosan nanoparticles for delivery of curcuminoid and its in vitro evaluation in glioma cells. *Int. J. Biol. Macromol.* **2015**, *72*, 1391–1401. [CrossRef]

115. Mirgani, M.T.; Isacchi, B.; Sadeghizadeh, M.; Marra, F.; Bilia, A.R.; Mowla, S.J.; Najafi, F.; Babaei, E. Dendrosomal curcumin nanoformulation downregulates pluripotency genes via miR-145 activation in U87MG glioblastoma cells. *Int. J. Nanomed.* **2014**, *9*, 403–417.

116. Kumar, A.; Ahuja, A.; Ali, J.; Baboota, S. Curcumin-loaded lipid nanocarrier for improving bioavailability, stability and cytotoxicity against malignant glioma cells. *Drug Deliv.* **2016**, *23*, 214–229. [CrossRef]

117. Nasr, M. Development of an optimized hyaluronic acid-based lipidic nanoemulsion co-encapsulating two polyphenols for nose to brain delivery. *Drug Deliv.* **2016**, *23*, 1444–1452. [CrossRef] [PubMed]

118. Vaz, G.R.; Hädrich, G.; Bidone, J.; Rodrigues, J.L.; Falkembach, M.C.; Putaux, J.L.; Hort, M.A.; Monserrat, J.M.; Varela Junior, A.S.; Teixeira, H.F.; et al. Development of Nasal Lipid Nanocarriers Containing Curcumin for Brain Targeting. *J. Alzheimer's Dis.* **2017**, *59*, 961–974. [CrossRef] [PubMed]

*Biomolecules* **2019**, *9*, 56

119. Singh, A.K.; Jiang, Y.; Gupta, S.; Younus, M.; Ramzan, M. Anti-Inflammatory Potency of Nano-Formulated Puerarin and Curcumin in Rats Subjected to the Lipopolysaccharide-Induced Inflammation. *J. Med. Food* **2013**, *16*, 899–911. [CrossRef] [PubMed]

120. Cheng, K.K.; Chan, P.S.; Fan, S.; Kwan, S.M.; Yeung, K.L.; Wáng, Y.X.J.; Chow, A.H.L.; Wu, E.X.; Baum, L. Curcumin-conjugated magnetic nanoparticles for detecting amyloid plaques in Alzheimer's disease mice using magnetic resonance imaging (MRI). *Biomaterials* **2015**, *44*, 155–172. [CrossRef] [PubMed]

121. Ghorbani, M.; Bigdeli, B.; Jalili-baleh, L.; Baharifar, H.; Akrami, M.; Dehghani, S.; Goliaei, B.; Amani, A.; Lotfabadi, A.; Rashedi, H.; et al. Curcumin-lipoic acid conjugate as a promising anticancer agent on the surface of gold-iron oxide nanocomposites: A pH-sensitive targeted drug delivery system for brain cancer theranostics. *Eur. J. Pharm. Sci.* **2018**, *114*, 175–188. [CrossRef] [PubMed]

122. Naserzadeh, P.; Hafez, A.A.; Abdorahim, M.; Abdollahifar, M.A.; Shabani, R.; Peirovi, H.; Simchi, A.; Ashtari, K. Curcumin loading potentiates the neuroprotective efficacy of $Fe_3O_4$ magnetic nanoparticles in cerebellum cells of schizophrenic rats. *Biomed. Pharmacother.* **2018**, *108*, 1244–1252. [CrossRef] [PubMed]

123. Fang, J.H.; Chiu, T.L.; Huang, W.C.; Lai, Y.H.; Hu, S.H.; Chen, Y.Y.; Chen, S.Y. Dual-Targeting Lactoferrin-Conjugated Polymerized Magnetic Polydiacetylene-Assembled Nanocarriers with Self-Responsive Fluorescence/Magnetic Resonance Imaging for in vivo Brain Tumor Therapy. *Adv. Healthc. Mater.* **2016**, *5*, 688–695. [CrossRef]

124. Lazar, A.N.; Mourtas, S.; Youssef, I.; Parizot, C.; Dauphin, A.; Delatour, B.; Antimisiaris, S.G.; Duyckaerts, C. Curcumin-conjugated nanoliposomes with high affinity for Aβ deposits: Possible applications to Alzheimer disease. *Nanomed. Nanotechnol. Biol. Med.* **2013**, *9*, 712–721. [CrossRef]

125. Li, W.; Zhou, M.; Xu, N.; Hu, Y.; Wang, C.; Li, D.; Liu, L.; Li, D. Comparative analysis of protective effects of curcumin, curcumin-β-cyclodextrin nanoparticle and nanoliposomal curcumin on unsymmetrical dimethyl hydrazine poisoning in mice. *Bioengineered* **2016**, *7*, 334–341. [CrossRef]

126. Citron, M. Alzheimer's disease: Strategies for disease modification. *Nat. Rev. Drug Discov.* **2010**, *9*, 387–398. [CrossRef]

127. Ballatore, C.; Lee, V.M.-Y.; Trojanowski, J.Q. Tau-mediated neurodegeneration in Alzheimer's disease and related disorders. *Nat. Rev. Neurosci.* **2007**, *8*, 663–672. [CrossRef] [PubMed]

128. Djiokeng Paka, G.; Doggui, S.; Zaghmi, A.; Safar, R.; Dao, L.; Reisch, A.; Klymchenko, A.; Roullin, V.G.; Joubert, O.; Ramassamy, C. Neuronal Uptake and Neuroprotective Properties of Curcumin-Loaded Nanoparticles on SK-N-SH Cell Line: Role of Poly(lactide-co-glycolide) Polymeric Matrix Composition. *Mol. Pharm.* **2016**, *13*, 391–403. [CrossRef] [PubMed]

129. Barbara, R.; Belletti, D.; Pederzoli, F.; Masoni, M.; Keller, J.; Ballestrazzi, A.; Vandelli, M.A.; Tosi, G.; Grabrucker, A.M. Novel Curcumin loaded nanoparticles engineered for Blood-Brain Barrier crossing and able to disrupt Aβ aggregates. *Int. J. Pharm.* **2017**, *526*, 413–424. [CrossRef] [PubMed]

130. Huang, N.; Lu, S.; Liu, X.-G.; Zhu, J.; Wang, Y.-J.; Liu, R.-T. PLGA nanoparticles modified with a BBB-penetrating peptide co-delivering Aβ generation inhibitor and curcumin attenuate memory deficits and neuropathology in Alzheimer's disease mice. *Oncotarget* **2017**, *8*, 81001–81013. [PubMed]

131. Siddique, Y.H.; Khan, W.; Singh, B.R.; Naqvi, A.H. Synthesis of Alginate-Curcumin Nanocomposite and Its Protective Role in Transgenic *Drosophila* Model of Parkinson's Disease. *ISRN Pharmacol.* **2013**, *2013*, 794582. [CrossRef] [PubMed]

132. Bollimpelli, V.S.; Kumar, P.; Kumari, S.; Kondapi, A.K. Neuroprotective effect of curcumin-loaded lactoferrin nano particles against rotenone induced neurotoxicity. *Neurochem. Int.* **2016**, *95*, 37–45. [CrossRef] [PubMed]

133. Zhang, N.; Yan, F.; Liang, X.; Wu, M.; Shen, Y.; Chen, M.; Xu, Y.; Zou, G.; Jiang, P.; Tang, C.; et al. Localized delivery of curcumin into brain with polysorbate 80-modified cerasomes by ultrasound-targeted microbubble destruction for improved Parkinson's disease therapy. *Theranostics* **2018**, *8*, 2264–2277. [CrossRef] [PubMed]

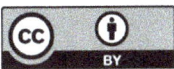

*biomolecules*

MDPI

*Article*

# NP-Scout: Machine Learning Approach for the Quantification and Visualization of the Natural Product-Likeness of Small Molecules

Ya Chen [1], Conrad Stork [1], Steffen Hirte [1] and Johannes Kirchmair [1,2,3,*]

[1]   Center for Bioinformatics (ZBH), Department of Informatics, Faculty of Mathematics, Informatics and
      Natural Sciences, Universität Hamburg, 20146 Hamburg, Germany; chen@zbh.uni-hamburg.de (Y.C.);
      stork@zbh.uni-hamburg.de (C.S.); steffen.hirte@studium.uni-hamburg.de (S.H.)
[2]   Department of Chemistry, University of Bergen, 5007 Bergen, Norway
[3]   Computational Biology Unit (CBU), Department of Informatics, University of Bergen, 5008 Bergen, Norway
*    Correspondence: johannes.kirchmair@uib.no or kirchmair@zbh.uni-hamburg.de; Tel.: +47-5558-3464

Received: 4 December 2018; Accepted: 21 January 2019; Published: 24 January 2019

**Abstract:** Natural products (NPs) remain the most prolific resource for the development of small-molecule drugs. Here we report a new machine learning approach that allows the identification of natural products with high accuracy. The method also generates similarity maps, which highlight atoms that contribute significantly to the classification of small molecules as a natural product or synthetic molecule. The method can hence be utilized to (i) identify natural products in large molecular libraries, (ii) quantify the natural product-likeness of small molecules, and (iii) visualize atoms in small molecules that are characteristic of natural products or synthetic molecules. The models are based on random forest classifiers trained on data sets consisting of more than 265,000 to 322,000 natural products and synthetic molecules. Two-dimensional molecular descriptors, MACCS keys and Morgan2 fingerprints were explored. On an independent test set the models reached areas under the receiver operating characteristic curve (AUC) of 0.997 and Matthews correlation coefficients (MCCs) of 0.954 and higher. The method was further tested on data from the Dictionary of Natural Products, ChEMBL and other resources. The best-performing models are accessible as a free web service at http://npscout.zbh.uni-hamburg.de/npscout.

**Keywords:** natural products; natural product-likeness; machine learning; random forest; classification; similarity maps; visualization; molecular fingerprints; web service

---

## 1. Introduction

Natural products (NPs) continue to be the most prolific resource for drug leads [1–4]. A recent analysis found that over 60% of all small-molecule drugs approved between 1981 and 2014 are genuine NPs, NP analogs or their derivatives, or compounds containing an NP pharmacophore [5]. NPs are characterized by enormous structural and physicochemical diversity [6–8]. Some of the regions in chemical space covered by NPs are not, or only rarely, populated by synthetic molecules (SMs) [7,9]. The structural complexity of many NPs exceeds that of compounds found in conventional synthetic libraries for screening, in particular with respect to stereochemical aspects, molecular shape, and ring systems [10–18].

The primary bottleneck of NP research is the scarcity of materials for testing. In a recent study, we showed that the molecular structures of more than 250,000 NPs have been deposited in public databases, and that only approximately 10% of these are readily obtainable from commercial providers and other sources [19].

Given the fact that NPs exhibit a wide range of biological activities that are of immediate relevance to human health, new avenues that would make NP research more effective are being explored, in particular, research involving computational approaches [2]. For example, computational methods have been employed successfully for the identification of bioactive NPs [20–22] and their bio-macromolecular targets [23–26]. They have also been successfully utilized for the design of simple synthetic, bioactive mimetics of NPs [27–29]. In this context, computational methods for quantifying the NP-likeness of compounds can be valuable tools to guide the de novo generation of NP mimetics and optimize the NP-likeness of lead compounds. Such methods may also be useful for identifying genuine NPs in commercial compound libraries, which often also contain SMs [19]. This can be valuable in the context of library design and for the prioritization of compounds for experimental testing.

The best-known in-silico approach for identifying NPs is the NP-likeness score developed by Ertl et al. [30]. The NP-likeness score is a Bayesian measure that quantifies a compound's similarity with the structural space of NPs based on structural fragments. As such, the model can identify sub-structures characteristic to NPs. The method has been re-implemented, with some modifications, in various platforms (e.g., [31–33]). Among them is the Natural-Product-Likeness Scoring System [31], which allows the calculation of the NP-likeness score (with some modifications). The Natural-Product-Likeness Scoring System also allows the use of customized data sets for training. An alternative approach for quantifying NP-Likeness, following a similar modeling strategy, but based on extended connectivity fingerprints (ECFPs), was reported by Yu [34]. Also a rule-based approach has been reported [35].

In this work, we present the development and validation of new machine learning models for the discrimination of NPs and SMs. To the best of our knowledge, these models are trained on the largest collection of known NPs that have been employed for the development of such classifiers. Among further developments, we present the utilization of similarity maps [36] for the visualization of atoms of a molecule, which are characteristic for NPs or SMs, according to the models.

## 2. Materials and Methods

### 2.1. Data Preparation

NPs were compiled from several physical and virtual NP databases (see Results for details). The chemical structures were parsed directly from SMILES notation, where available. Alternatively, chemical structures stored in chemical table files (e.g., SDF) were parsed with RDKit [37] and converted into SMILES. Minor components of salts were removed by the method described in ref. [38]. Any compounds with a molecular weight below 150 Da or above 1500 Da, and any compounds consisting of elements other than H, B, C, N, O, F, Si, P, S, Cl, Se, Br, or I were filtered. The "canonicalize" method, which was implemented in the "tautomer" class of MolVS [39], was used for neutralizing the molecular structures and merging tautomers. After the removal of duplicate SMILES (ignoring stereochemistry), the processed NP reference data set consisted of a total of 201,761 NPs.

SMs were compiled from the "in-stock" subset of ZINC [40,41]. In a first step, 500,000 compounds of ZINC were picked by random selection from the complete "in-stock" subset and pre-processed following the identical protocol used for the NP databases. After generating unique, canonicalized SMILES, any molecules present in the NP reference data set were removed from the SM data set (as determined by the comparison of canonicalized SMILES). Then, random sampling was used to compile a reference data set of SMs of identical size as the NP reference data set (i.e., 201,761 compounds).

The Dictionary of Natural Products (DNP) [42] and the ChEMBL database [43,44] were pre-processed following the identical protocol outlined for the NP and SM data sets. The ChEMBL sub-set of molecules, published in the Journal of Natural Products, was retrieved directly from ChEMBL [43,45]. The natural products subset of ZINC was downloaded from the ZINC website [46].

### 2.2. Principal Component Analysis

Fifteen two-dimensional molecular descriptors calculated with the Molecular Operating Environment (MOE) [47] were used for principle component analysis (PCA): MW (Weight), log

$P$ (log $P$ (o/w)), topological polar surface area (TPSA), number of hydrogen bond acceptors (a_acc), number of hydrogen bond donors (a_don), number of heavy atoms (a_heavy), fraction of rotatable bonds (b_rotR), number of nitrogen atoms (a_nN), number of oxygen atoms (a_nO), number of acidic atoms (a_acid), number of basic atoms (a_base), sum of formal charges (FCharge), number of aromatic atoms (a_aro) and number of chiral centers (chiral), and number of rings (rings).

*2.3. Model Building*

Prior to model building, the preprocessed NP and SM reference data sets were merged, resulting in a total of 403,522 data records. The merged data set was then randomly split into a training set of 322,817 and a test set of 80,705 compounds (ratio of 4:1). In fingerprint space, structurally distinct molecules may have identical fingerprints. For this reason, de-duplication, based on fingerprints, was separately performed for all NPs and all SMs in the training data. Any fingerprints present in both the NP and SM subsets were removed, in order to avoid conflicting class labels. This procedure resulted in a training set of 156,119 NPs and 161,378 SMs represented by Morgan2 fingerprints, and in a training set of 108,393 NPs and 157,162 SMs represented by MACCS keys.

Morgan2 fingerprints (1024 bits) [48,49] and MACCS keys (166 bits) were calculated with RDKit, and 206 two-dimensional physicochemical property descriptors were calculated with MOE. Random forest classifiers (RFCs) were generated with scikit-learn [50,51] using default settings, except for "n_estimators", which was set to "100", and "class_weight", which was set to "balanced".

The NP-likeness calculator [30,31,52] was trained on atom signatures derived from the identical NP and SM data sets, used for training the RFCs. Subsequently, the NP-likeness score was calculated for each molecule in the test set, according to the atom signatures. All calculations used a signature height of 3, resulting in scores ranging from −3 to 3. Molecules with a score greater than 0.0 were labeled as NPs, and molecules with a score lower, or equal to 0.0 were labeled as SMs. NP class probabilities (and AUCs) were derived by normalizing these scores to a range from 0.0 to 1.0.

*2.4. Similarity Maps*

Similarity maps were computed with the RDKit [37] Chem.Draw.SimilarityMaps module based on RFCs derived from Morgan2 fingerprints (1024 bits).

**3. Results**

*3.1. Compilation of Data Sets for Model Development*

An NP reference data set of 201,761 unique NPs was compiled from 18 virtual NP libraries and nine physical NP databases. The reference data set is identical to that compiled as part of our previous work [8], with two amendments: First, the compounds of the DNP [42] were not included in the data set, as they serve as an external test set in this work, and second, the recently published Natural Products Atlas database [53] was added as a new data source. An overview of the NP data sources utilized in this work is provided in Table 1. The table also reports the number of molecules that are contained in the individual databases prior to, and after, data preprocessing. This is a procedure that includes the removal of salt components and stereochemical information, the filtering of molecules composed of uncommon elements, and with a molecular weight (MW) below 150 Da or above 1500 Da, and the removal of duplicate molecules (see Methods for details). An equal amount (i.e., 201,761) of synthetic organic molecules (SMs) was collected from the "in-stock" subset of ZINC [41] by random selection.

**Table 1.** Size of the individual data sets prior to and after data preprocessing.

| Name [1] | Number of Molecules in SMILES Notation Successfully Parsed with RDKit | Number of Unique Molecules After Data Preprocessing | Scientific Literature and/or Online Presence |
|---|---|---|---|
| UNPD | 229,140 | 161,228 | [54,55] |
| TCM Database@Taiwan | 56,325 | 45,422 | [56,57] |
| NP Atlas | 20,010 | 18,358 | [53] |
| TCMID | 13,188 | 10,918 | [58,59] |
| TIPdb | 8838 | 7620 | [60–62] |
| Ambinter and Greenpharma NPs | 7905 | 6680 | [63,64] |
| AnalytiCon Discovery MEGx | 4315 | 4063 | [65] |
| NANPDB | 6841 | 3734 | [66,67] |
| StreptomeDB | 3990 | 3353 | [68,69] |
| NPs of PubChem Substance Database | 3533 | 2638 | [70,71] |
| NuBBE | 1856 | 1637 | [72,73] |
| Pi Chemicals NPs | 1783 | 1511 | [74] |
| NPCARE | 1613 | 1479 | [75,76] |
| NPACT | 1516 | 1376 | [77,78] |
| InterBioScreen NPs | 1359 | 1116 | [79] |
| AfroDb | 954 | 865 | [80,81] |
| TargetMol Natural Compound Library | 850 | 745 | [82] |
| HIM | 1284 | 641 | [83,84] |
| SANCDB | 623 | 588 | [85,86] |
| UEFS Natural Products | 493 | 469 | via ZINC [40,87] |
| p-ANAPL | 538 | 456 | [88] |
| NCI/NIH DTP NP set IV | 419 | 394 | [89] |
| HIT | 707 | 362 | [90,91] |
| AfroCancer | 388 | 352 | [92,93] |
| AfroMalariaDB | 265 | 250 | [94,95] |
| AK Scientific NPs | 242 | 177 | [96] |
| Selleck Chemicals NPs | 173 | 163 | [97] |
| **NP data set TOTAL** | - | **201761** | |

[1] UNPD: the Universal Natural Products Database; TCM Database@Taiwan: the Traditional Chinese Medicine Database@Taiwan; NP Atlas: the Natural Products Atlas; TCMID: the Traditional Chinese Medicine Integrated Database; TIPdb: the Taiwan Indigenous Plant Database; NANPDB: the Northern African Natural Products Database; StreptomeDB: Streptome Database; NuBBE: Nuclei of Bioassays, Ecophysiology and Biosynthesis of Natural Products Database; NPCARE: Database of Natural Products for Cancer Gene Regulation; NPACT: the Naturally Occurring Plant-based Anti-Cancer Compound-Activity-Target Database; AfroDb: NPs from African medicinal plants; HIM: the Herbal Ingredients in-vivo Metabolism Database; UEFS Natural Products: the natural products database of the State University of Feira De Santana; p-ANAPL: the Pan-African Natural Products Library; NCI/NIH DTP NP set IV: the NP (plated) set IV of the Developmental Therapeutic Program of the National Cancer Institute/National Institutes of Health; HIT, the Herbal Ingredients' Targets Database; AfroCancer, the African Anticancer Natural Products Library; AfroMalariaDB, the African Antimalarial Natural Products Library.

## 3.2. Analysis of the Physicochemical Properties of Natural Products and Synthetic Molecules

Prior to model development, we compared the chemical space covered by the 201,761 unique NPs, and the equal number of unique SMs, using principal component analysis (PCA), based on 15 relevant physicochemical properties (see Methods for details). The score plot in Figure 1 shows that the chemical space of SMs is essentially a sub-space of NPs.

NPs have on average a higher MW than SMs (506 Da vs 384 Da) and a larger proportion of heavy compounds (38% vs. 10% of all molecules have a MW greater than 500 Da; Figure 2a). SMs have a narrower distribution of calculated log *P* values as compared to NPs (Figure 2b) but their averages are comparable (3.31 versus 3.25). SMs and NPs show clear differences in the entropy of element distributions in molecules, with NPs having, on average, a lower entropy than SMs (1.39 versus 1.63; Figure 2c). NPs tend to have more chiral centers (mean 6.66 vs. 0.75; Figure 2d), substantially fewer nitrogen atoms than SMs (mean 0.76 vs. 2.94; Figure 2e), and more oxygen atoms (mean 7.39 vs. 2.88; Figure 2f) [7,10,12–15,17].

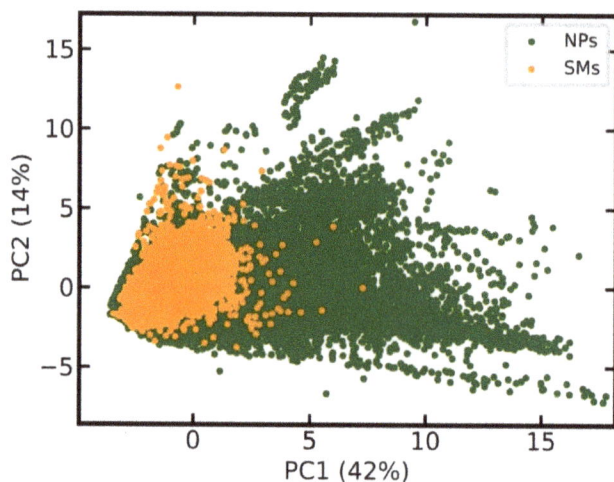

**Figure 1.** Comparison of the chemical space covered by natural products (NPs) and synthetic organic molecules (SMs). The score plot is based on the principle component analysis (PCA) of all molecules in the data set, characterized by 15 calculated physicochemical properties. PCA was performed on the full data sets. For the sake of clarity, only a randomly selected 10% of all data points are reported in the score plot. The percentage of the total variance explained by the first two principal components is reported in the respective axis labels.

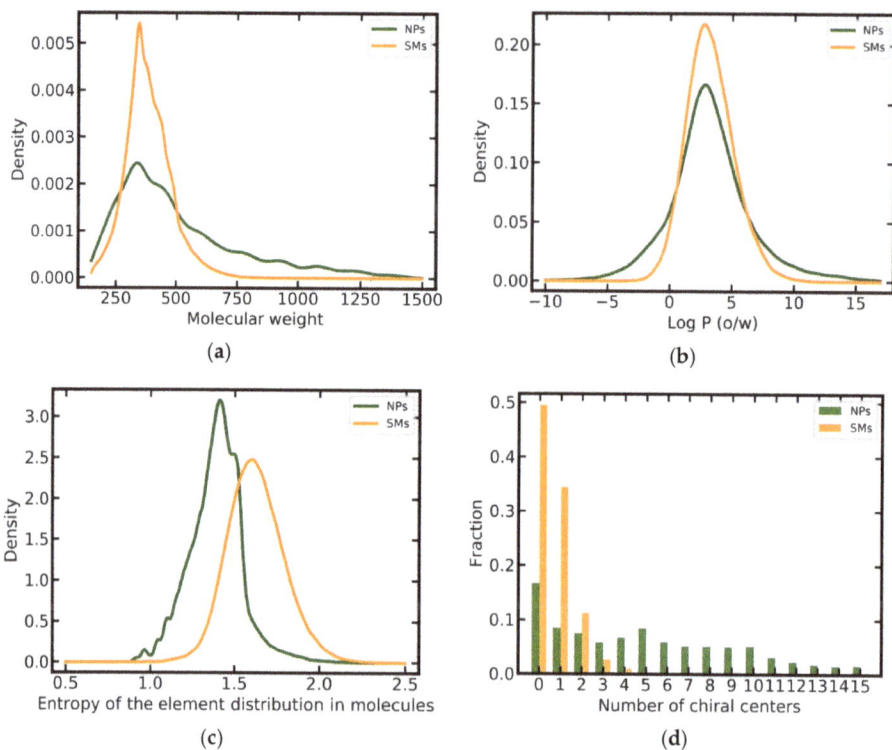

**Figure 2.** *Cont.*

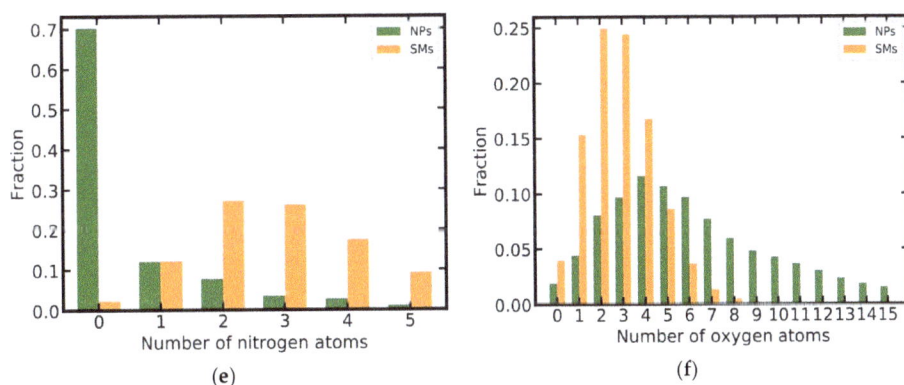

**Figure 2.** Distributions of key physicochemical properties among NPs and SMs: (**a**) Molecular weight; (**b**) log *P* (o/w); (**c**) entropy of the element distribution in molecules; (**d**) number of chiral centers; (**e**) number of nitrogen atoms; (**f**) number of oxygen atoms.

## 3.3. Model Development and Selection

Random forest classifiers [98] were trained on three different descriptor sets: 206 two-dimensional physicochemical property descriptors calculated with MOE [47], Morgan2 fingerprints (1024 bits) [48,49] calculated with RDKit [37], and MACCS keys (166 bits), also calculated with RDKit. Model performance was characterized utilizing the Matthews correlation coefficient (MCC) [99] and area under the receiver operating characteristic curve (AUC). The MCC is one of the most robust measures for evaluating the performance of binary classifiers, as it considers the proportion of all classes in the confusion matrix (i.e., true positives, false positives, true negatives, and false negatives). The AUC was used to measure how well the models are able to rank NPs early in a list.

As reported in Table 2, the models derived from any of the three descriptor sets performed very well. The AUC values, that were obtained during 10-fold cross-validation, were between 0.996 and 0.997; the MCC values were 0.950 or higher. No noticeable increase in performance was obtained by the further increase in the number of estimators (n_estimators) and the optimization of the maximum fraction of features considered per split (max_features; data not shown). Therefore, we chose to use 100 estimators, and the square root of the number of features, as the most suitable setup for model generation.

**Table 2.** Performance of models derived from different descriptors or fingerprints.

| Test Method | Metric [1] | MOE Two-Dimensional Descriptors | Morgan2 Fingerprints (1024 Bits) | MACCS Keys | NP-Likeness Calculator |
|---|---|---|---|---|---|
| 10-fold cross-validation | AUC | 0.997 | 0.997 | 0.996 | / |
| | MCC | 0.953 | 0.958 | 0.950 | / |
| Independent test set | AUC | 0.997 | 0.997 | 0.997 | 0.997 |
| | MCC | 0.954 | 0.960 | 0.960 | 0.959 |

[1] AUC: area under the receiver operating characteristic curve: MCC: Matthews correlation coefficient.

## 3.4. Model Validation

In a first step, the performance of the selected models was tested on an independent test set. The AUC and MCC values, that were obtained for the selected models on this independent test set, are comparable with those obtained for the 10-fold cross-validation: AUC values were 0.997 for models based on any of the three types of descriptors and MCC values were 0.954 or higher.

Given the fact that the type of descriptor, used for model generation, did not have a substantial impact on model performance, we opted to select the model based on MACCS keys as the primary model for further experiments, because of its low complexity and good interpretability. This model achieved a very good separation of NPs and SMs for the independent test set, as shown in Figure 3a. Approximately 63% of all NPs were assigned an NP class probability of 1.0, whereas 51% SMs were assigned an NP class probability of 0.0. Only approximately 1% of all compounds were assigned values close to the decision threshold of 0.5 (i.e., between 0.4 and 0.6).

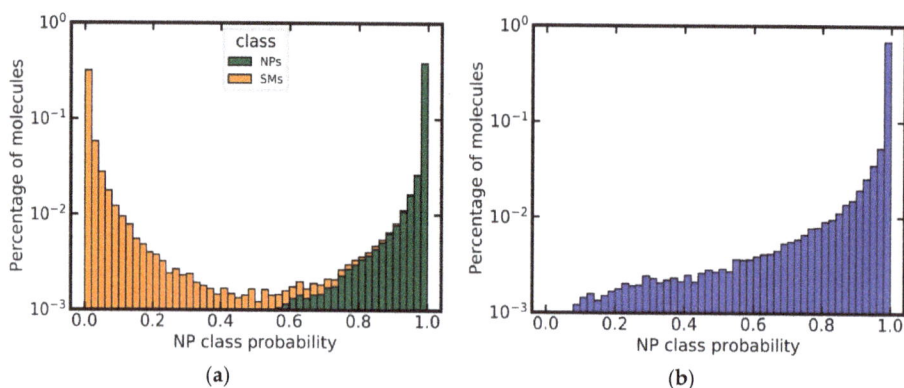

**Figure 3.** Predicted NP class probabilities distributions for (**a**) the independent test set (stacked histogram), (**b**) the DNP (after the removal of any compounds present in the training set). Note that the y-axis is in logarithmic scale.

The model's ability to identify NPs was also tested using the DNP as an external validation set. By definition, the DNP should consist exclusively of NPs. After the removal of any molecules present in the training data (based on canonicalized SMILES), the preprocessed DNP consisted of 60,502 compounds. Approximately 95% of these compounds were predicted as NPs by the model, demonstrating the model's capacity to identify NPs with high sensitivity (Figure 3b).

*3.5. Comparison of Model Performance with the NP-Likeness Calculator*

We compared the performance of the model derived from MACCS keys to the NP-likeness calculator (based on the Natural-Product-Likeness Scoring System; see Introduction), which we trained and tested on the identical data sets used for the development of our models. On the independent test set, the NP-likeness calculator performed equally well as our model, with an AUC of 0.997 and an MCC of 0.959 (Table 2). Approximately 95% of all compounds of the DNP were classified as NPs (i.e., having assigned an NP-likeness score greater than 0; see Figure S1), which is comparable to the classification obtained with our model based on MACCS keys.

*3.6. Analysis of Class Probability Distributions for Different Data Sets*

In addition to the above experiments, we used the model based on MACCS keys for profiling the ChEMBL database and a subset thereof. The ChEMBL database [44] primarily contains SMs, and 87% of all compounds stored in ChEMBL were predicted as such (Figure 4a). Interestingly, 42,949 molecules (~3%) were assigned an NP class probability of 1.0, and therefore likely are NPs. This finding is in agreement with our previous study, which identified approximately 40,000 NPs in the ChEMBL database, by overlapping the database with a comprehensive set of known NPs [19].

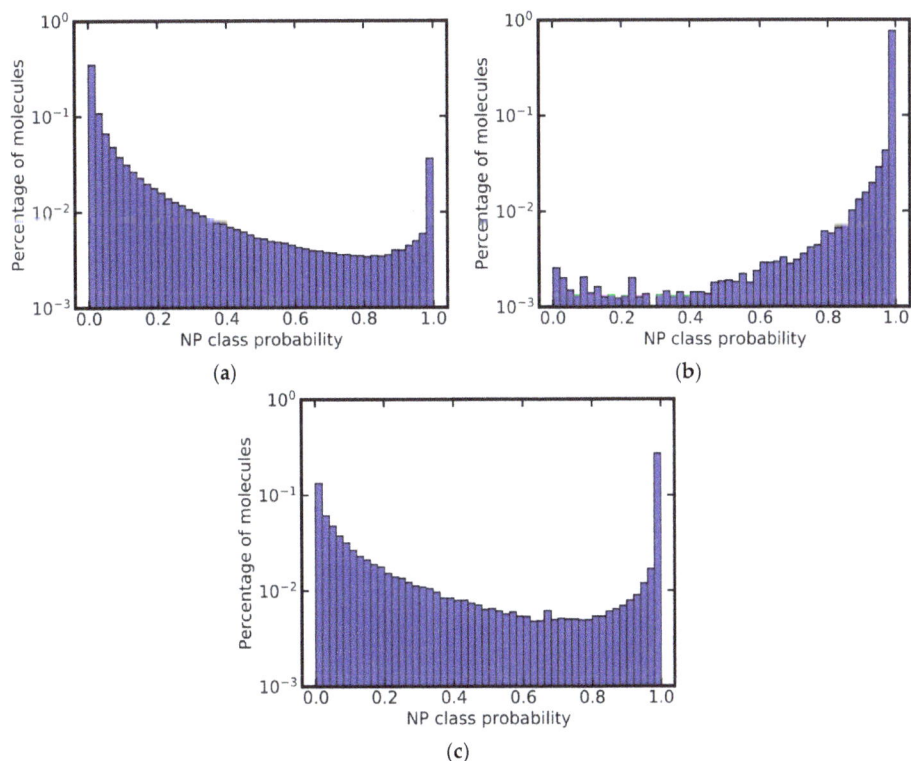

**Figure 4.** Predicted NP class probability distributions for (**a**) the ChEMBL database, (**b**) a subset of the ChEMBL database composed of molecules originating from the Journal of Natural Products, and (**c**) the natural products subset of ZINC. Note that the y-axis is in logarithmic scale.

A subset of the ChEMBL database containing molecules originating from the Journal of Natural Products [45] has been used as a source of genuine NPs to train models for the prediction of NP-likeness [31]. Our model based on MACCS keys predicts a small percentage of the molecules (less than 4%) in this data set as not NP-like (Figure 4b). Closer inspection of the compounds predicted as not NP-like reveals that these are, for example, SMs used as positive controls in biochemical assays. They include the drugs celecoxib, glibenclamide and linezolid, all of which are predicted with an NP class probability of 0.0. This experiment demonstrates that the classifiers can be used as powerful tools for the identification of NPs or SMs in mixed data sets with high accuracy.

A second example of a data set that by its name is assumed to consist exclusively of NPs is the natural products subset of ZINC [46]. The class probability distribution calculated for this subset however is similar to that obtained for the complete ChEMBL, indicating the presence of a substantial number of SMs (including NP derivatives and NP analogs) in this subset (Figure 4c): Only approximately 43% of all compounds in the NPs subset of ZINC were classified as NPs; around 23% were assigned an NP class probability of 1.0.

*3.7. Analysis of Discriminative Features of Natural Products and Synthetic Molecules*

The most discriminative features were determined, based on the feature_importances_ attributes computed with scikit-learn (see Methods for details). For the classifier based on MOE two-dimensional molecular descriptors, the three most important features were the number of nitrogen atoms (a large fraction of NPs has no nitrogen atom; see Figure 2e), the entropy of the element distribution in molecules (NPs have on average lower element distribution entropy than SMs; see Figure 2c), and the number of unconstrained chiral centers (NPs have on average more chiral centers than SMs; see Figure 2d). An overview of the ten most important features is provided in Table 3.

**Table 3.** Feature importance for the random forest classifier based on MOE two-dimensional descriptors.

| Identifier Used by MOE | Feature Importance [1] | Description |
|---|---|---|
| a_nN | 0.103 | Number of nitrogen atoms. |
| a_ICM | 0.051 | Entropy of the element distribution in the molecule. |
| chiral_u | 0.045 | Number of unconstrained chiral centers. |
| GCUT_SLOGP_0 | 0.045 | Descriptor derived from graph distance adjacency matrices utilizing atomic contribution to log $P$. |
| SlogP_VSA0 | 0.044 | Surface area descriptor taking into account the contributions of individual atoms to log $P$. |
| chiral | 0.042 | Number of chiral centers. |
| GCUT_SLOGP_3 | 0.036 | Descriptor derived from graph distance adjacency matrices utilizing atomic contribution to log $P$. |
| a_nO | 0.025 | The number of oxygen atoms. |
| GCUT_PEOE_0 | 0.025 | Descriptor derived from graph distance adjacency matrices utilizing partial equalization of orbital electronegativities charges. |
| SlogP_VSA1 | 0.024 | Surface area descriptor taking into account the contributions of individual atoms to log $P$. |

[1] From the feature_importances_ attribute of the classifier based on MOE two-dimensional descriptors. The higher, the more important the feature is.

For the classifier based on MACCS keys, the 15 most important features are reported in Figure 5. In agreement with the differences observed in the physiochemical property distributions of NPs versus SMs (see Analysis of the Physicochemical Properties of Natural Products and Synthetic Molecules), the most important MACCS keys describe the presence or absence of nitrogen atoms, such as key 161, matching molecules containing at least one nitrogen atom, key 142, matching molecules with at least two nitrogen atoms, and keys 117, 158, 122, 156, 75, 110, 133, 92 and 80, matching molecules containing specific nitrogen-containing substructures. Also several oxy gen-containing substructures are among the most important features, such as keys 139, 117, 110, 92.

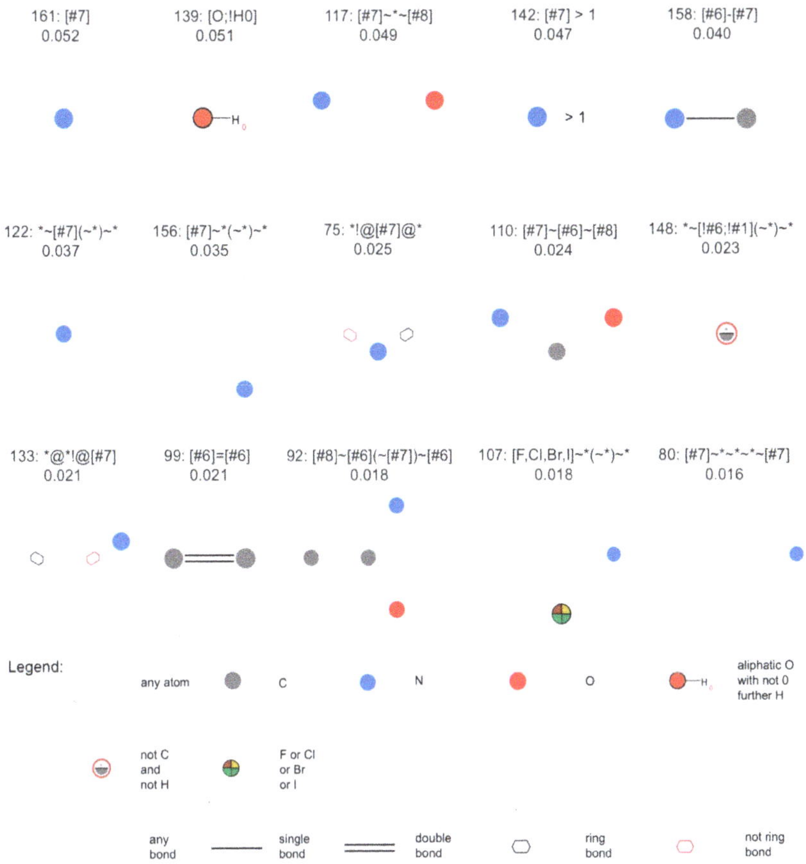

**Figure 5.** The 15 most relevant MACCS keys, sorted by decreasing feature importance. Above each diagram, the first line reports the index of the respective MACCS key and its SMARTS pattern. The second line reports the feature importance (feature_importances_ attribute). The figure was produced with SMARTSviewer [100,101].

## 3.8. Similarity Maps

Similarity maps [36] allow the visualization of the atomic contribution of molecular fingerprints and can be extended to visualize the "atomic weights" of the predicted probability of the machine learning model. During several test runs with different Morgan fingerprint, radii, and bit vector lengths, we identified a radius of 2 and a bit vector length of 1024 bits as the most suitable setup for generating fine-grained similarity maps. The examples of similarity maps, generated with this descriptor, and the random forest approach, are reported in Table 4 for representative molecules, none of which have been part of model training. In this similarity maps, green highlights mark atoms contributing to the classification of a molecule as NP, whereas orange highlights mark atoms contributing to the classification of a molecule as SM. As expected, the similarity maps for the NP arglabin are mostly green, whereas for the synthetic drugs, bilastine and perampanel, are mostly orange. For NP derivatives and mimetics, the similarity maps are more heterogeneous and show green, as well as orange areas. The thrombin receptor antagonist vorapaxar is a derivative of the piperidine alkaloid himbacine. Vorapaxar shares a decahydronaphtho[2,3-c]furan-1(3H)-one scaffold with himbacine, but has the piperidine ring replaced by a pyridine, besides other modifications. The similarity map generated for vorapaxar shows that the model correctly identifies the decahydronaphtho[2,3-c]furan-1(3H)-one as NP-like, whereas it associates the modified areas with synthetic molecules. In the case of empagliflozin, which mimics the flavonoid phlorozin, the model correctly recognizes the C-glycosyl moiety as NP-like, whereas other atoms in the molecule are associated with synthetic molecules.

**Table 4.** Examples of similarity maps generated by the NP classifier based on Morgan2 fingerprints.

| Similarity Map [1] | Name | Source [2] | NP Class Probability | Disease Indication | Year Introduced |
|---|---|---|---|---|---|
| | arglabin | N | 1.0 | anticancer | 1999 |
| | cefonicid sodium | ND | 0.34 | antibacterial | 1984 |
| | dutaseride | ND | 0.18 | benign prostatic hypertrophy | 2001 |
| | vorapaxar | ND | 0.30 | coronary artery disease | 2014 |
| | empagliflozin | S*/NM | 0.67 | antidiabetic (diabetes 2) | 2014 |
| | belinostat | S*/NM | 0.09 | anticancer | 2014 |
| | febuxostat | S/NM | 0.19 | hyperuricemia | 2009 |
| | zalcitabine | S* | 0.46 | antiviral | 1992 |

**Table 4.** *Cont.*

| Similarity Map [1] | Name | Source [2] | NP Class Probability | Disease Indication | Year Introduced |
|---|---|---|---|---|---|
| 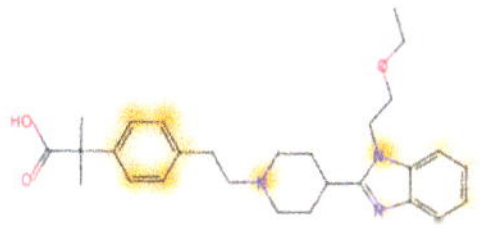 | bilastine | S | 0.17 | antihistamine | 2011 |
| 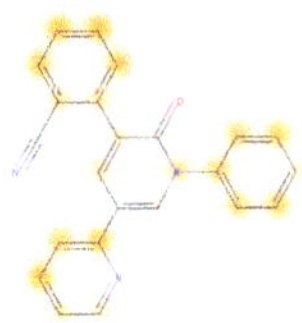 | perampanel | S | 0.16 | antiepileptic | 2012 |

[1] Green highlights mark atoms contributing to the classification of a molecule as NP, whereas orange highlights mark atoms contributing to the classification of a molecule as SM. [2] N: Unaltered NP; ND: NP derivative; S*: Synthetic drug (NP pharmacophore); S: Synthetic drug; NM: Mimic of NP. Definitions according to ref [5].

### 3.9. NP-Scout Web Service

A web service named "NP-Scout" is accessible free of charge via http://npscout.zbh.uni-hamburg. de/npscout. It features the random forest model, based on MACCS keys for the computation of NP class probabilities and the random forest model, based on Morgan2 fingerprints (with 1024 bits) for the generation of similarity maps.

Users can submit molecular structures for calculation, by entering SMILES, uploading a file with SMILES or a list of SMILES, or drawing the molecule with the JavaScript Molecule Editor (JSME) [102]. The results page (Figure 6) presents the calculated NP class probabilities and similarity maps of submitted molecules in a tabular format. The results can be downloaded in CSV file format. Calculations of the NP class probabilities and the similarity maps take few seconds per compound and approximately 15 min for 1000 compounds. Users may utilize a unique link provided upon job submission to return to the website after all calculations have been completed.

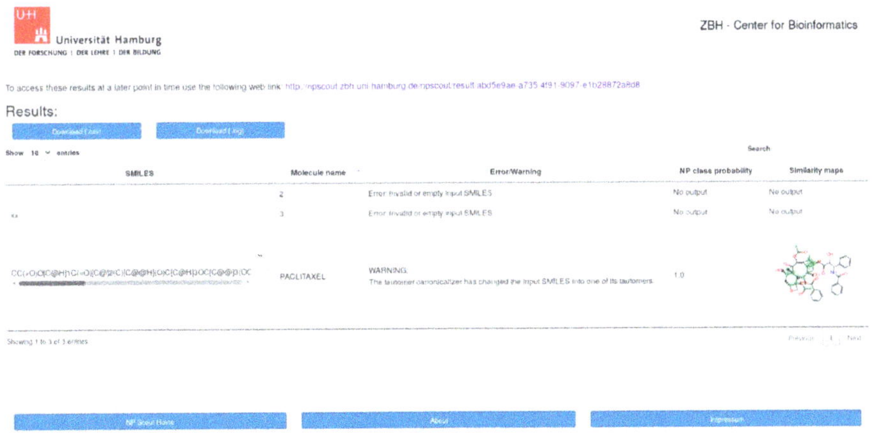

**Figure 6.** Screenshot of the result page of NP-Scout.

## 4. Conclusions

In this work, we introduced a pragmatic machine learning approach for the discrimination of NPs and SMs and for the quantification of NP-likeness. As shown by validation experiments using independent and external testing data, the models reach a very high level of accuracy. An interesting and relevant new aspect of this work is the utilization of similarity maps to visualize atoms in molecules making decisive contributions to the assignment of compounds to either class. A free web service for the classification of small molecules and the visualization of similarity maps is available at http://npscout.zbh.uni-hamburg.de/npscout.

**Supplementary Materials:** The following are available online at http://www.mdpi.com/2218-273X/9/2/43/s1, Figure S1: Distribution of calculated NP-likeness scores for the DNP (after removal of any compounds present in the training set).

**Author Contributions:** Conceptualization, Y.C. and J.K.; methodology, Y.C. and J.K.; software, Y.C., C.S., and S.H.; validation, Y.C.; formal analysis, Y.C; investigation, Y.C., C.S., and S.H.; resources, J.K.; data curation, Y.C.; writing—original draft preparation, Y.C., C.S., S.H., and J.K.; visualization, Y.C. and S.H.; supervision, J.K.; project administration, J.K.; funding acquisition, Y.C. and J.K.

**Funding:** Y.C. is supported by the China Scholarship Council, grant number 201606010345. C.S. and J.K. are supported by the Deutsche Forschungsgemeinschaft (DFG, German Research Foundation), project number KI 2085/1-1. J.K. is also supported by the Bergens Forskningsstiftelse (BFS, Bergen Research Foundation), grant number BFS2017TMT01.

**Acknowledgments:** Gerd Embruch from the Center of Bioinformatics (ZBH) of the Universität Hamburg is thanked for his technical support with the web service.

**Conflicts of Interest:** The authors declare no conflict of interest. The funders had no role in the design of the study; in the collection, analyses, or interpretation of data; in the writing of the manuscript, and in the decision to publish the results.

## References

1. Cragg, G.M.; Newman, D.J. Biodiversity: A continuing source of novel drug leads. *J. Macromol. Sci. Part A Pure Appl. Chem.* **2005**, *77*, 7–24. [CrossRef]
2. Rodrigues, T.; Reker, D.; Schneider, P.; Schneider, G. Counting on natural products for drug design. *Nat. Chem.* **2016**, *8*, 531–541. [CrossRef] [PubMed]
3. Harvey, A.L.; Edrada-Ebel, R.; Quinn, R.J. The re-emergence of natural products for drug discovery in the genomics era. *Nat. Rev. Drug Discov.* **2015**, *14*, 111–129. [CrossRef]
4. Shen, B. A new golden age of natural products drug discovery. *Cell* **2015**, *163*, 1297–1300. [CrossRef] [PubMed]
5. Newman, D.J.; Cragg, G.M. Natural products as sources of new drugs from 1981 to 2014. *J. Nat. Prod.* **2016**, *79*, 629–661. [CrossRef] [PubMed]
6. Grabowski, K.; Baringhaus, K.-H.; Schneider, G. Scaffold diversity of natural products: Inspiration for combinatorial library design. *Nat. Prod. Rep.* **2008**, *25*, 892–904. [CrossRef]
7. Ertl, P.; Schuffenhauer, A. Cheminformatics analysis of natural products: Lessons from nature inspiring the design of new drugs. *Prog. Drug Res.* **2008**, *66*, 219–235.
8. Chen, Y.; de Lomana, M.G.; Friedrich, N.-O.; Kirchmair, J. Characterization of the chemical space of known and Readily Obtainable Natural Products. *J. Chem. Inf. Model.* **2018**, *58*, 1518–1532. [CrossRef]
9. Chen, H.; Engkvist, O.; Blomberg, N.; Li, J. A comparative analysis of the molecular topologies for drugs, clinical candidates, natural products, human metabolites and general bioactive compounds. *Med. Chem. Commun.* **2012**, *3*, 312–321. [CrossRef]
10. Camp, D.; Garavelas, A.; Campitelli, M. Analysis of physicochemical properties for drugs of natural origin. *J. Nat. Prod.* **2015**, *78*, 1370–1382. [CrossRef]
11. Koch, M.A.; Schuffenhauer, A.; Scheck, M.; Wetzel, S.; Casaulta, M.; Odermatt, A.; Ertl, P.; Waldmann, H. Charting biologically relevant chemical space: A structural classification of natural products (SCONP). *Proc. Natl. Acad. Sci. USA* **2005**, *102*, 17272–17277. [CrossRef] [PubMed]
12. Stratton, C.F.; Newman, D.J.; Tan, D.S. Cheminformatic comparison of approved drugs from natural product versus synthetic origins. *Bioorg. Med. Chem. Lett.* **2015**, *25*, 4802–4807. [CrossRef] [PubMed]

13. Wetzel, S.; Schuffenhauer, A.; Roggo, S.; Ertl, P.; Waldmann, H. Cheminformatic analysis of natural products and their chemical space. *CHIMIA Int. J. Chem.* **2007**, *61*, 355–360. [CrossRef]

14. López-Vallejo, F.; Giulianotti, M.A.; Houghten, R.A.; Medina-Franco, J.L. Expanding the medicinally relevant chemical space with compound libraries. *Drug Discov. Today* **2012**, *17*, 718–726. [CrossRef]

15. Feher, M.; Schmidt, J.M. Property distributions: Differences between drugs, natural products, and molecules from combinatorial chemistry. *J. Chem. Inf. Comput. Sci.* **2003**, *43*, 218–227. [CrossRef] [PubMed]

16. Clemons, P.A.; Bodycombe, N.E.; Carrinski, H.A.; Wilson, J.A.; Shamji, A.F.; Wagner, B.K.; Koehler, A.N.; Schreiber, S.L. Small molecules of different origins have distinct distributions of structural complexity that correlate with protein binding profiles. *Proc. Natl. Acad. Sci. USA* **2010**, *107*, 18787–18792. [CrossRef] [PubMed]

17. Henkel, T.; Brunne, R.M.; Müller, H.; Reichel, F. Statistical investigation into the structural complementarity of natural products and synthetic compounds. *Angew. Chem. Int. Ed. Engl.* **1999**, *38*, 643–647. [CrossRef]

18. Lee, M.L.; Schneider, G. Scaffold architecture and pharmacophoric properties of natural products and trade drugs: Application in the design of natural product-based combinatorial libraries. *J. Comb. Chem.* **2001**, *3*, 284–289. [CrossRef]

19. Chen, Y.; de Bruyn Kops, C.; Kirchmair, J. Data resources for the computer-guided discovery of bioactive natural products. *J. Chem. Inf. Model.* **2017**, *57*, 2099–2111. [CrossRef]

20. Rupp, M.; Schroeter, T.; Steri, R.; Zettl, H.; Proschak, E.; Hansen, K.; Rau, O.; Schwarz, O.; Müller-Kuhrt, L.; Schubert-Zsilavecz, M.; et al. From machine learning to natural product derivatives that selectively activate transcription factor PPARγ. *ChemMedChem* **2010**, *5*, 191–194. [CrossRef]

21. Maindola, P.; Jamal, S.; Grover, A. Cheminformatics based machine learning models for AMA1-RON2 abrogators for inhibiting Plasmodium falciparum erythrocyte invasion. *Mol. Inform.* **2015**, *34*, 655–664. [CrossRef] [PubMed]

22. Chagas-Paula, D.A.; Oliveira, T.B.; Zhang, T.; Edrada-Ebel, R.; Da Costa, F.B. Prediction of anti-inflammatory plants and discovery of their biomarkers by machine learning algorithms and metabolomic studies. *Planta Med.* **2015**, *81*, 450–458. [CrossRef] [PubMed]

23. Reker, D.; Perna, A.M.; Rodrigues, T.; Schneider, P.; Reutlinger, M.; Mönch, B.; Koeberle, A.; Lamers, C.; Gabler, M.; Steinmetz, H.; et al. Revealing the macromolecular targets of complex natural products. *Nat. Chem.* **2014**, *6*, 1072–1078. [CrossRef] [PubMed]

24. Rodrigues, T.; Sieglitz, F.; Somovilla, V.J.; Cal, P.M.S.D.; Galione, A.; Corzana, F.; Bernardes, G.J.L. Unveiling (−)-englerin A as a modulator of L-type calcium channels. *Angew. Chem. Int. Ed. Engl.* **2016**, *55*, 11077–11081. [CrossRef] [PubMed]

25. Merk, D.; Grisoni, F.; Friedrich, L.; Gelzinyte, E.; Schneider, G. Computer-assisted discovery of retinoid X receptor modulating natural products and isofunctional mimetics. *J. Med. Chem.* **2018**, *61*, 5442–5447. [CrossRef] [PubMed]

26. Schneider, P.; Schneider, G. De-orphaning the marine natural product (±)-marinopyrrole A by computational target prediction and biochemical validation. *Chem. Commun.* **2017**, *53*, 2272–2274.

27. Merk, D.; Grisoni, F.; Friedrich, L.; Schneider, G. Tuning artificial intelligence on the de novo design of natural-product-inspired retinoid X receptor modulators. *Commun. Chem.* **2018**, *1*, 68.

28. Friedrich, L.; Rodrigues, T.; Neuhaus, C.S.; Schneider, P.; Schneider, G. From complex natural products to simple synthetic mimetics by computational de novo design. *Angew. Chem. Int. Ed. Engl.* **2016**, *55*, 6789–6792. [CrossRef]

29. Grisoni, F.; Merk, D.; Consonni, V.; Hiss, J.A.; Tagliabue, S.G.; Todeschini, R.; Schneider, G. Scaffold hopping from natural products to synthetic mimetics by holistic molecular similarity. *Commun. Chem.* **2018**, *1*, 44.

30. Ertl, P.; Roggo, S.; Schuffenhauer, A. Natural product-likeness score and its application for prioritization of compound libraries. *J. Chem. Inf. Model.* **2008**, *48*, 68–74. [CrossRef]

31. Jayaseelan, K.V.; Moreno, P.; Truszkowski, A.; Ertl, P.; Steinbeck, C. Natural product-likeness score revisited: An open-source, open-data implementation. *BMC Bioinform.* **2012**, *13*, 106. [CrossRef] [PubMed]

32. Jayaseelan, K.V.; Steinbeck, C. Building blocks for automated elucidation of metabolites: Natural product-likeness for candidate ranking. *BMC Bioinform.* **2014**, *15*, 234. [CrossRef] [PubMed]

33. RDKit NP_Score. Available online: https://github.com/rdkit/rdkit/tree/master/Contrib/NP_Score (accessed on 27 November 2018).

34. Yu, M.J. Natural product-like virtual libraries: Recursive atom-based enumeration. *J. Chem. Inf. Model.* **2011**, *51*, 541–557. [CrossRef] [PubMed]

35. Zaid, H.; Raiyn, J.; Nasser, A.; Saad, B.; Rayan, A. Physicochemical properties of natural based products versus synthetic chemicals. *Open Nutraceuticals J.* **2010**, *3*, 194–202. [CrossRef]

36. Riniker, S.; Landrum, G.A. Similarity maps—A visualization strategy for molecular fingerprints and machine-learning methods. *J. Cheminform.* **2013**, *5*, 43. [CrossRef] [PubMed]

37. RDKit Version 2017.09.3: Open-source cheminformatics software. Available online: http://www.rdkit.org (accessed on 22 May 2018).

38. Stork, C.; Wagner, J.; Friedrich, N.-O.; de Bruyn Kops, C.; Šícho, M.; Kirchmair, J. Hit Dexter: A machine-learning model for the prediction of frequent hitters. *ChemMedChem* **2018**, *13*, 564–571. [CrossRef]

39. MolVs Version 0.1.1. Available online: https://github.com/mcs07/MolVS (accessed on 12 July 2018).

40. Sterling, T.; Irwin, J.J. ZINC 15-Ligand discovery for everyone. *J. Chem. Inf. Model.* **2015**, *55*, 2324–2337. [CrossRef]

41. ZINC "in-stock" subset. ZINC15. Available online: http://zinc15.docking.org/ (accessed on 21 August 2018).

42. *Dictionary of Natural Products*, version 19.1; Chapman & Hall/CRC: London, UK, 2010.

43. Bento, A.P.; Gaulton, A.; Hersey, A.; Bellis, L.J.; Chambers, J.; Davies, M.; Krüger, F.A.; Light, Y.; Mak, L.; McGlinchey, S.; et al. The ChEMBL bioactivity database: An update. *Nucleic Acids Res.* **2014**, *42*, D1083–D1090. [CrossRef]

44. ChEMBL Version 24_1. Available online: https://www.ebi.ac.uk/chembl/ (accessed on 30 July 2018).

45. ChEMBL Version 23. Available online: https://www.ebi.ac.uk/chembl (accessed on 6 June 2017).

46. Natural products subset of ZINC. ZINC15. Available online: http://zinc15.docking.org/substances/subsets/ (accessed on 7 November 2018).

47. *Molecular Operating Environment (MOE)*, version 2016.08; Chemical Computing Group: Montreal, QC, Canada, 2016.

48. Morgan, H.L. The generation of a unique machine description for chemical structures-A technique developed at Chemical Abstracts Service. *J. Chem. Doc.* **1965**, *5*, 107–113. [CrossRef]

49. Rogers, D.; Hahn, M. Extended-connectivity fingerprints. *J. Chem. Inf. Model.* **2010**, *50*, 742–754. [CrossRef]

50. Pedregosa, F.; Varoquaux, G.; Gramfort, A.; Michel, V.; Thirion, B.; Grisel, O.; Blondel, M.; Prettenhofer, P.; Weiss, R.; Dubourg, V.; et al. Scikit-learn: Machine learning in Python. *J. Mach. Learn. Res.* **2011**, *12*, 2825–2830.

51. Scikit-Learn: Machine Learning in Python. version 0.19.1.

52. Natural Product Likeness Calculator Version 2.1. Available online: https://sourceforge.net/projects/np-likeness/ (accessed on 5 October 2018).

53. Natural Products Atlas. Available online: https://www.npatlas.org/ (accessed on 20 August 2018).

54. Gu, J.; Gui, Y.; Chen, L.; Yuan, G.; Lu, H.-Z.; Xu, X. Use of natural products as chemical library for drug discovery and network pharmacology. *PLoS ONE* **2013**, *8*, e62839. [CrossRef]

55. Universal Natural Products Database (UNPD). Available online: http://pkuxxj.pku.edu.cn/UNPD (accessed on 17 October 2016).

56. Chen, C.Y.-C. TCM Database@Taiwan: The world's largest traditional Chinese medicine database for drug screening in silico. *PLoS ONE* **2011**, *6*, e15939. [CrossRef] [PubMed]

57. TCM Database@Taiwan. Available online: http://tcm.cmu.edu.tw (accessed on 17 October 2016).

58. Xue, R.; Fang, Z.; Zhang, M.; Yi, Z.; Wen, C.; Shi, T. TCMID: Traditional Chinese medicine integrative database for herb molecular mechanism analysis. *Nucleic Acids Res.* **2013**, *41*, D1089–D1095. [CrossRef] [PubMed]

59. Traditional Chinese Medicine Integrated Database (TCMID). Available online: www.megabionet.org/tcmid (accessed on 19 October 2016).

60. Lin, Y.-C.; Wang, C.-C.; Chen, I.-S.; Jheng, J.-L.; Li, J.-H.; Tung, C.-W. TIPdb: A database of anticancer, antiplatelet, and antituberculosis phytochemicals from indigenous plants in Taiwan. *Sci. World J.* **2013**, *2013*, 736386. [CrossRef]

61. Tung, C.-W.; Lin, Y.-C.; Chang, H.-S.; Wang, C.-C.; Chen, I.-S.; Jheng, J.-L.; Li, J.-H. TIPdb-3D: The three-dimensional structure database of phytochemicals from Taiwan indigenous plants. *Database* **2014**, *2014*, bau055. [CrossRef] [PubMed]

62. Taiwan Indigenous Plant Database (TIPdb). Available online: http://cwtung.kmu.edu.tw/tipdb (accessed on 19 October 2016).
63. Ambinter. Available online: www.ambinter.com (accessed on 2 June 2017).
64. GreenPharma. Available online: www.greenpharma.com (accessed on 2 June 2017).
65. AnalytiCon Discovery. Available online: www.ac-discovery.com (accessed on 14 November 2017).
66. Ntie-Kang, F.; Telukunta, K.K.; Döring, K.; Simoben, C.V.; A Moumbock, A.F.; Malange, Y.I.; Njume, L.E.; Yong, J.N.; Sippl, W.; Günther, S. NANPDB: A resource for natural products from Northern African sources. *J. Nat. Prod.* **2017**, *80*, 2067–2076. [CrossRef]
67. Northern African Natural Products Database (NANPDB). Available online: www.african-compounds.org/nanpdb (accessed on 5 April 2017).
68. Klementz, D.; Döring, K.; Lucas, X.; Telukunta, K.K.; Erxleben, A.; Deubel, D.; Erber, A.; Santillana, I.; Thomas, O.S.; Bechthold, A.; et al. StreptomeDB 2.0—An extended resource of natural products produced by streptomycetes. *Nucleic Acids Res.* **2015**, *44*, D509–D514. [CrossRef]
69. StreptomeDB. Available online: http://132.230.56.4/streptomedb2/ (accessed on 13 April 2017).
70. Ming, H.; Tiejun, C.; Yanli, W.; Stephen, B.H. Web search and data mining of natural products and their bioactivities in PubChem. *Sci. China Chem.* **2013**, *56*, 1424–1435.
71. Natural products subset. PubChem Substance Database. Available online: http://ncbi.nlm.nih.gov/pcsubstance (accessed on 7 April 2017).
72. Pilon, A.C.; Valli, M.; Dametto, A.C.; Pinto, M.E.F.; Freire, R.T.; Castro-Gamboa, I.; Andricopulo, A.D.; Bolzani, V.S. NuBBE: An updated database to uncover chemical and biological information from Brazilian biodiversity. *Sci. Rep.* **2017**, *7*, 7215. [CrossRef]
73. Núcleo de Bioensaios, Biossíntese e Ecofisiologia de Produtos Naturais (NuBBE). Available online: http://nubbe.iq.unesp.br/portal/nubbedb.html (accessed on 19 April 2017).
74. PI Chemicals. Available online: www.pipharm.com (accessed on 5 May 2017).
75. Choi, H.; Cho, S.Y.; Pak, H.J.; Kim, Y.; Choi, J.-Y.; Lee, Y.J.; Gong, B.H.; Kang, Y.S.; Han, T.; Choi, G.; et al. NPCARE: Database of natural products and fractional extracts for cancer regulation. *J. Cheminform.* **2017**, *9*, 2. [CrossRef] [PubMed]
76. Database of Natural Products for Cancer Gene Regulation (NPCARE). Available online: http://silver.sejong.ac.kr/npcare (accessed on 20 February 2017).
77. Mangal, M.; Sagar, P.; Singh, H.; Raghava, G.P.S.; Agarwal, S.M. NPACT: Naturally Occurring Plant-based Anti-cancer Compound-Activity-Target database. *Nucleic Acids Res.* **2013**, *41*, D1124–D1129. [CrossRef] [PubMed]
78. Naturally Occurring Plant-based Anti-cancer Compound-Activity-Target database (NPACT). Available online: http://crdd.osdd.net/raghava/npact (accessed on 13 April 2017).
79. InterBioScreen. Available online: www.ibscreen.com (accessed on 14 November 2017).
80. Ntie-Kang, F.; Zofou, D.; Babiaka, S.B.; Meudom, R.; Scharfe, M.; Lifongo, L.L.; Mbah, J.A.; Mbaze, L.M.; Sippl, W.; Efange, S.M.N. AfroDb: A select highly potent and diverse natural product library from African medicinal plants. *PLoS ONE* **2013**, *8*, e78085. [CrossRef] [PubMed]
81. AfroDb. Available online: http://african-compounds.org/about/afrodb (accessed on 18 October 2016).
82. TargetMol. Available online: www.targetmol.com (accessed on 17 May 2017).
83. Kang, H.; Tang, K.; Liu, Q.; Sun, Y.; Huang, Q.; Zhu, R.; Gao, J.; Zhang, D.; Huang, C.; Cao, Z. HIM-herbal ingredients in-vivo metabolism database. *J. Cheminform.* **2013**, *5*, 28. [CrossRef] [PubMed]
84. Herbal Ingredients In-Vivo Metabolism database (HIM). Available online: http://binfo.shmtu.edu.cn:8080/him (accessed on 13 April 2017).
85. Hatherley, R.; Brown, D.K.; Musyoka, T.M.; Penkler, D.L.; Faya, N.; Lobb, K.A.; Tastan Bishop, Ö. SANCDB: A South African natural compound database. *J. Cheminform.* **2015**, *7*, 29. [CrossRef] [PubMed]
86. South African Natural Compound Database (SANCDB). Available online: http://sancdb.rubi.ru.ac.za (accessed on 8 February 2017).
87. UEFS Natural Products Catalog. ZINC15. Available online: http://zinc15.docking.org (accessed on 26 May 2017).
88. Ntie-Kang, F.; Amoa Onguéné, P.; Fotso, G.W.; Andrae-Marobela, K.; Bezabih, M.; Ndom, J.C.; Ngadjui, B.T.; Ogundaini, A.O.; Abegaz, B.M.; Meva'a, L.M. Virtualizing the p-ANAPL library: A step towards drug discovery from African medicinal plants. *PLoS ONE* **2014**, *9*, e90655. [CrossRef]

89. Natural Products Set IV of the Developmental Therapeutic Program of the National Cancer Institute/National Institutes of Health. Available online: http://dtp.cancer.gov/organization/dscb/obtaining/available_plates.htm (accessed on 20 October 2016).

90. Ye, H.; Ye, L.; Kang, H.; Zhang, D.; Tao, L.; Tang, K.; Liu, X.; Zhu, R.; Liu, Q.; Chen, Y.Z.; et al. HIT: Linking herbal active ingredients to targets. *Nucleic Acids Res.* **2011**, *39*, D1055–D1059. [CrossRef]

91. Herbal Ingredients' Targets database (HIT). Available online: http://lifecenter.sgst.cn/hit (accessed on 13 April 2017).

92. Ntie-Kang, F.; Nwodo, J.N.; Ibezim, A.; Simoben, C.V.; Karaman, B.; Ngwa, V.F.; Sippl, W.; Adikwu, M.U.; Mbaze, L.M. Molecular modeling of potential anticancer agents from African medicinal plants. *J. Chem. Inf. Model.* **2014**, *54*, 2433–2450. [CrossRef]

93. AfroCancer. Available online: http://african-compounds.org/about/afrocancer (accessed on 10 February 2017).

94. Onguéné, P.A.; Ntie-Kang, F.; Mbah, J.A.; Lifongo, L.L.; Ndom, J.C.; Sippl, W.; Mbaze, L.M. The potential of anti-malarial compounds derived from African medicinal plants, part III: An *in silico* evaluation of drug metabolism and pharmacokinetics profiling. *Org. Med. Chem. Lett.* **2014**, *4*, 6. [CrossRef]

95. AfroMalariaDB. Available online: http://african-compounds.org/about/afromalariadb (accessed on 10 February 2017).

96. Natural products subset of AK Scientific. AK Scientific. Available online: www.aksci.com (accessed on 19 April 2017).

97. Natural products of Selleck Chemicals. Selleck Chemicals. Available online: www.selleckchem.com (accessed on 14 November 2017).

98. Breiman, L. Random forests. *Machine Learning* **2001**, *45*, 5–32. [CrossRef]

99. Matthews, B.W. Comparison of the predicted and observed secondary structure of T4 phage lysozyme. *Biochim. Biophys. Acta* **1975**, *405*, 442–451. [CrossRef]

100. Schomburg, K.; Ehrlich, H.-C.; Stierand, K.; Rarey, M. From structure diagrams to visual chemical patterns. *J. Chem. Inf. Model.* **2010**, *50*, 1529–1535. [CrossRef] [PubMed]

101. SMARTSview. Available online: http://smartsview.zbh.uni-hamburg.de/ (accessed on 30 November 2018).

102. Bienfait, B.; Ertl, P. JSME: A free molecule editor in JavaScript. *J. Cheminform.* **2013**, *5*, 24. [CrossRef] [PubMed]

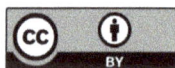

*biomolecules*

MDPI

*Article*

# Flavonoids as Putative Epi-Modulators: Insight into Their Binding Mode with BRD4 Bromodomains Using Molecular Docking and Dynamics

Fernando D. Prieto-Martínez * and José L. Medina-Franco *

Facultad de Química, Departamento de Farmacia, Universidad Nacional Autónoma de México,
Avenida Universidad 3000, Mexico City 04510, Mexico
* Correspondence: fprieto@comunidad.unam.mx (F.D.P.-M.); medinajl@unam.com.mx (J.L.M.-F.);
  Tel.: +52-55-5622-3899 (J.L.M.-F.).

Received: 22 June 2018; Accepted: 18 July 2018; Published: 23 July 2018

**Abstract:** Flavonoids are widely recognized as natural polydrugs, given their anti-inflammatory, antioxidant, sedative, and antineoplastic activities. Recently, different studies showed that flavonoids have the potential to inhibit bromodomain and extraterminal (BET) bromodomains. Previous reports suggested that flavonoids bind between the Z and A loops of the bromodomain (ZA channel) due to their orientation and interactions with P86, V87, L92, L94, and N140. Herein, a comprehensive characterization of the binding modes of fisetin and the biflavonoid, amentoflavone, is discussed. To this end, both compounds were docked with BET bromodomain 4 (BRD4) using four docking programs. The results were post-processed with protein–ligand interaction fingerprints. To gain further insight into the binding mode of the two natural products, the docking results were further analyzed with molecular dynamics simulations. The results showed that amentoflavone makes numerous contacts in the ZA channel, as previously described for flavonoids and kinase inhibitors. It was also found that amentoflavone can potentially make contacts with non-canonical residues for BET inhibition. Most of these contacts were not observed with fisetin. Based on these results, amentoflavone was experimentally tested for BRD4 inhibition, showing activity in the micromolar range. This work may serve as the basis for scaffold optimization and the further characterization of flavonoids as BET inhibitors.

**Keywords:** docking; epigenetics; epi-informatics; molecular interactions; molecular dynamics; natural products; flavonoids

## 1. Introduction

Epigenetics has arisen as the missing link in the biogenesis of disease. Histone modifications have a significant effect on the fate of certain genes. Current research is primarily focused on the writing and erasing mechanisms of the epigenome. There are many examples of this in the literature [1], one of the most prominent being histone acetylation. Acetylation is regulated by two main systems: histone acetyl transferases (HATs) and histone deacetylases (HDACs) [2]. Histone deacetylases have been studied thoroughly by means of pharmacophore modeling [3], molecular docking [4], and molecular dynamics (MD) [5]. These efforts contributed to the identification and development of two FDA-approved HDAC inhibitors, the most notable being a natural product, romidepsin [6].

Readers are epi-enzymes whose function is to recognize certain modifications and their patterns on histones [7]. Therefore, reader enzymes are interesting molecular targets for a better understanding of epigenetics. Bromodomains are 120-residue proteins that were first discovered on the brahma (*brm*) gene of the *Drosophila* genus [8]. Later, it was confirmed as a common motif in most eukaryotic organisms. As of today, 62 isoforms were identified and are classified in eight families [9]. Family II, known as the bromodomain and extraterminal domain (BET), is extensively studied, as shown in Figure 1. This family includes bromodomain 2 (BRD2), BRD3, BRD4, and bromodomain testis-specific (BRDT) isoforms, each with their respective first and second domains (BD1 and BD2). Figure 2 shows the active site of bromodomains, which comprises three main hotspots: the WPF shelf, a region exclusive to BET bromodomains, a hydrophobic triad comprised by tryptophan, proline and phenylalanine (residues 80 to 83), and the ZA channel, located between the Z and A loops (residues 85 through 96), often seen as a frontier region with mixed contacts (mainly hydrophobic). The third hotspot is the Ac-binding pocket, responsible for reading histones and their $\varepsilon$-*N*-acetylated lysine residues (Kac). This hotspot is defined by a "tandem checkpoint" made by N140 and Y97 [10].

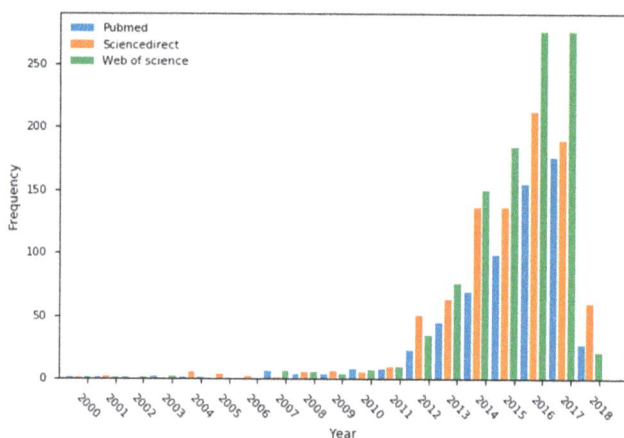

**Figure 1.** Frequency of the "bromodomain" keyword in three major search engines during the past 18 years.

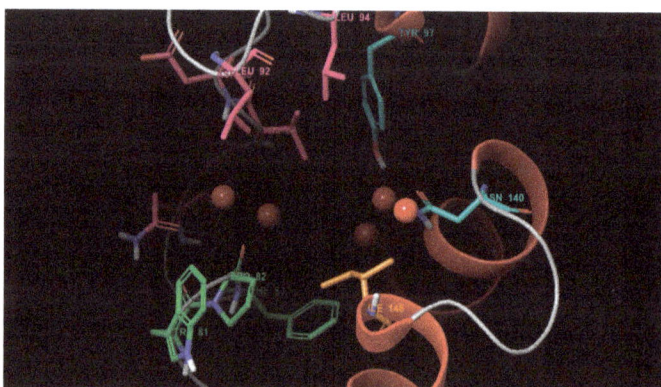

**Figure 2.** Binding pocket of bromodomain and extraterminal domain (BET) bromomains. The main structural features are the WPF shelf (green), ZA channel (pink), an Ac-pocket (cyan), and the gatekeeper (orange). Red spheres represent structural waters found with BET isoforms.

Additionally, evidence of structural water molecules was shown on a double bridge with ligands and Y97 [11]. Generally speaking, the role of water in binding is a dividing issue for drug design [12]. For example, structure-based design often ignores it or recognizes few instances of its importance [13]. Because of this, early approaches to ligand design followed a water-displacement strategy [14]. Nonetheless, a slow but steady paradigm shift came with increasing evidence of water-based stabilization in binding kinetics [15] and target selectivity [16]. One of the main problems in this approach is the increased difficulty of modeling of such phenomena, i.e., identifying "crucial waters" [17,18]. For bromodomains, recent studies showed that the network of structural waters in the ZA channel plays a significant role in binding [19,20] and this topic served as a case study for the development of novel methods in the field [21].

Bromodomain inhibition is currently at an impasse [22], as chemotypes are not diverse enough to make more robust models and approaches toward their pharmacology. Hence, current efforts are focused on the synthesis and identification of plausible and novel inhibitors [23]. As part of this effort, quinazolones were proposed as novel inhibitors of BETs. An interesting property of these ligands is their selectivity toward BD2 [24]. Later, it was found that some kinase inhibitors can bind to bromodomains [25], e.g., flavopiridol. Figure 3a illustrates the quintessential BRD inhibitors. These results led to the hypothesis of flavonoids as putative modulators of bromodomains; nonetheless, this possibility was only explored in recent studies [26].

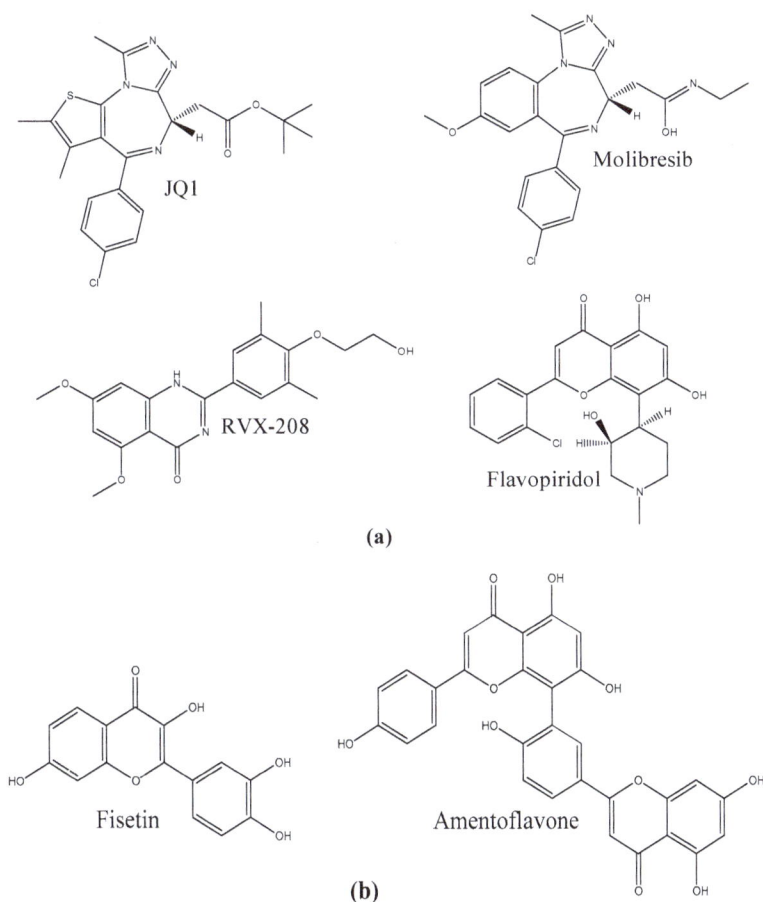

**Figure 3.** Chemical structures of (**a**) reference ligands for BET inhibition, and (**b**) flavonoids studied in this work.

Flavonoids are one of the most well-known natural products, often regarded as major scaffolds in medicinal chemistry [27]. Flavonoids showed antioxidant [28], anti-inflammatory [29], and sedative [30] effects in various studies. Moreover, flavonoid scaffolds present the outstanding potential of being chemoprotective agents toward cancer [31]. Consequently, flavonoids are often seen as quintessential nutraceuticals; e.g., the average intake of flavonoids in the United States is around 1 g/day [32]. Finally, it was suggested that flavonoids may interact significantly with the epigenome; however, as of today, this is limited to writing and eraser epi-enzymes [33].

Fisetin, shown in Figure 3b, is a dietary flavonoid found in a broad array of vegetables such as strawberry, apple, grape, onion, and cucumber [34], and is considered a health-promoting compound [35]. Studies showed that fisetin is capable of blocking cell proliferation on many cancer lines [36]. One of the most interesting aspects of its pharmacology is its capacity to modulate nuclear factor kappa B (NF-κB) [37]. Fisetin is capable of doing this through the mitogen-activated protein kinase (MAPK) pathway and tumor necrosis factor (TNF)-blocking, downregulating pro-inflammatory genes [38]. Of note, recent studies showed the role of BRD4 in the recruitment of NF-κβ [39]. Thus, bromodomains were also studied for their role in chronic diseases like diabetes [40] and psoriasis [41]. Amentoflavone (Figure 3b) is a biflavonoid produced from two apigenin units. It is commonly found in *Ginko biloba, Hypericum perforatum, Biophytum sensitivum,* and *Nandina domestica* [42]. Like fisetin, amentoflavone was also identified as an NF-κβ modulator [43], thus giving rise to its capacity to reduce inflammation.

Computational methods are valuable approaches to solving chemical problems. Molecular docking, for example, allows the simulation of protein–ligand binding. Despite its simplifications and limitations, docking yields significant results used for binding-mode predictions [44]. Molecular dynamics is gaining increasing attention with regards to the elucidation of ligand binding and protein behavior [45].

Since amentoflavone and fisetin were identified as putative ligands of BRD4 in two independent studies [46,47], a comprehensive characterization of the putative binding profile of both flavonoids with BRD4 is presented herein. The binding profile was carried out with consensus docking and molecular dynamics. Based on the computational results, amentoflavone was experimentally tested for activity as BRD4 inhibitor, showing activity in the micromolar range. These results further support the activity of flavonoids as putative epi-modulators.

## 2. Materials and Methods

### 2.1. Protein Preparation

An ensemble of 14 structures for the BET isoform, BRD4, was selected from the Protein Data Bank (PBD). Full details are presented in Table S1 of the Supplementary Materials. Selection criteria were based on their resolutions (<1.8 Å) and $R$-values (<0.25). Additional criteria were the structural similarity between the co-crystal ligand and the flavonoid scaffold, and the ability of the ligand to form hydrogen bonds with the binding pocket. All protein–ligand complexes were prepared with the Quickprep module of the MOE software [48]. Energy minimization was carried with the Amber 14: EHT force field (using Amber 14 forcefield [49] for protein parametrization and Extended Hückel Theory for ligands [50]). Complexes were visually inspected to ensure that key interactions were kept.

### 2.2. Molecular Docking

Docking was carried out using four programs: Autodock Vina [51], LeDock [52], MOE (v.2018.01), and PLANTS [53]. The rationale for selecting these programs was their performance and different scoring functions for consensus (vide infra). Protein inputs were kept from the preparation step and were validated with their respective native ligands. Details are provided in Table S2 of the Supplementary Materials. Amentoflavone and fisetin were parameterized with the Amber 14: EHT force field for the MOE software, and a charge reassignment was done with the LeDock, Vina, and PLANTS programs. The charge used for these programs was calculated with the MOPAC 2016 software [54] using PM6-D3H4X, as this correction was shown to enhance docking performance [55]. The docking poses were post-processed using protein–ligand interaction fingerprints (PLIF) as available in the MOE software. Docking poses were analyzed for clustering, based on the most common interactions found across the four programs.

*2.3. Molecular Dynamics*

Molecular dynamics simulations were carried out using Desmond [56] for both BRD4 (see Supplementary Materials, Figures S2, S3, and S6, and Table S12) and BRD4 ligand complexes. The complex used was the top ranked pose from the MOE software with consensus interactions. Complexes were then submitted to the System Builder utility in Maestro to assign a buffered 10 Å × 10 Å × 10 Å orthorhombic box using the transferable intermolecular potential with 3 points (TIP3P) water model and the OPLS_2005 force field. The system was neutralized, and a 0.15 M concentration of NaCl was added. Further details can be found in the Supplementary Materials, Figure S1. The production time for MD was set at 100 ns. The simulation was repeated three times. Electrostatics were computed using the Particle Mesh Ewald algorithm with a 9 Å cut-off, and constraints were enforced by the M-SHAKE algorithm [57]. Integration was done every 1.2 fs, with the recording interval set to 50 ps. The trajectories were then analyzed using the Simulation Interaction Diagram, Simulation Event Analysis, and Simulation Quality Analysis utilities in Maestro.

*2.4. Experimental Testing of Amentoflavone*

Amentoflavone was purchased from Sigma-Aldrich (St. Louis, MO, USA), and was tested for BRD4 tandem (BD1 + BD2) binding by means of AlphaScreen [58], using an H4 peptide (1–21) K5/8/12/16 Ac. Experimental work was performed by the Reaction Biology Corp., providing 2-mg samples to obtain duplicate dose-response curves beginning at a 100-µM concentration, following a three-fold dilution. The positive control for the test was the JQ-1 compound. The half maximal inhibitory concentration ($IC_{50}$) values were obtained from the curves, and the Hill slope for amentoflavone was calculated.

## 3. Results

*3.1. Molecular Docking*

Table 1 summarizes the docking scores for amentoflavone and fisetin as computed with the four docking programs (the raw docking scores for each protein used are reported in the Supplementary Materials, Tables S4–S11). Figure 4 shows the consensus PLIF found for both compounds.

**Table 1.** Summary statistics of docking scores for the programs used.

| Molecule | Summary Stats * | Autodock VINA (kcal/mol) | LeDock (kcal/mol) | MOE (kcal/mol) | PLANTS |
|---|---|---|---|---|---|
| Amentoflavone | Min | −10.5 | −7.9 | −9.0 | −102.1 |
| | 1Q | −9.5 | −7.3 | −7.9 | −89.4 |
| | Avg | −9.2 | −7.0 | −7.6 | −86.9 |
| | 3Q | −9.0 | −6.8 | −7.2 | −84.0 |
| | Max | −8.2 | −6.3 | −6.4 | −77.4 |
| | SD | 0.46 | 0.34 | 0.54 | 4.6 |
| Fisetin | Min | −8.6 | −6.0 | −7.4 | −79.6 |
| | 1Q | −8.2 | −5.6 | −6.5 | −73.2 |
| | Avg | −7.9 | −5.4 | −6.2 | −71.0 |
| | 3Q | −7.7 | −5.3 | −6.0 | −68.9 |
| | Max | −7.1 | −4.7 | −5.6 | −65.0 |
| | SD | 0.31 | 0.24 | 0.39 | 2.94 |

* Min: Minimum; 1Q: First quartile; Avg: Average; 3Q: Third quartile; Max: Maximum; and SD: Standard deviation values.

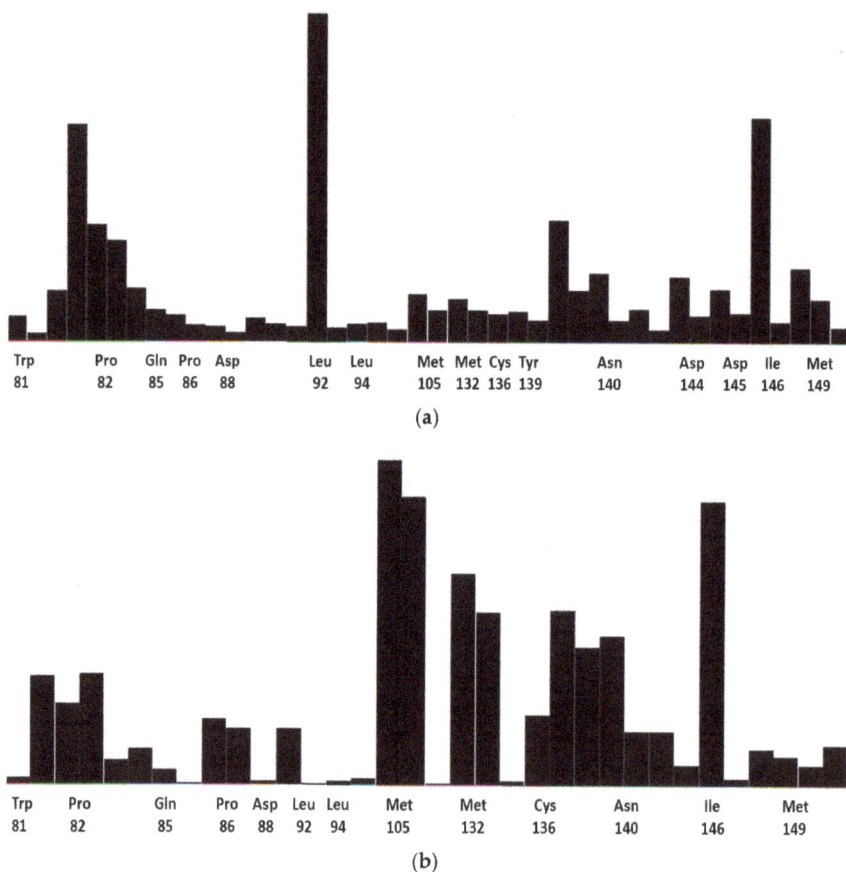

**Figure 4.** Consensus protein–ligand interaction fingerprint obtained from a consensus analysis of the docking with the Autodock Vina, LeDock, MOE, and PLANTS programs. (**a**) Amentoflavone; (**b**) Fisetin.

*3.2. Molecular Dynamics*

The overall quality of the MD simulations was measured with the corresponding utilities in Maestro. Energy, potential energy, temperature, pressure, and volume values were computed (results are shown in Figures S4 and S5, and Tables S13 and S14 in the Supplementary Materials). Once complex stability was assessed, the root-mean-square deviation (RMSD) values for backbone, Cα, side chains, and ligand were computed, as shown in Figure 5a,b. This measure shows the global deviation of atoms to a reference status (frame 0); usually, values below 5.0 Å can be considered as valid [59].

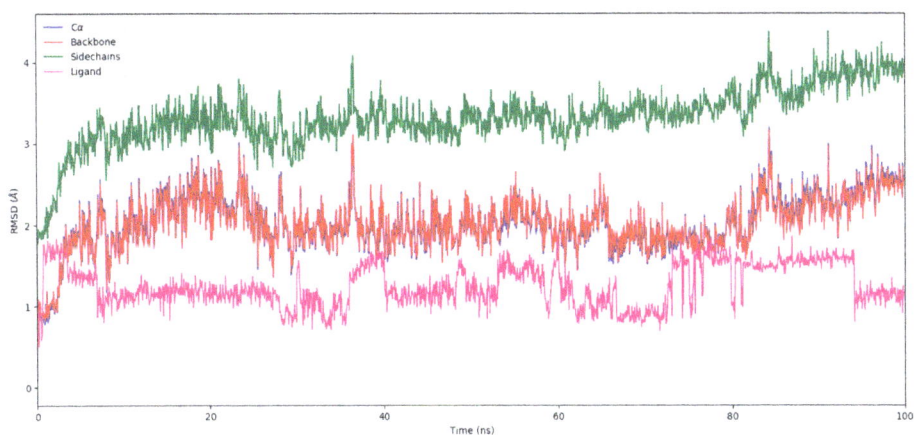

(a)

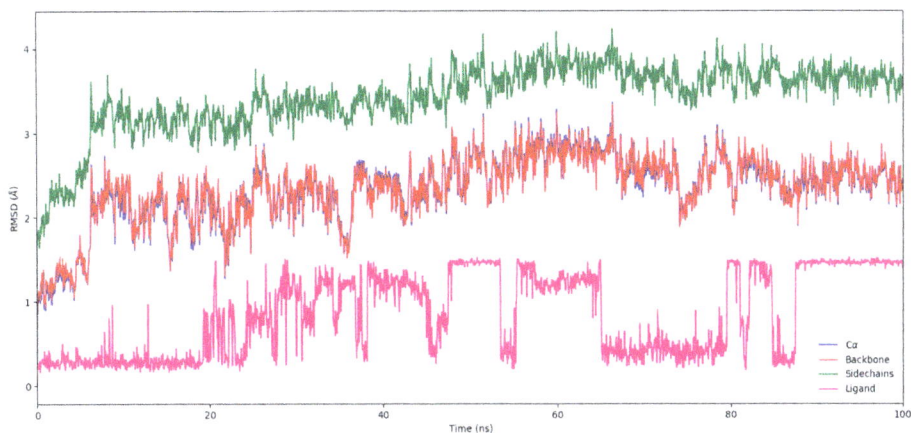

(b)

**Figure 5.** Root-mean-square deviation (RMSD) values for the protein backbone, alpha carbons, side chains, and ligand. (**a**) Amentoflavone; (**b**) Fisetin.

Root-mean-square fluctuation (RMSF) was also calculated, as shown in Figure 6a,b. These values show the general movement of each residue across the total simulation time. In this figure, the ligand contacts are shown as green lines matching the residue index, while the orange lines indicate protein secondary structures (helices, in this case). See Figure S6 in the Supplementary Materials for further details.

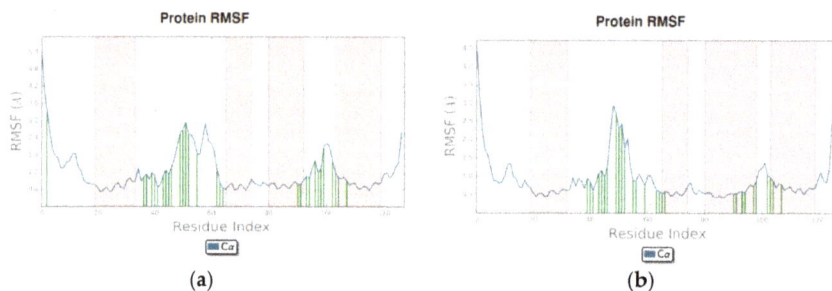

**Figure 6.** Root-mean-square fluctuation (RMSF) values based on alpha carbons; ligand contacts are presented in green, and protein helices in orange. (**a**) Amentoflavone; (**b**) Fisetin.

Figures 7 and 8 show the protein–ligand contact analysis for the MD simulations. Protein–ligand contacts can be interpreted as "dynamic PLIFs", showing the population of contacts during the simulation. Plots at the bottom of both figures represent the number of contacts and their density, i.e., a darker shade of orange indicates more than one contact in that frame. These plots also show the type of contact mapped to the structure of the ligand.

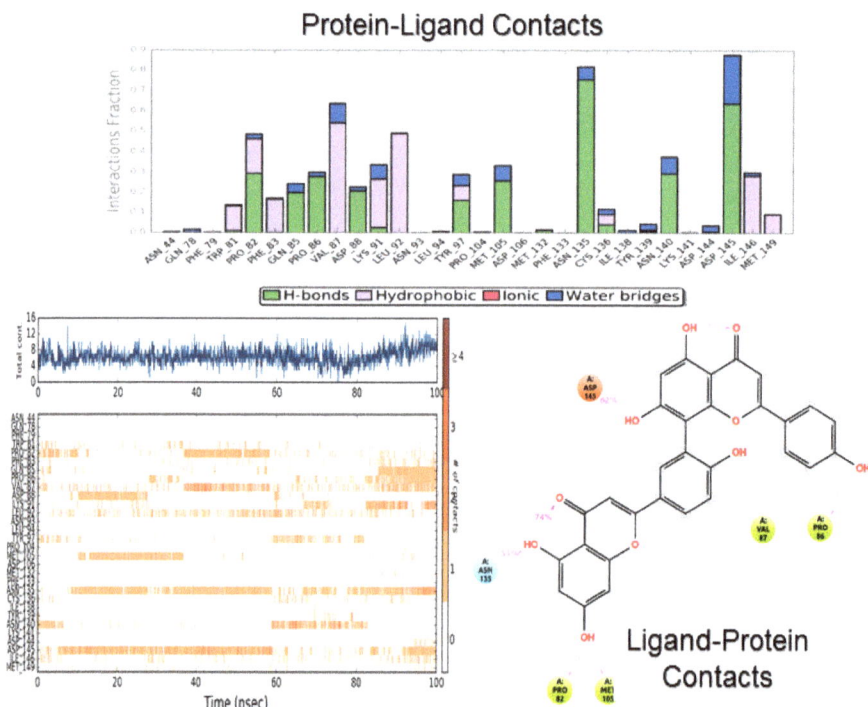

**Figure 7.** Protein–ligand contact analysis for amentoflavone during the molecular dynamics (MD) simulation.

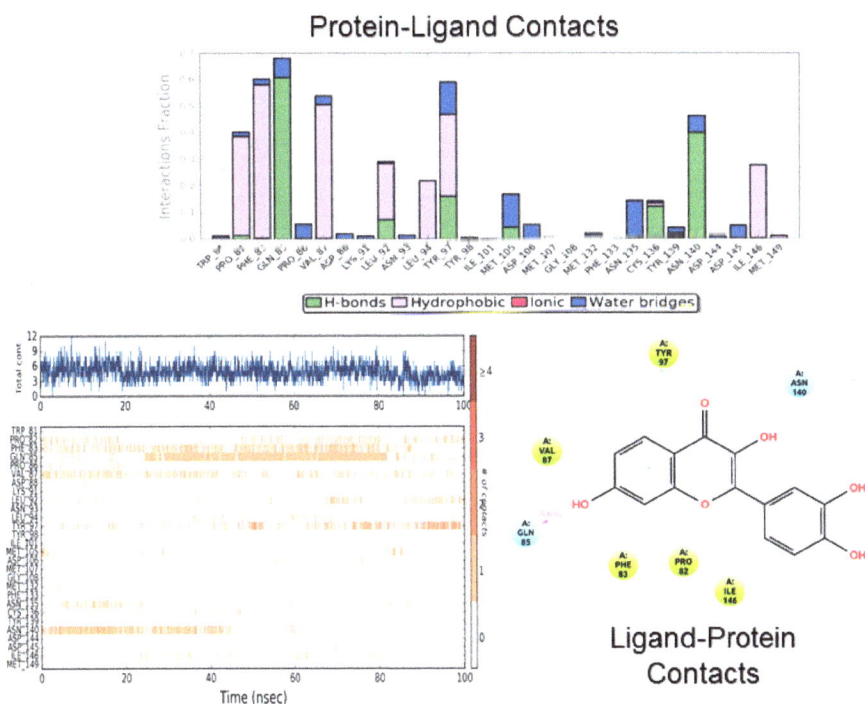

**Figure 8.** Protein–ligand contact analysis for fisetin during the MD simulation.

Figure 9a,b show other ligand properties during the MD simulations. These include the radius of gyration, intramolecular hydrogen bonding, van der Waals (VdW) surface area, solvent-accessible surface area, and polar surface area. Of note, if a ligand is not capable of intramolecular hydrogen bonding, this plot appears empty.

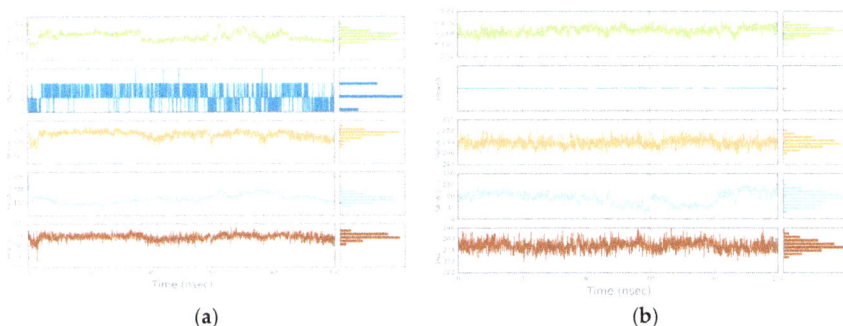

(a)

(b)

**Figure 9.** Ligand properties during the 100-ns simulations. (**a**) Amentoflavone; (**b**) Fisetin.

Figure 10a,b show the energy values for dihedral angles (line plot), which account for torsional analysis. The histogram shows the density of probability of that torsion, while the dial on the left shows the rotation of that bond during the simulation (the beginning is marked by the center). The plots in Figure 10 allow determining whether or not a given ligand undergoes torsional strain during binding.

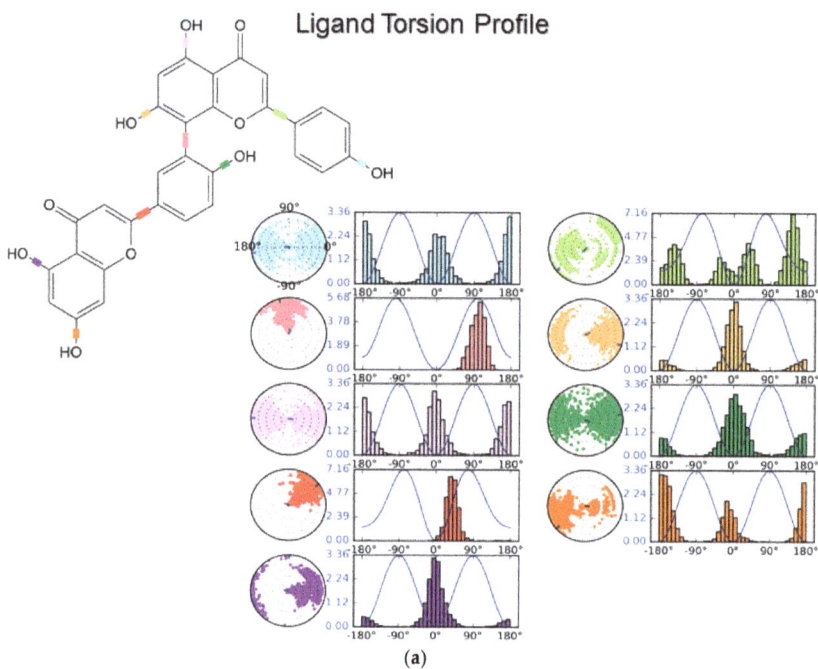

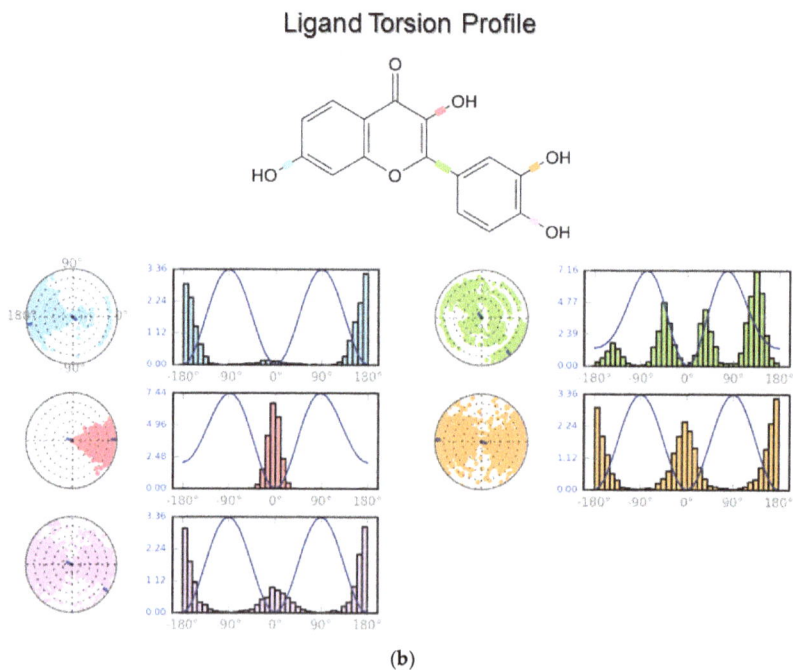

Figure 10. Torsional analysis of ligand conformations during the 100-ns simulations. (a) Amentoflavone; (b) Fisetin. The colors represent the different rotatable bonds of the ligands. Values on the Y-axis are in kcal/mol.

### 3.3. Binding Assay of Amentoflavone

Table 2 summarizes the experimentally determined activity of amentoflavone.

**Table 2.** Values for the half maximal inhibitory concentration ($IC_{50}$) and the Hill slope of amentoflavone, as obtained using AlphaScreen [†] against the bromodomain 4 (BRD4) tandem.

|                   | DATA 1 | DATA 2 |
| ----------------- | ------ | ------ |
| $IC_{50}$ (µM)    | 36.1   | 30.4   |
| Hill slope        | −2.5   | −1.9   |

[†] As mentioned in the Methods section, experimental characterization was performed with the Reaction Biology application using the AlphaScreen assay.

## 4. Discussion

### 4.1. Molecular Docking

Bromodomain inhibitors may be classified into two broad categories: KAc-mimicking and non-mimicking, the former being the most prominent [60]. Flavonoids belong to this category as their carbonyl groups are their main anchor toward Asn140 and Tyr97 [46]. Nonetheless, as shown in Figure 4, these interactions are not as populated as might be expected. Certainly, this may seem negative, as the Ac-pocket is the main anchor for bromodomain inhibition. Nonetheless, the exclusion of molecules based solely on this criterion was questioned [61].

Because of this, an integral approach based on ensemble docking and consensus scoring was conducted, as a means of correctly assessing the probability of a given interaction. Ensemble docking is a common technique used to account for protein flexibility [62], and was applied successfully to several workflows [63]. Consensus scoring, on the other hand, significantly increases the rate of hit identification [64]. However, the rate of success has a strong dependence on the selected programs for consensus. Consequently, a naïve choice leads to an overestimation of weighted terms if similar parameters in scoring functions are used [65]. Hence, we selected the docking software based on searching-algorithm capabilities and scoring-function diversity. Briefly, the rationale for each selection is presented hereunder.

- Autodock VINA: It has a well-established performance against several protein families; additionally, its empirical scoring function has a significant correlation with experimental values [66]. Finally, its hybrid search algorithm optimized by local search allows a better sampling of the free-energy landscape [67].
- LeDock: Its search algorithm based on simulated annealing provides a significant clustering of poses. In addition, it was implemented successfully in virtual screening campaigns for BET bromodomains [52].
- MOE: Its docking algorithm allows for induced-fit search. Furthermore, its force-field-based scoring function (using AMBER parameters with generalized Born/volume integral (GB/VI) solvation) considers the solvation contributions to ligand binding [68].
- PLANTS: It provides a notable sampling of side-chain flexibility. Also, its searching algorithm (based on metaheuristics) and its empirical scoring function have a well-established performance [69].

Additionally, knowledge-based filtering was used to improve consensus results. This method takes advantage of PLIFs to identify trends in binding while selecting poses with "canonical" interactions [47]. Of note, the interactions of both flavonoids with Asn140 show a similar shift in MD simulations, which suggests a good sampling of our ensemble, and a notable performance of the protocol presented herein.

Based on the docking scores, both amentoflavone and fisetin are comparable to currently known inhibitors (see Supplementary Materials, Table S3). To the best of our knowledge, there are no studies or data showing a correlation of docking scores with experimental binding energies of bromodomain inhibitors. While such analysis goes beyond the scope of this work, we provided reference values obtained from the literature (see Supplementary Materials, Table S2).

Notably, docking scores calculated with LeDock were lower when compared to the scores computed with other programs. Nevertheless, this same trend was observed for reference inhibitors. This result was mostly due to the scoring function, as it was shown that, while accurate for identifying correct binding poses, energy values assigned to them are often underestimated [70].

Additionally, the difference in score values for both compounds is significant. Roughly, these values suggest that amentoflavone could be three times more potent than fisetin. Arguably, this may be due to the bigger size of amentoflavone and the higher number of hydroxyl groups giving it more anchors toward BRD4. However, average scoring values rank them with a virtual $IC_{50}$ of around 1–5 µM, based on scaffold similarity and reference values.

Amentoflavone showed mainly hydrophobic contacts with the WPF shelf (Pro81) and the ZA channel (Leu92). Fisetin on the other hand, showed more contacts with residues Met105 and Met132. Previous reports of docking indicate that flavonoids have a notable preference toward these residues [26]; in the case of fisetin, affinity for Cys136 was also observed [46]. This hints to flavonoids having a significant affinity toward different residues beyond the Ac-pocket, while their aromatic characteristics gives them selectivity for the WPF shelf.

Interestingly, the consensus PLIF (Figure 4) shows that amentoflavone made fewer contacts than fisetin. Moreover, the population of Asn140 bonding was significantly reduced for amentoflavone. In contrast, the MD simulations of both compounds showed a similar interaction profile, whereby the fraction is higher for amentoflavone (0.9 vs. 0.7). The Asn140-interaction fraction was similar for both flavonoids (around 0.4). Tyr97 on the other hand, made a stronger and more lasting interaction with fisetin by means of pi stacking and hydrogen bonding. This may be due to the size of amentoflavone and its orientation in the protein cavity, evidenced by the contacts with "non-canonical" residues. An example of this was Asp145, a contact with amentoflavone with a rather small population. However, this contact was identified as significant, as it provides ligand stabilization and water-network interactions [71].

*4.2. Molecular Dynamics*

As stated, MD simulations were conducted to contrast docking results, and to provide further insight into the binding mode of flavonoids. Based on the protein RMSD values, BRD4 remained stable enough during the simulation with both flavonoids. The ligand RMSD values, on the other hand, showed higher deviations at times. This could suggest that both ligands underwent conformational changes during the simulation, i.e., they had two binding modes.

Therefore, torsional profiling plots assisted in this interpretation (Figure 10), as these provided the spatial and energetic distributions of bond torsions during the simulation, showing that both flavonoids were mostly strained in two main conformations. This could imply that fisetin changes its conformation more quickly than amentoflavone, due to a rotation of its catechol ring. However, this observation differs from a previous report [37], which suggested that fisetin keeps a restrained conformation when bound to BRD4. The main reason for this may be related to the use of different force fields (OPLS_2005 vs. OPLS3). On this matter, it is noteworthy that other ligand properties (Figure 9) showed similar trend values for fisetin to those in the previous study.

Amentoflavone, on the other hand, kept a restrained conformation of its shared phenol ring. This behavior can be related to atropisomerism features present on the biflavonoid. Based on these results, it can be hypothesized that amentoflavone activity on BETs is mediated by atropisomerism. Of course, stability studies of amentoflavone and its atropisomers are required to confirm this hypothesis. However, such techniques and focus were beyond the aims of this work. It suffices to say that, even though such phenomena may be common in bioflavonoids, their recognition in medicinal chemistry is often overlooked [72]. Moreover, the interest in atropisomerism is recently increasing [73]. Thus, we believe that knowledge of this feature could improve novel ligand designs, giving a paradigm shift mostly needed for these targets.

The RMSF plots (Figure 6) also showed that the protein–ligand complexes remained consistently stable, and the main secondary structures were four α-helices, which confirms a correct sampling of the system. These plots also showed that the main contacts in both flavonoids were with the ZA channel, with high fluctuations of these residues during the simulation. Interestingly, when these protein ligand contacts were analyzed, different interaction profiles arose for both flavonoids.

Amentoflavone clearly made more contacts with the ZA channel as the MD simulation went on. Also, its presence in the cavity made a significant impact on the secondary structure of the protein, increasing the helical portion of this region (Figure S6 in the Supporting Materials). As stated above, this may be related to the bigger size of the structure. However, based on the "contact mixture" this could also be related to the strained conformation of the molecule, allowing a more favorable angle toward hydrogen bonding and the hydrophobic interactions.

Again, the contact with Asp145 is remarkable; in this case, it was the most populated contact in the MD simulations with amentoflavone. Also, the presence of water bridges with this residue proved significant, a feature recently observed by other groups [71]. Furthermore, this residue is present only in BRD4 BD1, providing specific contact with histone H3 via hydrogen bonding, an interaction not present with inhibitors such as JQ-1 [74]. This would suggest that amentoflavone can be selective for the first domain of BRD4. This is noteworthy, considering molecular similarity toward RVX-208 would suggest selectivity for BRD4 BD2.

### 4.3. Experimental Evaluation

Based on the results of molecular docking and dynamics, it was decided to acquire a sample, and to experimentally test amentoflavone as a BRD4 inhibitor. Fisetin was not considered for testing due to a previous report of quercetin showing an $IC_{50}$ of 38 μM [58]. With this value as reference, our efforts focused on the biflavonoid scaffold. It is very positive that amentoflavone showed significant binding for BRD4, with an $IC_{50}$ in the micromolar range. Indeed, it was more potent when compared to a flavonoid monomer (38 vs. 30 μM). Additionally, its Hill slope value could indicate that amentoflavone is indeed selective for one domain of BRD4. However, more testing is required, i.e., binding assays for separate domains of BRD4.

Furthermore, this experimental confirmation provides further evidence of flavonoids as general chemoprotective agents. One of the main concerns about the use of flavonoids as nutraceutics is their putative toxicity, as fisetin and other flavonoid monomers inhibit DNA topoisomerases [75] and actin polymerization [36]. Biflavonoids, on the other hand, do not present this feature; however, they were reported as potentially mutagenic [76]. Nonetheless, such negative effects are only present at concentrations between 100 and 250 μM [77,78]. As such, based on the $IC_{50}$ values of both quercetin and amentoflavone, flavonoids have significant potential as epi-nutraceutics.

Summarizing, the work presented here serves as a remarkable proof of concept for both the flavonoids as epi-modulators and the computational methods used herein. Putting the results together, amentoflavone showed the characteristic contacts previously reported for flavonoids, i.e., strong contacts with the ZA region, in addition to novel predicted interactions with Asp145 and the water network. Biological tests supported the hypothesis of binding and the plausible selectivity.

Despite the fact that flavonoids have small room for optimization and break Lipinski's rule of five, their true potential is as chemoprotective agents. As previously mentioned, this finding further advances the field of nutriepigenomics. Moreover, it is remarkable that these natural products provide pharmacophoric templates for novel inhibitors of an epigenetic target.

## 5. Conclusions

Amentoflavone is a natural product with several associated biological effects. Its ability to block NF-κβ is the key for its anti-inflammatory potential. BETs were identified as NF-κβ promoters, with JQ-1 being highly effective in psoriasis models. Previously, a similar effect was reported for amentoflavone. Based on these results and other reports, we conducted a binding characterization of this ligand, and compared it to fisetin, another flavonoid with reports of putative activity. We presented a consensus docking methodology which allowed binding characterization and hit selection. Certainly, such an approach is impractical for large virtual-screening campaigns. However, based on the performance and results presented, it provides a powerful tool for pose selection, as supported by the MD results.

The simulations conducted herein indicated that amentoflavone can make numerous contacts in the ZA channel, as previously described for flavonoids and kinase inhibitors. It was also determined that amentoflavone can potentially make contacts with "non-canonical" residues for BET inhibition, e.g., Met105, Asn135, Cys136, and Asp145. Most of these contacts were not observed with fisetin (except for Cys136). Based on the analysis of torsional values, it is plausible that this behavior was due to the atropisomerism present in the molecule. As a first step toward testing this hypothesis, the in vitro inhibition of BRD4 was evaluated. The experimental evaluation showed that amentoflavone was indeed active in the micromolar range, with plausible selectivity against one domain in the BRD4 tandem.

Perspectives of this work include the experimental testing of fisetin and the contrast of its result with molecular modeling predictions. Additionally, for amentoflavone, specific tests for BD1 and BD2 are required to confirm its selectivity. Finally, we consider that these results, while preliminary, offer a new paradigm for inhibitor design, as well as characteristics for novel modulation of BETs.

**Supplementary Materials:** The following are available online at http://www.mdpi.com/2218-273X/8/3/61/s1. Figure S1: Relaxation protocol and MD workflow used in this work, Table S1: BRD4 PDBIDs used for cross-docking studies Figure S2: Simulation Quality parameters for the BRD4 protein for 100 ns, Table S2: IC$_{50}$ and experimental binding energy values and of reference ligands for BRD4 inhibition as reported on the literature, Figure S3: RMSD values for BRD4 protein for 100ns, Table S3: Scoring values for reference ligands as obtained by the docking software used herein, Figure S4: Simulation Quality parameters for the BRD4 protein with fisetine for 100 ns, Table S4: Scoring values obtained with LeDock for amentoflavone per protein-ligand complex of the ensemble, Figure S5: Simulation Quality parameters for the BRD4 protein with amentoflavone for 100 ns, Table S5: Scoring values obtained with MOE for amentoflavone per protein-ligand complex of the ensemble, Figure S6: Secondary structure of BRD4 as observed for 100 ns. A) BRD4 without ligand. B) amentoflavone. C) fisetin., Table S6: Scoring values obtained with PLANTS for amentoflavone per protein-ligand complex of the ensemble, Table S7: Scoring values obtained with Vina for amentoflavone per protein-ligand complex of the ensemble, Table S8: Scoring values obtained with LeDock for fisetin per protein-ligand complex of the ensemble, Table S9: Scoring values obtained with MOE for fisetin per protein-ligand complex of the ensemble, Table S10: Scoring values obtained with PLANTS for protein-ligand complex of the ensemble, Table S11: Scoring values obtained with Vina for fisetin per protein-ligand complex of the ensemble, Table S12: Summary values for quality measures for the BRD4 protein, Table S13: Summary values for quality measures BRD4 protein with fisetine, Table S14: Summary values for quality measures BRD4 protein with amentoflavone.

**Author Contributions:** Conceptualization, F.D.P.-M. Methodology, F.D.P.-M. Formal analysis, F.D.P.-M. Investigation, F.D.P.-M. and J.L.M.-F. Resources, J.L.M.-F. Writing—original draft preparation, F.D.P.-M. Writing—review and editing, J.L.M.-F. Supervision, J.L.M.-F. Project administration, J.L.M.-F. Funding acquisition, J.L.M.-F.

**Funding:** This research was funded by the Consejo Nacional de Ciencia y Tecnologia, grant number 282785.

**Acknowledgments:** F.D.P.-M. acknowledges the PhD scholarship from CONACyT No. 660465/576637. The authors would like to thank Joaquín Barroso-Flores (Centro Conjunto de Investigación en Química Sustentable, Instituto de Química, UNAM) and Durbis Castillo-Pazos (Universidad Nacional Autónoma del Estado de México) for the suggestion of software used for MD. Additionally, discussions with Marcelino Arciniega (Instituto de Fisiología Celular, UNAM) were highly valuable to this work. The authors are grateful for the support given by the Programa de Apoyo a la Investigación y el Posgrado (PAIP) grant 5000–9163, Facultad de Química, UNAM; and by the Programa de Apoyo a Proyectos de Investigación e Innovación Tecnológica (PAPIIT) grant IA203718, UNAM. The authors are grateful for the computational resources granted by the Dirección General de Cómputo y de Tecnologías de Información y Comunicación (DGTIC), project grant LANCAD-UNAM-DGTIC-335 that

*Biomolecules* **2018**, *8*, 61

allowed the use of the Miztli supercomputer at UNAM. We also thank the Programa de Nuevas Alternativas de Tratamiento para Enfermedades Infecciosas (NUATEI-IIB-UNAM).

**Conflicts of Interest:** The authors declare no conflict of interest. The funders had no role in the design of the study; in the collection, analyses, or interpretation of data; in the writing of the manuscript, and in the decision to publish the results.

## References

1.  Cabaye, A.; Nguyen, K.T.; Liu, L.; Pande, V.; Schapira, M. Structural diversity of the epigenetics pocketome. *Proteins Struct. Funct. Bioinform.* **2015**, *83*, 1316–1326. [CrossRef] [PubMed]
2.  Eberharter, A.; Becker, P.B. Histone acetylation: A switch between repressive and permissive chromatin. Second in review on chromatin dynamics. *EMBO Rep.* **2002**, *3*, 224–229. [CrossRef] [PubMed]
3.  Kalyaanamoorthy, S.; Chen, Y.P.P. Energy based pharmacophore mapping of HDAC inhibitors against class i HDAC enzymes. *Biochim. Biophys. Acta Proteins Proteomics* **2013**, *1834*, 317–328. [CrossRef]
4.  Ortore, G.; Colo, F.D.; Martinelli, A. Docking of Hydroxamic Acids into HDAC1 and HDAC8: A Rationalization of Activity Trends and Selectivities. *J. Chem. Inf. Model.* **2009**, *49*, 2774–2785. [CrossRef] [PubMed]
5.  Hassanzadeh, M.; Bagherzadeh, K.; Amanlou, M. A comparative study based on docking and molecular dynamics simulations over HDAC-tubulin dual inhibitors. *J. Mol. Graph. Model.* **2016**, *70*, 170–180. [CrossRef] [PubMed]
6.  VanderMolen, K.M.; McCulloch, W.; Pearce, C.J.; Oberlies, N.H. Romidepsin (Istodax, NSC 630176, FR901228, FK228, depsipeptide): A natural product recently approved for cutaneous T-cell lymphoma. *J. Antibiot. (Tokyo)* **2011**, *64*, 525–531. [CrossRef] [PubMed]
7.  Arrowsmith, C.H.; Bountra, C.; Fish, P.V.; Lee, K.; Schapira, M. Epigenetic protein families: a new frontier for drug discovery. *Nat. Rev. Drug Discov.* **2012**, *11*, 384–400. [CrossRef] [PubMed]
8.  Berkovits, B.D.; Wolgemuth, D.J. The Role of the Double Bromodomain-Containing BET Genes During Mammalian Spermatogenesis. *Curr. Top. Dev. Biol.* **2013**, *102*, 293–326. [CrossRef] [PubMed]
9.  Hewings, D.S.; Rooney, T.P.C.; Jennings, L.E.; Hay, D.A.; Schofield, C.J.; Brennan, P.E.; Knapp, S.; Conway, S.J. Progress in the Development and Application of Small Molecule Inhibitors of Bromodomain–Acetyl-lysine Interactions. *J. Med. Chem.* **2012**, *55*, 9393–9413. [CrossRef] [PubMed]
10. Ferri, E.; Petosa, C.; McKenna, C.E. Bromodomains: Structure, function and pharmacology of inhibition. *Biochem. Pharmacol.* **2016**, *106*, 1–18. [CrossRef] [PubMed]
11. Brand, M.; Measures, A.M.; Wilson, B.G.; Cortopassi, W.A.; Alexander, R.; Höss, M.; Hewings, D.S.; Rooney, T.P.C.; Paton, R.S.; Conway, S.J. Small Molecule Inhibitors of Bromodomain–Acetyl-lysine Interactions. *ACS Chem. Biol.* **2015**, *10*, 22–39. [CrossRef] [PubMed]
12. Ladbury, J.E. Just add water! The effect of water on the specificity of protein-ligand binding sites and its potential application to drug design. *Chem. Biol.* **1996**, *3*, 973–980. [CrossRef]
13. Plumridge, T.H.; Waigh, R.D. Water structure theory and some implications for drug design. *J. Pharm. Pharmacol.* **2002**, *54*, 1155–1179. [CrossRef] [PubMed]
14. Crawford, T.D.; Tsui, V.; Flynn, E.M.; Wang, S.; Taylor, A.M.; Côté, A.; Audia, J.E.; Beresini, M.H.; Burdick, D.J.; Cummings, R.; et al. Diving into the Water: Inducible Binding Conformations for BRD4, TAF1(2), BRD9, and CECR2 Bromodomains. *J. Med. Chem.* **2016**, *59*, 5391–5402. [CrossRef] [PubMed]
15. Pan, A.C.; Borhani, D.W.; Dror, R.O.; Shaw, D.E. Molecular determinants of drug-receptor binding kinetics. *Drug Discov. Today* **2013**, *18*, 667–673. [CrossRef] [PubMed]
16. Huggins, D.J.; Sherman, W.; Tidor, B. Rational approaches to improving selectivity in drug design. *J. Med. Chem.* **2012**, *55*, 1424–1444. [CrossRef] [PubMed]
17. Ross, G.A.; Morris, G.M.; Biggin, P.C. Rapid and accurate prediction and scoring of water molecules in protein binding sites. *PLoS ONE* **2012**, *7*, e32036. [CrossRef] [PubMed]
18. García-Sosa, A.T.; Firth-Clark, S.; Mancera, R.L. Including tightly-bound water molecules in de novo drug design. exemplification through the in silico generation of poly(ADP-ribose)polymerase ligands. *J. Chem. Inf. Model.* **2005**, *45*, 624–633. [CrossRef] [PubMed]

19. Shadrick, W.R.; Slavish, P.J.; Chai, S.C.; Waddell, B.; Connelly, M.; Low, J.A.; Tallant, C.; Young, B.M.; Bharatham, N.; Knapp, S.; et al. Exploiting a water network to achieve enthalpy-driven, bromodomain-selective BET inhibitors. *Bioorgan. Med. Chem.* **2018**, *26*, 25–36. [CrossRef] [PubMed]
20. Bharatham, N.; Slavish, P.J.; Young, B.M.; Shelat, A.A. The role of ZA channel water-mediated interactions in the design of bromodomain-selective BET inhibitors. *J. Mol. Graph. Model.* **2018**, *81*, 197–210. [CrossRef] [PubMed]
21. Geist, L.; Mayer, M.; Cockcroft, X.L.; Wolkerstorfer, B.; Kessler, D.; Engelhardt, H.; McConnell, D.B.; Konrat, R. Direct NMR Probing of Hydration Shells of Protein Ligand Interfaces and Its Application to Drug Design. *J. Med. Chem.* **2017**, *60*, 8708–8715. [CrossRef] [PubMed]
22. Prieto-Martínez, F.D.; Fernandez-de Gortari, E.; Méndez-Lucio, O.; Medina-Franco, J.L. A chemical space odyssey of inhibitors of histone deacetylases and bromodomains. *RSC Adv.* **2016**, *6*, 56225–56239. [CrossRef]
23. Galdeano, C.; Ciulli, A. Selectivity on-target of bromodomain chemical probes by structure-guided medicinal chemistry and chemical biology. *Future Med. Chem.* **2016**, *8*, 1655–1680. [CrossRef] [PubMed]
24. Kharenko, O.A.; Gesner, E.M.; Patel, R.G.; Norek, K.; White, A.; Fontano, E.; Suto, R.K.; Young, P.R.; McLure, K.G.; Hansen, H.C. RVX-297-a novel BD2 selective inhibitor of BET bromodomains. *Biochem. Biophys. Res. Commun.* **2016**, *477*, 62–67. [CrossRef] [PubMed]
25. Ember, S.W.J.; Zhu, J.Y.; Olesen, S.H.; Martin, M.P.; Becker, A.; Berndt, N.; Georg, G.I.; Schonbrunn, E. Acetyl-lysine binding site of bromodomain-containing protein 4 (BRD4) interacts with diverse kinase inhibitors. *ACS Chem. Biol.* **2014**, *9*, 1160–1171. [CrossRef] [PubMed]
26. Dhananjayan, K. Molecular Docking Study Characterization of Rare Flavonoids at the Nac-Binding Site of the First Bromodomain of BRD4 (BRD4 BD1). *J. Cancer Res.* **2015**, *2015*, 1–15. [CrossRef]
27. Singh, M.; Kaur, M.; Silakari, O. Flavones: An important scaffold for medicinal chemistry. *Eur. J. Med. Chem.* **2014**, *84*, 206–239. [CrossRef] [PubMed]
28. Perry, N.S.L.; Bollen, C.; Perry, E.K.; Ballard, C. Salvia for dementia therapy: Review of pharmacological activity and pilot tolerability clinical trial. *Pharmacol. Biochem. Behav.* **2003**, *75*, 651–659. [CrossRef]
29. Hwang, S.-L.; Shih, P.-H.; Yen, G.-C. Citrus Flavonoids and Effects in Dementia and Age-Related Cognitive Decline. In *Diet and Nutrition in Dementia and Cognitive Decline*; Elsevier: Cambridge, MA, USA, 2015; pp. 869–878, ISBN 9780124079397.
30. Fernández, S.P.; Wasowski, C.; Paladini, A.C.; Marder, M. Synergistic interaction between hesperidin, a natural flavonoid, and diazepam. *Eur. J. Pharmacol.* **2005**, *512*, 189–198. [CrossRef] [PubMed]
31. Thilakarathna, W.W.; Langille, M.G.; Rupasinghe, H.V. Polyphenol-based prebiotics and synbiotics: potential for cancer chemoprevention. *Curr. Opin. Food Sci.* **2018**, *20*, 51–57. [CrossRef]
32. Khan, N.; Syed, D.N.; Ahmad, N.; Mukhtar, H. Fisetin: A Dietary Antioxidant for Health Promotion. *Antioxid. Redox Signal.* **2013**, *19*, 151–162. [CrossRef] [PubMed]
33. Vasantha Rupasinghe, H.P.; Nair, S.V.G.; Robinson, R.A. *Chemopreventive Properties of Fruit Phenolic Compounds and Their Possible Mode of Actions*, 1st ed.; Elsevier: Amsterdam, The Netherlands, 2014; Volume 42, ISBN 9780444632814.
34. Sung, B.; Pandey, M.K.; Aggarwal, B.B. Fisetin, an Inhibitor of Cyclin-Dependent Kinase 6, Down-Regulates Nuclear Factor-B-Regulated Cell Proliferation, Antiapoptotic and Metastatic Gene Products through the Suppression of TAK-1 and Receptor-Interacting Protein-Regulated IκBα Kinase Activation. *Mol. Pharmacol.* **2007**, *71*, 1703–1714. [CrossRef] [PubMed]
35. Syed, D.N.; Adhami, V.M.; Khan, N.; Khan, M.I.; Mukhtar, H. Exploring the molecular targets of dietary flavonoid fisetin in cancer. *Semin. Cancer Biol.* **2016**, *40–41*, 130–140. [CrossRef] [PubMed]
36. Sundarraj, K.; Raghunath, A.; Perumal, E. A review on the chemotherapeutic potential of fisetin: In vitro evidences. *Biomed. Pharmacother.* **2018**, *97*, 928–940. [CrossRef] [PubMed]
37. Kashyap, D.; Sharma, A.; Sak, K.; Tuli, H.S.; Buttar, H.S.; Bishayee, A. Fisetin: A bioactive phytochemical with potential for cancer prevention and pharmacotherapy. *Life Sci.* **2018**, *194*, 75–87. [CrossRef] [PubMed]
38. Rengarajan, T.; Yaacob, N.S. The flavonoid fisetin as an anticancer agent targeting the growth signaling pathways. *Eur. J. Pharmacol.* **2016**, *789*, 8–16. [CrossRef] [PubMed]
39. Nadeem, A.; Al-Harbi, N.O.; Al-Harbi, M.M.; El-Sherbeeny, A.M.; Ahmad, S.F.; Siddiqui, N.; Ansari, M.A.; Zoheir, K.M.A.; Attia, S.M.; Al-Hosaini, K.A.; et al. Imiquimod-induced psoriasis-like skin inflammation is suppressed by BET bromodomain inhibitor in mice through RORC/IL-17A pathway modulation. *Pharmacol. Res.* **2015**, *99*, 248–257. [CrossRef] [PubMed]

40. Coletta, D.K. Genetic and Epigenetics of Type 2 Diabetes. In *Pathobiology of Human Disease*; Elsevier: Amsterdam, The Netherlands, 2014; pp. 467–476, ISBN 9780123864567.

41. Mele, D.A.; Salmeron, A.; Ghosh, S.; Huang, H.-R.; Bryant, B.M.; Lora, J.M. BET bromodomain inhibition suppresses TH17-mediated pathology. *J. Exp. Med.* **2013**, *210*, 2181–2190. [CrossRef] [PubMed]

42. Burkard, M.; Leischner, C.; Lauer, U.M.; Busch, C.; Venturelli, S.; Frank, J. Dietary flavonoids and modulation of natural killer cells: implications in malignant and viral diseases. *J. Nutr. Biochem.* **2017**, *46*, 1–12. [CrossRef] [PubMed]

43. Catarino, M.D.; Talhi, O.; Rabahi, A.; Silva, A.M.S.; Cardoso, S.M. The Antiinflammatory Potential of Flavonoids. In *Studies in Natural Products Chemistry*; Elsevier: Amsterdam, The Netherlands, 2016; Volume 48, pp. 65–99, ISBN 9780444636027.

44. Onawole, A.T.; Sulaiman, K.O.; Adegoke, R.O.; Kolapo, T.U. Identification of potential inhibitors against the Zika virus using consensus scoring. *J. Mol. Graph. Model.* **2017**, *73*, 54–61. [CrossRef] [PubMed]

45. Śledź, P.; Caflisch, A. Protein structure-based drug design: from docking to molecular dynamics. *Curr. Opin. Struct. Biol.* **2018**, *48*, 93–102. [CrossRef] [PubMed]

46. Raj, U.; Kumar, H.; Varadwaj, P.K. Molecular docking and dynamics simulation study of flavonoids as BET bromodomain inhibitors. *J. Biomol. Struct. Dyn.* **2016**, *1102*, 1–12. [CrossRef] [PubMed]

47. Prieto-Martínez, F.D.; Medina-Franco, J.L. Charting the Bromodomain BRD4: Towards the Identification of Novel Inhibitors with Molecular Similarity and Receptor Mapping. *Lett. Drug Des. Discov.* **2018**, *15*, 1–10. [CrossRef]

48. *Molecular Operating Environment (MOE), 2013.08*; Chemical Computing Group ULC: Montreal, QC, Canada, 2018.

49. Case, D.A.; Babin, V.; Berryman, J.; Betz, R.; Cai, Q.; Cerutti, D.S.; Cheatham, T.; Darden, T.; Duke, R.; Gohlke, H.; et al. *AMBER 14*, University of California: San Francisco, CA, USA, 2014.

50. Gerber, P.R.; Müller, K. MAB, a generally applicable molecular force field for structure modelling in medicinal chemistry. *J. Comput. Aided. Mol. Des.* **1995**, *9*, 251–268. [CrossRef] [PubMed]

51. Trott, O.; Olson, A.J. AutoDock Vina: Improving the speed and accuracy of docking with a new scoring function, efficient optimization, and multithreading. *J. Comput. Chem.* **2009**, *31*. [CrossRef] [PubMed]

52. Unzue, A.; Zhao, H.; Lolli, G.; Dong, J.; Zhu, J.; Zechner, M.; Dolbois, A.; Caflisch, A.; Nevado, C. The "gatekeeper" Residue Influences the Mode of Binding of Acetyl Indoles to Bromodomains. *J. Med. Chem.* **2016**, *59*, 3087–3097. [CrossRef] [PubMed]

53. Korb, O.; Stützle, T.; Exner, T.E. Empirical scoring functions for advanced Protein-Ligand docking with PLANTS. *J. Chem. Inf. Model.* **2009**, *49*, 84–96. [CrossRef] [PubMed]

54. Stewart, J.J.P. Application of the PM6 method to modeling the solid state. *J. Mol. Model.* **2008**, *14*, 499–535. [CrossRef] [PubMed]

55. Hostaš, J.; Řezáč, J.; Hobza, P. On the performance of the semiempirical quantum mechanical PM6 and PM7 methods for noncovalent interactions. *Chem. Phys. Lett.* **2013**, *568–569*, 161–166. [CrossRef]

56. Bowers, K.; Chow, E.; Xu, H.; Dror, R.; Eastwood, M.; Gregersen, B.; Klepeis, J.; Kolossvary, I.; Moraes, M.; Sacerdoti, F.; et al. Scalable Algorithms for Molecular Dynamics Simulations on Commodity Clusters. In Proceedings of the 2006 ACM/IEEE SC Conference on Supercomputing (SC'06), Tampa, FL, USA, 11–17 November 2006.

57. Kräutler, V.; van Gusteren, W.F.; Hünenberger, P.H. A fast SHAKE algorithm to solve distance constraints for small molecules in molecular dynamics simulations. *J. Comput. Chem.* **2001**, *22*, 501–508. [CrossRef]

58. Andrews, F.H.; Singh, A.R.; Joshi, S.; Smith, C.A.; Morales, G.A.; Garlich, J.R.; Durden, D.L.; Kutateladze, T.G. Dual-activity PI3K–BRD4 inhibitor for the orthogonal inhibition of MYC to block tumor growth and metastasis. *Proc. Natl. Acad. Sci. USA* **2017**, *114*, E1072–E1080. [CrossRef] [PubMed]

59. Sargsyan, K.; Grauffel, C.; Lim, C. How Molecular Size Impacts RMSD Applications in Molecular Dynamics Simulations. *J. Chem. Theory Comput.* **2017**, *13*, 1518–1524. [CrossRef] [PubMed]

60. Romero, F.A.; Taylor, A.M.; Crawford, T.D.; Tsui, V.; Côté, A.; Magnuson, S. Disrupting Acetyl-Lysine Recognition: Progress in the Development of Bromodomain Inhibitors. *J. Med. Chem.* **2016**, *59*, 1271–1298. [CrossRef] [PubMed]

61. Ran, T.; Zhang, Z.; Liu, K.; Lu, Y.; Li, H.; Xu, J.; Xiong, X.; Zhang, Y.; Xu, A.; Lu, S.; et al. Insight into the key interactions of bromodomain inhibitors based on molecular docking, interaction fingerprinting, molecular dynamics and binding free energy calculation. *Mol. Biosyst.* **2015**, *11*, 1295–1304. [CrossRef] [PubMed]

62. Korb, O.; Olsson, T.S.G.; Bowden, S.J.; Hall, R.J.; Verdonk, M.L.; Liebeschuetz, J.W.; Cole, J.C. Potential and Limitations of Ensemble Docking. *J. Chem. Inf. Model.* **2012**, 1262–1274. [CrossRef] [PubMed]
63. Evangelista, W.; Weir, R.L.; Ellingson, S.R.; Harris, J.B.; Kapoor, K.; Smith, J.C.; Baudry, J. Ensemble-based docking: From hit discovery to metabolism and toxicity predictions. *Bioorganic Med. Chem.* **2016**, *24*, 4928–4935. [CrossRef] [PubMed]
64. Tuccinardi, T.; Poli, G.; Romboli, V.; Giordano, A.; Martinelli, A. Extensive consensus docking evaluation for ligand pose prediction and virtual screening studies. *J. Chem. Inf. Model.* **2014**, *54*, 2980–2986. [CrossRef] [PubMed]
65. Kitchen, D.B.; Decornez, H.; Furr, J.R.; Bajorath, J. Docking and scoring in virtual screening for drug discovery: methods and applications. *Nat. Rev. Drug Discov.* **2004**, *3*, 935–949. [CrossRef] [PubMed]
66. Palestro, P.H.; Gavernet, L.; Estiu, G.L.; Bruno Blanch, L.E. Docking Applied to the Prediction of the Affinity of Compounds to P-Glycoprotein. *Biomed Res. Int.* **2014**, *2014*, 1–10. [CrossRef] [PubMed]
67. Ferreira, L.; dos Santos, R.; Oliva, G.; Andricopulo, A. Molecular Docking and Structure-Based Drug Design Strategies. *Molecules* **2015**, *20*, 13384–13421. [CrossRef] [PubMed]
68. Naïm, M.; Bhat, S.; Rankin, K.N.; Dennis, S.; Chowdhury, S.F.; Siddiqi, I.; Drabik, P.; Sulea, T.; Bayly, C.I.; Jakalian, A.; et al. Solvated Interaction Energy (SIE) for scoring protein-ligand binding affinities. 1. Exploring the parameter space. *J. Chem. Inf. Model.* **2007**, *47*, 122–133. [CrossRef] [PubMed]
69. Richter, L.; de Graaf, C.; Sieghart, W.; Varagic, Z.; Mörzinger, M.; de Esch, I.J.P.; Ecker, G.F.; Ernst, M. Diazepam-bound GABAA receptor models identify new benzodiazepine binding-site ligands. *Nat. Chem. Biol.* **2012**, *8*, 455–464. [CrossRef] [PubMed]
70. Wang, Z.; Sun, H.; Yao, X.; Li, D.; Xu, L.; Li, Y.; Tian, S.; Hou, T. Comprehensive evaluation of ten docking programs on a diverse set of protein-ligand complexes: The prediction accuracy of sampling power and scoring power. *Phys. Chem. Chem. Phys.* **2016**, *18*, 12964–12975. [CrossRef] [PubMed]
71. Hoffer, L.; Voitovich, Y.V.; Raux, B.; Carrasco, K.; Muller, C.; Fedorov, A.Y.; Derviaux, C.; Amouric, A.; Betzi, S.; Horvath, D.; et al. Integrated Strategy for Lead Optimization Based on Fragment Growing: The Diversity-Oriented-Target-Focused-Synthesis Approach. *J. Med. Chem.* **2018**. [CrossRef]
72. Waterman, M.J.; Nugraha, A.S.; Hendra, R.; Ball, G.E.; Robinson, S.A.; Keller, P.A. Antarctic Moss Biflavonoids Show High Antioxidant and Ultraviolet-Screening Activity. *J. Nat. Prod.* **2017**, *80*, 2224–2231. [CrossRef] [PubMed]
73. Glunz, P.W. Recent encounters with atropisomerism in drug discovery. *Bioorgan. Med. Chem. Lett.* **2018**, *28*, 53–60. [CrossRef] [PubMed]
74. Jung, M.; Philpott, M.; Müller, S.; Schulze, J.; Badock, V.; Eberspächer, U.; Moosmayer, D.; Bader, B.; Schmees, N.; Fernández-Montalván, A.; Haendler, B. Affinity map of bromodomain protein 4 (BRD4) interactions with the histone H4 tail and the small molecule inhibitor JQ1. *J. Biol. Chem.* **2014**, *289*, 9304–9319. [CrossRef] [PubMed]
75. Scotti, L.; Bezerra Mendonca, F.J.; Ribeiro, F.F.; Tavares, J.F.; da Silva, M.S.; Barbosa Filho, J.M.; Scotti, M.T. Natural Product Inhibitors of Topoisomerases: Review and Docking Study. *Curr. Protein Pept. Sci.* **2018**, *19*, 275–291. [CrossRef] [PubMed]
76. Cardoso, C.R.P.; de Syllos Cólus, I.M.; Bernardi, C.C.; Sannomiya, M.; Vilegas, W.; Varanda, E.A. Mutagenic activity promoted by amentoflavone and methanolic extract of Byrsonima crassa Niedenzu. *Toxicology* **2006**, *225*, 55–63. [CrossRef] [PubMed]
77. Lee, E.-J.; Shin, S.-Y.; Lee, J.-Y.; Lee, S.-J.; Kim, J.-K.; Yoon, D.-Y.; Woo, E.-R.; Kim, Y.-M. Cytotoxic Activities of Amentoflavone against Human Breast and Cervical Cancers are Mediated by Increasing of PTEN Expression Levels due to Peroxisome Proliferator-Activated Receptor γ Activation. *Bull. Korean Chem. Soc.* **2012**, *33*, 2219–2223. [CrossRef]
78. Grynberg, N.F.; Carvalho, M.G.; Velandia, J.R.; Oliveira, M.C.; Moreira, I.C.; Braz- Filho, R.; Echevarria, A. DNA topoisomerase inhibitors: Biflavonoids from Ouratea species. *Braz. J. Med. Biol. Res.* **2002**, *35*, 819–822. [CrossRef] [PubMed]

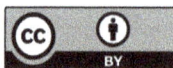

*biomolecules*

MDPI

*Article*

# In Silico Studies on Compounds Derived from *Calceolaria*: Phenylethanoid Glycosides as Potential Multitarget Inhibitors for the Development of Pesticides

**Marco A. Loza-Mejía \*, Juan Rodrigo Salazar \* and Juan Francisco Sánchez-Tejeda**

Benjamín Franklin 45, Cuauhtémoc, Mexico City 06140, Mexico; juansanchez@lasallistas.org
*   Correspondence: marcoantonio.loza@ulsa.mx (M.A.L.-M.); juan.salazar@ulsa.mx (J.R.S.);
    Tel.: +52-55-5278-9500 (M.A.L.-M. & J.R.S.)

Received: 28 September 2018; Accepted: 19 October 2018; Published: 23 October 2018

**Abstract:** An increasing occurrence of resistance in insect pests and high mammal toxicity exhibited by common pesticides increase the need for new alternative molecules. Among these alternatives, bioinsecticides are considered to be environmentally friendly and safer than synthetic insecticides. Particularly, plant extracts have shown great potential in laboratory conditions. However, the lack of studies that confirm their mechanisms of action diminishes their potential applications on a large scale. Previously, we have reported the insect growth regulator and insecticidal activities of secondary metabolites isolated from plants of the *Calceolaria* genus. Herein, we report an in silico study of compounds isolated from *Calceolaria* against acetylcholinesterase, prophenoloxidase, and ecdysone receptor. The molecular docking results are consistent with the previously reported experimental results, which were obtained during the bioevaluation of *Calceolaria* extracts. Among the compounds, phenylethanoid glycosides, such as verbascoside, exhibited good theoretical affinity to all the analyzed targets. In light of these results, we developed an index to evaluate potential multitarget insecticides based on docking scores.

**Keywords:** molecular docking; bioinsecticides; structure–activity relationship; phenylethanoid glycosides; *Calceolaria*; multitarget

## 1. Introduction

The continuous growth of the world population has created an enormous pressure to satisfy the global demand for agricultural products. The challenges include the depletion of soil fertility, the constant depredation of natural soils to convert them into agricultural ecosystems, and the ability of the arthropods to obtain resistance against traditional insecticidal controls.

Insecticides have been used for combating insect pests, mainly to increase the yield of food production among other agricultural products. From ancient times, there are records that describe the use of different types of products to combat insect pests [1]. It is known that various nonspecific agents have been used, such as sulfur and poisonous natural extracts, then organochlorines, organophosphates, carbamates, pyrethroids, and rotenoids, among others, and finally compounds, which are specifically designed and synthesized against enzymatic systems of arthropods.

The increasing need for agricultural goods has resulted in misutilization of insecticides, and this has led to the use of a higher concentration of insecticides or to the need for more toxic products. This has resulted in increased toxic effects on other beneficial organisms that coexist with pests in agroecosystems and on the bioaccumulation of higher concentrations of toxic insecticides in the bodies of predators or the final consumers, including humans. Despite these problems, the use of insecticides is needed to satisfy global demand for products. Thus, we can say that insecticides are a necessary evil. However, research must be carried out to identify better alternatives.

Among these alternatives, bioinsecticides enjoy a good reputation and are generally regarded as environmentally friendly and safer than synthetic insecticides [2]. For some years, many groups have conducted studies for biodirected phytochemical screening on plants toward the isolation and characterization of extracts and compounds that are useful as biocides. In most of published reports, authors investigate the effect of extracts or compounds against specific pest organisms, or against one or more isolated molecular targets, such as acetylcholinesterase (AChE) [3]. We use the extraordinary ability of plants to respond dynamically to herbivory through several molecular mechanisms, including the biosynthesis of defensive compounds to identify those with potential to be used for pest control. Those compounds can affect feeding, growth, and survival of insects and are widely distributed in nature [4]. The organic extracts prepared from the botanical material are a rich source of many classes of secondary metabolites. Many of them have been isolated via traditional chromatographic techniques and even used as active components in botanical pest management products, mainly rotenone, nicotine, strychnine, neem extracts, and essential oils [5]. Thus, the traditional methodology to discover new insecticides includes phytochemical work for the screening of microbial metabolites, terrestrial plants, algae, marine organisms, and so forth. Several factors make harder or more complicated the transition from synthetic insecticides to bioinsecticides. Specifically, the use of an extract generally does not offer guarantees of success in combating pests, and often, the insecticidal mechanisms involved are unknown or are too difficult to elucidate due to the complexity of mixtures of natural extracts [6].

However, less emphasis is given to pesticide-discovery efforts based upon natural products as templates for new structures via semisynthesis. In recent years, a renewed interest in obtaining biologically active compounds from natural sources has emerged, not only as a source of new molecules but also with innovative methodologies, including fragment-based design, high-throughput screening, and genetic engineering, towards the development of new pest-management products with low or absent toxicity towards nontarget insects and mammal organisms, low final concentrations caused by ambient degradability, and a relatively low cost compared with those compounds obtained via complete chemical synthesis [7].

Our group has conducted studies on the *Calceolaria* genus for the identification, isolation, and characterization of new bioinsecticides. The extracts and several secondary metabolites isolated from *Calceolaria* exhibit insect growth regulator (IGR) or insecticidal activities. The insecticidal activity was assayed against the fruit fly *(Drosophila melanogaster*, Diptera), yellow meal worm (*Tenebrio molitor*, Coleoptera: Tenebrionidae), and fall armyworm (*Spodoptera frugiperda*, J. E. Smith, Lepidoptera: Noctuidae), which are important insect pests in fruits, stored grains, and corn [8]. The experimental results indicate that some extracts and compounds isolated from *Calceolaria* interfere with sclerotization and molting processes, suggesting interaction with an ecdysone receptor [9]. Several of these extracts and compounds also act as enzymatic inhibitors against tyrosinase and protease enzymes [10], suggesting potential multitarget activity. Few examples of multitarget insecticides have been reported in the literature [11,12].

On the other hand, among the strategies used to find bioactive candidates, structure-based virtual screening (SBVS) has played a critical role, especially in the identification of potential chemotypes [13]. Docking-based virtual screening (DBVS) is probably the most widely used of these strategies. It involves docking of a library of ligands into a biological target and estimating the probability that a ligand will bind to the protein target by the application of a scoring algorithm, aiding in the identification of the most promising lead compounds for biological assays [14]. However, DBVS has some limitations: (a) the content and quality of the compound library has a profound effect on the success of DBVS, thus it is important to filter the library using the rule-of-five or other physicochemical filters, and (b) with the actual scoring functions, the prediction of correct binding poses is feasible but high accuracy prediction of binding affinity is still a challenge, thus there is little confidence on docking scores to rank potential ligands, particularly on those of the same structural frame [14,15].

Despite these limitations, DBVS has been successfully used in the identification of potential templates for new drug development [16–18]. Recently, some examples of the use of virtual screening and other computational chemistry tools in natural products research have been described [19–22].

With this in mind, we wanted to determine the potential use of compounds isolated from *Calceloraia* as leads in the discovery of multitarget insecticides using DBVS on some proteins recognized as targets for pesticides [12,23,24] and that could be targets for compounds present in *Calceolaria* extracts based on experimental results [9,25,26]: acetylcholinesterase (AChE), prophenoloxidase (PPO), and ecdysone receptor (EcR). Construction of a ligand library was based on compounds isolated and present in organic extracts with experimentally demonstrated pesticide activity aiming to identify potential structural templates that could be used in the development of new pesticides.

## 2. Materials and Methods

### 2.1. Ligand Construction

All of the ligands were chosen from a previously published review [27], which includes several compounds from different chemical families, including diterpenes, triterpenes, and naphthoquinones with a potential pesticidal activity, and some bioactive flavonoids and phenylethanoid glycosides as well. All of the structures were constructed using Spartan '10 for Windows, and these geometries were optimized using the MMFF force field. Then, these structures were exported to Molegro Virtual Docker 6.0.1 [28]; assignments of charges and ionization were based on standard templates as part of the Molegro software. A complete list of all ligands and their structures are presented in Supplementary Information.

### 2.2. Molecular Docking Studies

The docking studies were carried out based on the crystal structures of *Drosophila melanogaster* acetylcholinesterase (*Dm*AchE, PDB codes: 1DX4 [29] and 1QON [29]), *Heliothis virescens* ecdysone receptor (EcR, PDB code: 3IXP [30] and 2R40 [31]), and *Manduca sexta* prophenoloxidase (PPO, PDB code: 3HHS [32]). Two different structures from the Protein Data Bank (PDB) were selected to analyze repeatability of results, independent of the PDB structure selected. This was not possible for PPO as no other PDB structure has been reported. In addition, docking studies were carried out in human acetylcholinesterase (*h*AChE, PDB code: 4EY7 [33] and 4M0E [34]) to determine whether some of the compounds exhibited theoretical preference to the *Drosophila*/human enzyme. All structures were retrieved from the Protein Data Bank [35]. Docking studies were carried out using a previously reported methodology [36,37]. Briefly, all of the solvent molecules and cocrystallized ligands were removed from the structures. Molecular docking calculations for all of the compounds with each of the proteins were performed using Molegro Virtual Docker v. 6.0.1 [28]. Active sites of each enzyme were chosen as the binding sites and delimited with a 15 Å radius sphere centered on the cocrystallized ligand, except for the PPO structure, which has no cocrystallized ligand, and the sphere was centered on the active $Cu^{2+}$ ions. Standard software procedure was used. The assignments of charges on each protein were based on standard templates as part of the Molegro Virtual Docker program, and no other charges were necessary to be set. The Root Mean Square Deviation (RMSD) threshold for multiple cluster poses was set to <1.00 Å. The docking algorithm was set to 5000 maximum iterations with a simplex evolution population size of 50 and a minimum of 25 runs for each ligand. After docking, *MolDock Score* was calculated as the theoretical binding affinity. To assess the efficacy of this procedure, cocrystallized ligands were also docked to their respective receptors (except for PPO), the top-ranking score was recorded, and the RMSD of that pose from the corresponding crystal coordinates was computed. In all the cases, the RMSD was lower than 2 Å. For each enzyme, the 10 compounds with lower *MolDock scores* were selected for analyzing their docking poses to identify potential structural requirements for enzyme binding.

*2.3. Molecular Dynamics Simulations*

Molecular Dynamics (MD) simulations were carried out to observe differences that could account for potential selectivity of phenylpropanoids for *Dm*AChE over *h*AChE. Simulations were performed in YASARA Dynamics v.18.4.24 [38,39] using AMBER14 force field [40]. The initial structures for the MD simulation were obtained from the docking complexes of compound **87** with *Dm*AChE (PDB code: 1QON) and with *h*AChE (PDB code: 4M0E). Compound **87** (verbascoside) was selected, as it is the most studied compound of the phenylpropanoids derived from *Calceolaria*. Each complex was positioned into a water box with a size of 100 Å × 100 Å × 100 Å, with periodic boundary conditions. Temperature was set at 298 K, water density to 0.997 g/cm$^3$, and pH to 7.4. Sodium (Na$^+$) and chlorine (Cl$^-$) ions were included to provide conditions that simulate a physiological solution (NaCl 0.9%). Particle mesh Ewald algorithm was applied with a cut-off radius of 8 Å. A timestep of 2.5 fs was set. The simulation snapshots were recorded at intervals of 100 ps until a total simulation time of 30 ns. Results were analyzed with a script included as part of YASARA software and included RMSD, ligand binding energy variations (using MM-PBSA calculations), and distance of ligand 87 to Ser 283 (*Dm*AChE) or Ser 203 (*h*AChE), as these residues play a key role in acetylcholinesterase enzymatic activity. For *Dm*AChE, we considered the interaction between the primary alcohol group of the central glucopyranose ring with Ser 238, and for *h*AChE, the interaction between the hydroxyl group of the ferouyl residue with Ser 203. A similar procedure has been recently reported for the simulation of complexes of drugs with some proteins [41–43].

*2.4. Construction of the Virtual Multitarget Index and the Weighed Multi-Target Index*

The virtual Multitarget index of each compound was determined. To compare the multitarget index of the analyzed compounds, we propose a virtual multitarget index (*vMTi*), which was calculated for the three insect targets (EcR, PPO, and *Dm*AChE) using formula (1):

$$vMTi = \sum_{i=1}^{n} \frac{MD_i}{MDr} \tag{1}$$

where MDi corresponds to the *MolDock* score of the molecule in a specific target and MDr is the *MolDock* score of the reference ligand; we considered the compound with the lowest *MolDock* score (which has the highest theoretical affinity) for each target as the reference. Compounds with higher values have a higher multitarget index. However, binding to *h*AChE is an undesirable condition. To take this into consideration, we propose a weighed *MTi* (*wMTi*), which was calculated using formula 2, using an external coefficient *n*, which represents the desirability of binding to a specific target:

$$wMTi = \sum_{i=1}^{n} n\frac{MD_i}{MDr} \tag{2}$$

To calculate *wMTi*, we gave values of *n* = 0.3 to desirable targets (EcR, PPO, and *Dm*AChE) and *n* = −0.3 to *h*AChE.

In addition to these calculations, a contour plot was built with Minitab using PPO, *Dm*AChE, and EcR docking scores. This plot can help identify potential multitarget compounds because those compounds would appear in valleys since they would have lower *MolDock* scores.

## 3. Results

*3.1. Docking Studies Results*

Tables 1–3 show data for the 10 compounds with a lower average *MolDock score* in the ecdysone receptor (EcR), prophenoloxidase (PPO), and acetylcholinesterase (both *Dm*AchE and *h*AChE) docking study. A table with complete docking results is presented in Supplementary Information.

**Table 1.** *MolDock Scores* obtained in the ecdysone receptor (EcR) docking. Top 10 compounds with the better theoretical binding. PEG = Phenylethanoid glycosides.

| Ligand | Skeleton Type | Compound Name | PDB: 3IXP | PDB: 2R40 | Average *MolDock Scores* |
|--------|---------------|---------------|-----------|-----------|--------------------------|
| 88 | PEG | Calceolarioside C | −214.0 | −207.2 | −210.6 |
| 90 | PEG | Forsythoside A | −202.8 | −213.5 | −208.2 |
| 89 | PEG | Calceolarioside E | −184.7 | −212.5 | −198.6 |
| 92 | PEG | Isoarenarioside | −183.0 | −205.5 | −194.2 |
| 87 | PEG | Verbascoside | −197.4 | −184.1 | −190.8 |
| 86 | PEG | Calceolarioside A | −174.2 | −183.6 | −178.9 |
| 91 | PEG | Calceolarioside B | −162.1 | −176.7 | −169.4 |
| 93 | PEG | Calceolarioside D | −160.2 | −169.3 | −164.7 |
| 68 | Scopadulane | 3-Isovaleroyl-7-malonyloxy-thyrsiflorane | −147.2 | 157.1 | −152.2 |
| 45 | Isopimarane | 3-β-Isovaleroyl-18-hydroxy-7-α-malonyloxyent-isopimara-9(11), 15-diene | −150.2 | −151.5 | −150.8 |

**Table 2.** *MolDock Scores* obtained in the PPO docking. Top 10 compounds with the better theoretical binding. PEG = Phenylethanoid glycosides.

| Ligand | Skeleton | Compound Name | *MolDock* Score |
|--------|----------|---------------|-----------------|
| 86 | PEG | Calceolarioside A | −161.187 |
| 110 | Flavonoid | Kaempferol-7-methyl ether | −142.825 |
| 93 | PEG | Calceolarioside D | −142.017 |
| 109 | Flavonoid | Gossypetin-7,8,3′-trimethyl ether | −140.618 |
| 108 | Flavonoid | Herbacetin-8,4′-dimethyl ether | −138.595 |
| 88 | PEG | Calceolarioside C | −137.969 |
| 111 | Flavonoid | Kaempferol-4′-methyl ether | −137.519 |
| 104 | Flavonoid | Naringenin-4′-methyl ether | −137.451 |
| 107 | Flavonoid | Isoscutellarein-8,4′-dimethyl ether | −137.188 |

**Table 3.** *MolDock* scores obtained in the AChE docking study. Top 10 compounds with the better theoretical binding.

| Ligand | Compound Name | *Dm*AChE *MolDock* Scores | | | *h*AChE *MolDock* Scores | | | SR [1] |
|--------|---------------|---------------------------|--|--|--------------------------|--|--|----|
| | | PDB: 1DX4 | PDB: 1QON | Average Score | PDB: 4EY7 | PDB: 4M0E | Average Score | |
| 90 | Forsythoside A | −171.3 | −254.5 | −212.9 | −177.7 | −247.6 | −212.6 | 1.00 |
| 88 | Calceolarioside C | −174.0 | −251.6 | −212.8 | −145.7 | −217.7 | −181.7 | 1.17 |
| 87 | Verbascoside | −178.8 | −233.5 | −206.1 | −152.6 | −200.8 | −176.7 | 1.17 |
| 89 | Calceolarioside E | −169.0 | −239.1 | −204.0 | −116.7 | −209.0 | −162.8 | 1.25 |
| 93 | Calceolarioside D | −162.3 | −227.7 | −195.0 | −147.9 | −188.4 | −168.2 | 1.16 |
| 92 | Isoarenarioside | −141.1 | −244.8 | −193.0 | −165.1 | −208.0 | −186.6 | 1.03 |
| 86 | Calceolarioside A | −156.2 | −212.8 | −184.5 | −164.6 | −189.6 | −177.1 | 1.04 |
| 91 | Calceolarioside B | −128.0 | −210.5 | −169.2 | −137.9 | −183.9 | −160.9 | 1.05 |
| 44 | Isopimarane | −119.9 | −180.3 | −150.1 | −137.0 | −159.7 | −148.4 | 1.01 |
| 43 | Isopimarane | −127.3 | −164.5 | −145.9 | −150.2 | −154.6 | −152.4 | 0.96 |

[1] Selectivity ratio (SR) = Average docking score *Dm*AChE / Average docking score *h*AChE.

### 3.2. Molecular Dynamics Studies on Complexes of Verbascoside with DmAChE and hAChE

Figure 1a shows the comparison of the RMSD time profile for protein backbone atoms during the 30 ns simulation of the complexes of compound **87** and *Dm*AChE and *h*AChE. Both complexes have RMSD average values around 2 Å (RMSD = 2.13 Å for *Dm*AChE and RMSD = 1.88 Å for *h*AChE).

We also wanted to check if the distance of compound **87** (verbascoside) to the catalytic site of acetylcholinesterase variates during the simulation time. We selected the potential interactions to Ser 203 in *h*AChE or Ser 238 in *Dm*AChE predicted by molecular docking as described in Methodology. Figure 1b shows the variation of distances of compound **87** to these key serine residues along the simulation time. As seen in this figure, the distance to catalytic site diminished from 4.8 Å to 3.0 Å after 3 ns of simulation in the case of *Dm*AChE (average distance = 3.6 Å), while it maintained almost the same in *h*AChE (average distance = 5.21 Å).

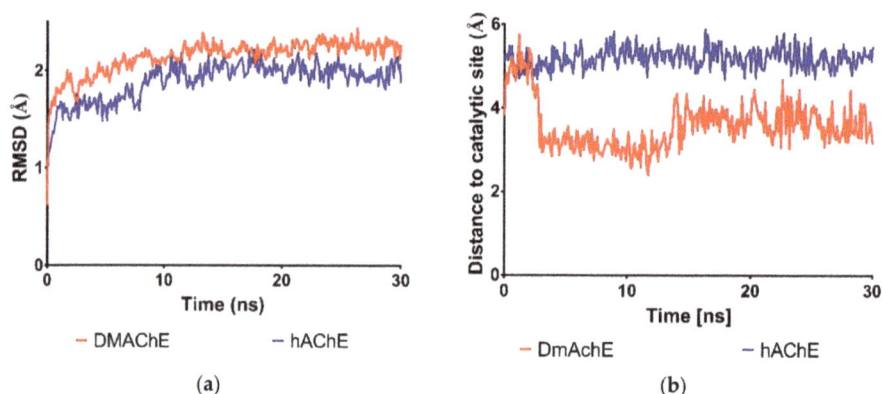

**Figure 1.** Plots of variations along time of Molecular Dynamics (MD) simulations of complexes of **87** with *Dm*AChE (red) and *h*AChE (blue). (**a**) The Root Mean Square Deviation (RMSD) of protein backbone; (**b**) distance of compound **87** to Ser 238 (*Dm*AChE) or Ser 203 (*h*AChE).

To estimate the difference in binding energy of compound **87** in its complex with *Dm*AChE and *h*AChE, MM-PBSA methods were applied. Ligand binding energy suggests better binding of compound **87** to *Dm*AChE (E = −131.5 kJ/mol) versus *h*AChE (E = −134.0 kJ/mol) as binding energy calculations implemented in YASARA Dynamics indicates that the higher the energy value, the better the binding.

*3.3. Construction of the Virtual Multitarget Index and the Weighed Multitarget Index*

Figure 2 shows a contour graphic that compares docking scores of the analyzed compounds on PPO, *Dm*AChE, and EcR. The zone in red corresponds to those molecules with high theoretical affinity against all the three molecular targets. Figure 3 shows the structure of the phenylpropanoids which resulted with the highest values of *vMTi* and *wMTi*. Table 4 shows a list of compounds with higher *vMti* and *wMTi* values; a full list is included in Supplementary Information.

**Table 4.** Compounds with higher *vMti* and *wMti* values. PEG = Phenylethanoid glycosides.

| Ligand | Skeleton | Compound Name | *vMTi* | *wMTi* |
|--------|----------|---------------|--------|--------|
| 88 | PEG | Calceolarioside C | 2.86 | 0.60 |
| 89 | PEG | Calceolarioside E | 2.67 | 0.57 |
| 86 | PEG | Calceolarioside A | 2.72 | 0.56 |
| 87 | PEG | Verbascoside | 2.67 | 0.55 |
| 93 | PEG | Calceolarioside D | 2.58 | 0.54 |
| 90 | PEG | Forsythoside A | 2.77 | 0.53 |
| 92 | PEG | Isoarenarioside | 2.64 | 0.53 |
| 91 | PEG | Calceolarioside B | 2.39 | 0.49 |
| 109 | Flavonoid | Gossypetin-7,8,3′-trimethyl ether | 2.05 | 0.43 |
| 110 | Flavonoid | Kaempferol-7-methyl ether | 2.03 | 0.43 |
| 77 | Labdane | 19-Malonyloxy-9-epi-ent-labda- 8(17), 12 Z, 14-triene | 2.04 | 0.42 |
| 45 | Isopimarane | 3-β-Isovaleroyl-18-hydroxy-7-α-malonyloxyent-isopimara-9(11), 15-diene | 2.13 | 0.42 |
| 3 | Abietane | 19-Malonyloxy-dehydroabietinol | 1.99 | 0.42 |
| 57 | Stemarane | 17-Acetoxy-19-malonyloxy-ent-stemar-13(14)-ene | 2.03 | 0.41 |
| 108 | Flavonoid | Herbacetin-8,4′-dimethyl ether | 1.92 | 0.40 |

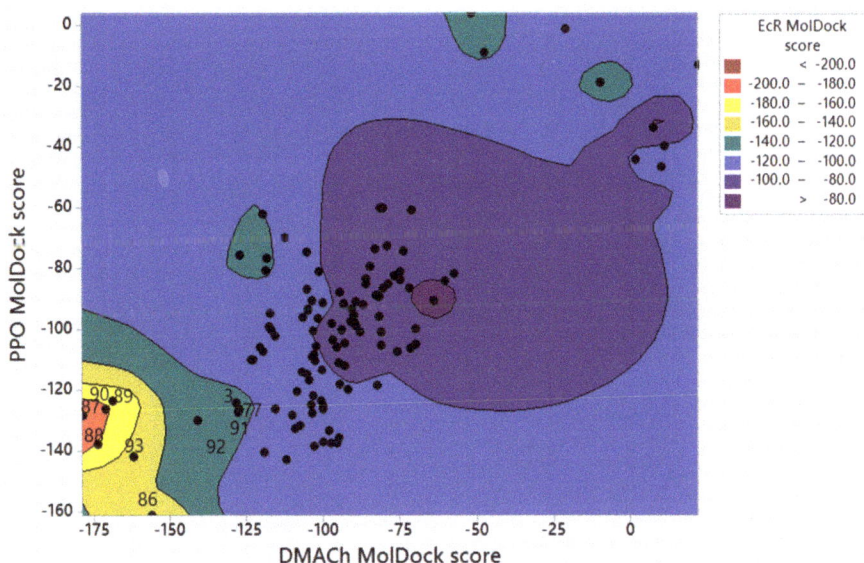

**Figure 2.** Contour plot correlating PPO, *Dm*AChE, and EcR docking scores. Zones in red-yellow indicate higher affinity to EcR than zones in purple or blue.

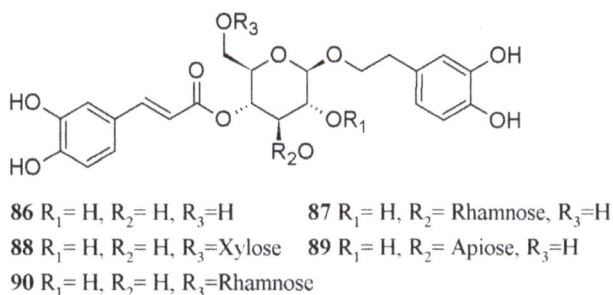

**86** R$_1$= H, R$_2$= H, R$_3$=H        **87** R$_1$= H, R$_2$= Rhamnose, R$_3$=H
**88** R$_1$= H, R$_2$= H, R$_3$=Xylose   **89** R$_1$= H, R$_2$= Apiose, R$_3$=H
**90** R$_1$= H, R$_2$= H, R$_3$=Rhamnose

**Figure 3.** Structures of phenylethanoid glycosides (compounds **86–90**) which exhibited the highest *vMTi* and *wMTi* values.

## 4. Discussion

### 4.1. Docking Studies on Ecdysone Receptor

Induction of molting in Arthropods coincides with a release of 20-hydroxyecdysone (20-E), a steroidal-type hormone. Prior to each of the larval molts, at pupariation, at pupation, and during metamorphosis, the hormone is released in carefully timed spurts, coinciding with major morphological transitions. Ecdysone receptor (EcR) exists in three isoforms. Each requires a partner during the heterodimerization, a *Drosophila* homolog of vertebrate RXR protein named ultraspiracle (USP) protein. Although ecdysone can bind to EcR on its own, binding is significantly augmented by the participation of USP. The interaction between EcR and ecdysone is a crucial event for the development of insects, which is why it represents an interesting molecular target against pest insects [44].

Table 1 shows data for the 10 compounds with a lower average *MolDock score* in the ecdysone receptor docking study. Phenylethanoid glycoside derivatives have better theoretical binding to EcR among the evaluated compounds. Among them, the results indicate that binding to EcR occurs through hydroxyl groups of caffeoyl and phenyl ethyl residues in similar fashion to 20-E (Figure 4a). Analysis of Figure 4a,b reveals that compound **87** (verbascoside, which is a major phenylethanoid glycoside present in *Calceolaria* extracts) adopted a J-shaped conformation in the binding site of EcR, which is similar to the conformation adopted by natural ligand of EcR, 20-E [31] and the interaction pattern is very similar between these compounds: phenylethanoid residue interacts through hydrogen bonds with Arg383 and Glu309 (in magenta in Figure 4a,b) like 2β and 3β hydroxyl groups of ring-A in 20-E, rhamnose residue interacts with Ala398 (in blue in Figure 3a,b) like C-6 ketone moiety in ring-B in 20-E, feruoyl residue interacts with Thr 343 and rhamnose residue with Thr 346 (also in blue in set of Figure 4) like 14-α hydroxyl group, and additional interactions between feruoyl residue and central glucose ring of verbascoside with Tyr 408 and Asn 504 (shown in yellow) are seen in a similar fashion for 25-OH group of side chain of 20-E. This interaction is notable because 20-E interacts with this residue via a water linkage [31], hence the interaction of verbascoside with Asn504 could increase affinity, as some studies have demonstrated that ligands designed to displace the water molecules exhibit higher affinity [45].

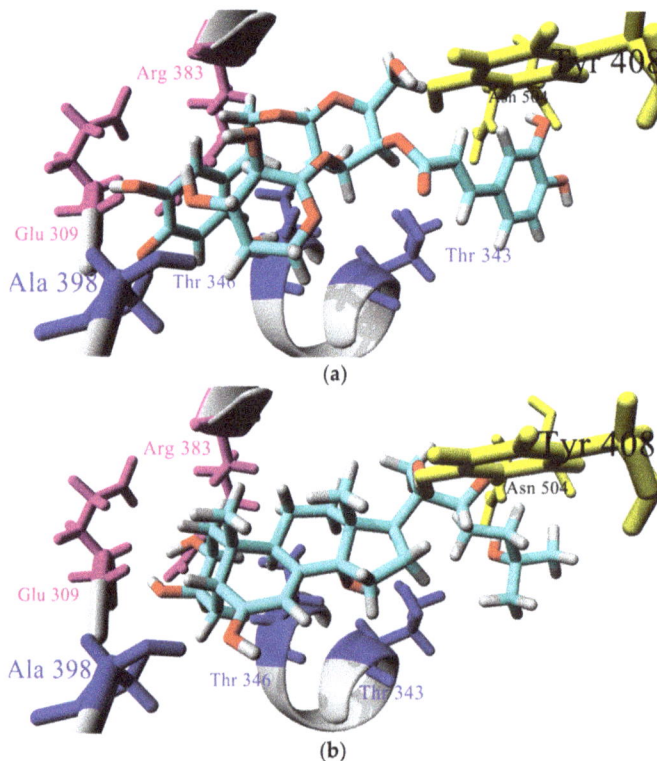

**Figure 4.** Comparison of (**a**) the docked pose of verbascoside (compound **87**) and (**b**) 20-E crystallized in the LBD of EcR (PDB:2R40).

Though there are no previous studies on phenylethanoid glycosides as EcR ligands, there is some experimental evidence that can support docking results. It has been previously reported that the ethyl acetate extract of *C. talcana*, of which verbascoside is its major component (compound **87**), caused a developmental disruption of *D. melanogaster* and *S. frugiperda* larvae. In addition, the authors of the study proposed verbascoside as a disruptor of ecdysteroid metabolism [26]. In another study, the incorporation of verbascoside in the artificial diet of the pest *Agrilus planipennis* caused a 100%

mortality at 45 mg/g of artificial diet [46] when testing the toxic effect of verbascoside against at least three different pest insect species. In addition, Harmatha and Dinan have reported that some polyhydroxylated stilbenoids have an antagonist EcR activity [47], and a previously reported pharmacophore model indicated that the presence of hydroxyl groups in an ecdysteroid template is important for EcR binding [48]. On the other hand, the presence of some other phenylethanoid glycosides, such as calceolarioside A, B, and C, in active extracts of *Calceolaria* as well as in *Fraxinus* spp. can be related to the strong larval molting disruption observed when the larvae of different species were exposed to extracts with high amounts of phenylethanoid glycosides or directly to different amounts of the isolated compounds [46]. All these experimental data strongly suggest that phenylpropanoid glycosides could be EcR ligands.

As described here, the effect of verbascoside and related phenylethanoid glycosides against the ecdysone receptor can explain only one of the multiple effects exerted by these compounds. The experimental evidence remarkably indicates that molting disruption exerted by phenylethanoid glycosides cannot be the only mechanism that explains the strong exerted insecticidal properties. The above information suggests a possible antagonist and multienzymatic inhibitory mechanism that phenylethanoid glycosides can exert, causing larvae disruption activity by acting as EcR antagonist in addition to other mechanisms.

*4.2. Docking Studies on Prophenoloxidase*

Melanization, a process performed by phenoloxidase (PO) and controlled by the prophenoloxidase (PPO) activation cascade, plays an important role in the invertebrate immune system in allowing a rapid response to pathogen infection. The activation of the PPO system, by the specific recognition of microorganisms by pattern-recognition proteins (PRPs), triggers a serine proteinase cascade, which eventually leads to the cleavage of the inactive PPO to the active PO that functions to produce melanin and toxic reactive intermediates. The importance of PPO–PO is due to cuticular sclerotization and defense against pathogens and parasites. PO catalyzes hydroxylation of monophenols to o-diphenols and oxidation of o-diphenols to quinones. Quinones take part in sclerotization and tanning of the cuticle and serve as precursors for synthesis of melanin [49,50]. Therefore, PPO is a very suitable molecular target for designing pesticide compounds.

Table 2 shows docking results from the PPO study. Among the compounds with better PPO binding, the best are flavonoids and phenylethanoid glycosides. The results are in agreement with several previous in vitro and in silico studies [10,51–55] in which most tyrosinase inhibitors possess a phenol moiety as the pharmacophore. Among them, flavonoids appear as effective competitive inhibitors of this enzyme. In addition, Karioti et al. [53] and Muñoz et al. [10] have reported tyrosinase inhibitory activities of some phenylethanoid glycosides, which have lower but comparable inhibitory activities compared with flavonols and flavones.

Hydroxyl groups of caffeoyl or phenylethyl residues have been proposed as essential structural requirements to display inhibitory activities against PPO because of their chelating properties. Figure 5 shows that phenylethanoid glycosides could bind to the PPO catalytic site through interaction with His residues, which are required to form a complex with copper ions. This is in agreement with the previously reported information that indicates verbascoside as a substrate for tyrosinase [10]. Among phenylethanoid glycosides, compounds **86** and **93** could bind better than other analogs. These compounds are monoglycosides, whereas other evaluated phenylethanoid glycosides are diglycosides, which is in agreement with previous reports that indicate the increase in the number of sugar units and the reduction of PPO inhibitory activity [53]. This observation could be explained in terms of the higher molecular volume of diglycosides that prevents them access to the active site as is shown Figure 5; the diglycoside compound **88** is shown in yellow and monoglycoside **86** is in cyan. From this figure, it can be concluded that it is possible that monoglycosides could bind closer to the catalytic site of PPO.

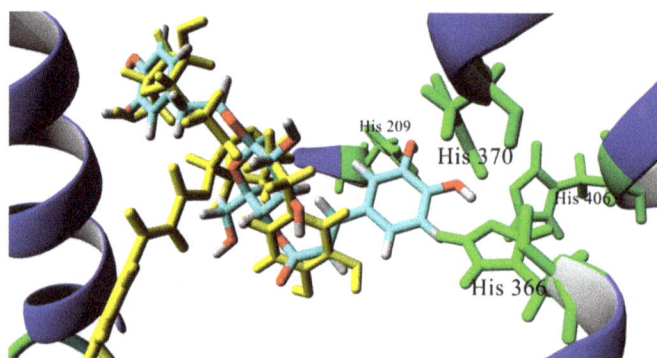

**Figure 5.** Overlap docking poses of compounds **86** (cyan) and **88** (yellow). Histidine residues of catalytic site are shown in green.

*4.3. Docking Studies and Molecular Dynamics Simulations on Drosophila and Human Acetylcholinesterase*

Acetylcholinesterase is a serine hydrolase that is vital for regulating the neurotransmitter acetylcholine in insects. This enzyme is an excellent molecular target for the development of insecticides [56,57]. The well-known active site has a deep and narrow gorge, with a catalytic site at the bottom and a peripheral site at the entrance. Acetylcholinesterase is a molecular target used to control insects that affect public health (e.g., mosquitoes, flies, cockroaches, among others) as well as those that affect agriculture and gardening (e.g., grasshoppers, aphids, caterpillars, among others) [58]. Current anticholinesterase insecticides work through phosphorylation of a serine residue at the AChE catalytic site, which disables the catalytic function and causes enzyme antagonism. Because this serine residue is also ubiquitous in AChEs of mammals and other species with cholinergic nerves, the use of anticholinesterase insecticides to target the serine residue causes serious off-target toxicity [59]. Therefore, it is necessary to evaluate in silico the affinity of molecules against the insect together with mammalian enzymes to determine whether there are some structural features that lead to design inhibitors specifically against insect enzymes.

Table 3 displays the *MolDock* scores of the top 10 compounds with better average docking scores for *Dm*AChE studies in PDB 1DX4 and 1QON structures. Data obtained during docking studies with *h*AChE (PDB structures 4EY7 and 4M0E) is also shown. Selectivity ratio versus *h*AChE was calculated with the average docking score obtained in both enzymes. Although some differences could be appreciated in docking scores values, the same tendency was observed in both *Dm*AChE structures and both *h*AChE structures as phenylethanoid glycosides are among the compounds with a better theoretical binding in the four docking studies. It has been reported that verbascoside and extracts containing other phenylethanoid glycosides are moderate inhibitors of AchE [25].

Figure 6a,b shows the predicted binding mode of verbascoside (compound **87**) in the active site of both *Dm*AChE and *h*AChE, respectively. In the case of the docking study carried out in *Dm*AChE, verbascoside and the rest of the analyzed PEGs adopted a Y-shaped conformation, with the central sugar core interacting with residues of the catalytic triad (colored in yellow in Figure 6a) and the phenylethoxy chain interacting with other residues within the bottom of the gorge. In the case of *h*AChE, the analyzed PEGs adopted a similar conformation, but the phenylethoxy chain did not reach the bottom of the gorge. An explanation to this is that PEGs interact with Asp74 through a hydrogen bond in *h*AChE, whereas this residue is absent in *Dm*AChE [60], limiting the access of PEGs to the catalytic triad, and this could explain the better theoretical affinity of PEGs to *Dm*AChE compared to *h*AChE.

To analyze additional differences that could account for potential selectivity of PGs to *Dm*AChE over *h*AChE, MD simulations were performed. The RMSD values could indicate the stability of the protein relative to its conformation. Figure 4 shows the comparison of the RMSD of the protein backbone profile during the 30 ns simulation of the complexes of compound **87** and *Dm*AChE and *h*AChE. Both complexes have RMSD values around 2Å (RMSD = 2.13 for *Dm*AChE and RMSD = 1.88 for *h*AChE), suggesting that both complexes are stable.

An important difference that was observed during visual analysis MD simulations was the variation of distance of verbascoside (compound **87**) to catalytic site in *Dm*AChE, as it appeared to move closer to key residues Glu 237 and Ser 238, while it seemed that compound **87** maintained a constant distance to equivalent residues Glu 202 and Ser 203 in *h*AChE complex. We confirmed this by measuring the distance of verbascoside to Ser 238 or Ser 203. As seen in Figure 2b, the distance to catalytic site diminished from 4.8 Å to 3.0 Å after 3 ns of simulation in the case of *Dm*AChE (average distance = 3.6 Å), while it maintained almost the same in *h*AChE (average distance = 5.21 Å). This could account for the better binding of **87** towards *Dm*AChE. This could be an important difference that could be useful to future design of selective inhibitors to *Dm*AChE based on the phenylethanoid glycoside template. Additionally, MM-PBSA calculations suggest that 87 binds better to *Dm*AChE (E = −131.5 kJ/mol) than to *h*AChE (E = −134.0 kJ/mol). Overall, we conclude that, based on molecular docking calculations and MD simulations, compound **87** is an interesting starting point for the design of selective *Dm*AchE inhibitors, an important factor to consider in terms of potential toxicity against human beings.

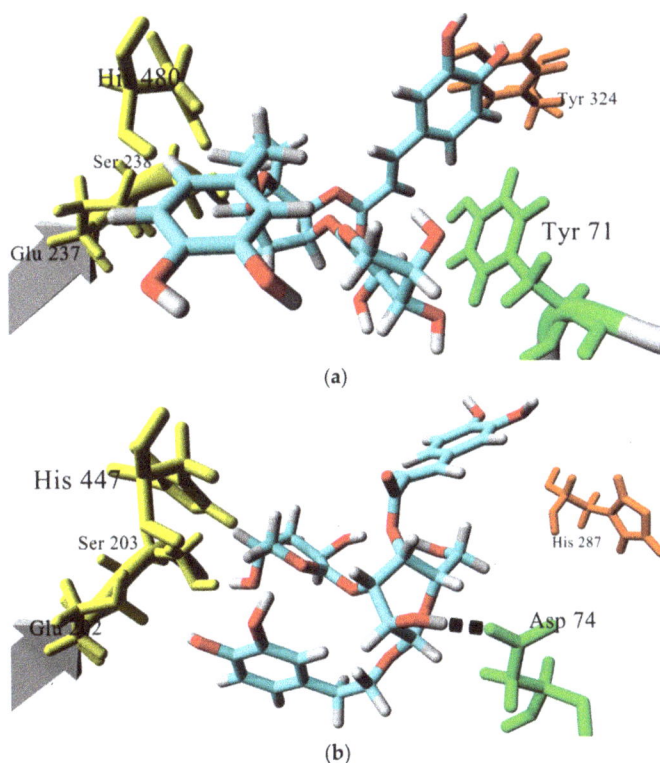

(a)

(b)

**Figure 6.** Comparison of the docking poses of compound **87** in *Dm*AChE (**a**) and *h*AChE (**b**). Catalytic residues are colored in yellow and residues at the entrance of the active site in orange. Tyr71/Asp 74 residues, which are different in each enzyme, are colored in green. Key hydrogen bond interaction of verbascoside to Asp 74 is shown in black.

*4.4. Virtual Multitarget Index and Weighed Multitarget Index*

A multitarget drug has been defined as the integration of multiple pharmacophores in one molecule with the purpose that it can have two or more simultaneous mechanisms of action [61]. Though the concept of multitarget drugs is an important research topic [62,63], there are few examples of the study of multitarget insecticides [12].

Computational tools like molecular docking and multitarget quantitative structure–activity relationship models (mt-QSAR) have been recently used for prediction and discovery of multitarget compounds [64–67]. However, the development of parameters to measure the multitarget index of a ligand is not an easy task. As described during the lapatinib discovery [68], the simple average of biological activity against several targets (or in our case, docking scores) can be misleading, because a compound with a promising average value of bioactivity on two or more targets could correspond to a multitarget compound or to a highly selective compound against only one target. Thus, a reference parameter and weighed coefficients for biological activities of interest should be included. Herein, we propose the use of contour graphics, such as the one shown in Figure 2, and a multitarget index (*vMTi*) to identify potential multitarget insecticides. In the contour plot of Figure 2, the docking scores in three targets of interest (EcR, PPO, and *Dm*AChE) are shown. Compounds that have shown greater theoretical affinity for the three targets will appear in the bottom left of the plot and inside the red and yellow contour areas. This would be a first criteria to identify potential multitarget compounds, because selective compounds would not appear in this area. As expected, the phenylethanoid glycosides appear in this area, but other compounds, such as abietane **3** and isopimarane **77**, can be considered to have potential multitarget properties.

Table 4 shows a list of compounds with higher *vMti* and *wMTi* values. In this table, phenylethanoid glycosides appear as compounds with a better multitarget profile. In addition, compounds **88**, **89**, and **87** (Figure 2) have not only high *vMTi* values, but also the highest *wMTi* due to their higher selectivity to *Dm*AChE than *h*AChE. Thus, these compounds are interesting candidates for the development and evaluation of safer multitarget insecticides.

## 5. Conclusions

Our results complement the experimental results obtained during *Calceolaria* extracts evaluation as biopesticides, and suggest that some of the compounds, such as the phenylethanoid family, can be used for the development of *multitarget* bioinsecticides. Based on the docking studies, it appears that verbascoside and other phenylethanoid glycosides could exert their bioactivity by modifying the activity of various receptors like EcR and enzymes like PPO and AChE, as was suggested and confirmed in previous experimental assays [25,26]. Theoretical affinity, together with *vMTi* and *wMTi*, can be useful for the rational design of *multitarget* bioinsecticides. Verbascoside appears as a good candidate for the development of a multitarget insecticide due to its prolific natural occurrence and its chemical and biological properties [69].

**Supplementary Materials:** The following are available online at http://www.mdpi.com/2218-273X/8/4/121/s1, Table S1: *MolDock* scores and multitarget index for all analyzed compounds, Table S2: MD simulation data.

**Author Contributions:** Conceptualization, M.A.L.-M. and J.R.S.; methodology, M.A.L.-M. and J.F.S.-T.; formal analysis, M.A.L.-M., J.R.S., and J.F.S.-T.; investigation, M.A.L.-M., J.R.S., and J.F.S.-T.; writing—original draft preparation, M.A.L.-M., J.R.S., and J.F.S.-T.; writing—review and editing, M.A.L.-M., J.R.S., and J.F.S.-T.; supervision, M.A.L.-M.; project administration, M.A.L.-M. and J.R.S.; funding acquisition, M.A.L.-M.

**Funding:** This research was funded by Universidad La Salle, grant number SAL 05/16.

**Acknowledgments:** The authors thank Dirección de Posgrado e Investigación of Universidad La Salle for access to additional computational resources.

**Conflicts of Interest:** The authors declare no conflict of interest. The funders had no role in the design of the study; in the collection, analyses, or interpretation of data; in the writing of the manuscript; or in the decision to publish the results.

## References

1. Panagiotakopulu, E.; Buckland, P.C.; Day, P.M. Natural Insecticides and Insect Repellents in Antiquity: A Review of the Evidence. *J. Archeol. Sci.* **1995**, *22*, 705–710. [CrossRef]
2. Sporleder, M.; Lacey, L.A. Biopesticides. In *Insect Pests of Potato*; Elsevier: Amsterdam, The Netherlands, 2013; pp. 463–497. ISBN 9780123868954.
3. Isman, M.B. Bridging the gap: Moving botanical insecticides from the laboratory to the farm. *Ind. Crops Prod.* **2017**, *110*, 10–14. [CrossRef]
4. War, A.R.; Paulraj, M.G.; Ahmad, T.; Buhroo, A.A.; Hussain, B.; Ignacimuthu, S.; Sharma, H.C. Mechanisms of Plant Defense against Insect Herbivores. *Plant Signal. Behav.* **2012**, *7*, 1306–1320. [CrossRef] [PubMed]
5. Miresmailli, S.; Isman, M.B. Botanical insecticides inspired by plant-herbivore chemical interactions. *Trends Plant Sci.* **2014**, *19*, 29–35. [CrossRef] [PubMed]
6. Isman, M.B.; Grieneisen, M.L. Botanical insecticide research: Many publications, limited useful data. *Trends Plant Sci.* **2014**, *19*, 140–145. [CrossRef] [PubMed]
7. Schrader, K.K.; Andolfi, A.; Cantrell, C.L.; Cimmino, A.; Duke, S.O.; Osbrink, W.; Wedge, D.E.; Evidente, A. A survey of phytotoxic microbial and plant metabolites as potential natural products for pest management. *Chem. Biodivers.* **2010**, *7*, 2261–2280. [CrossRef] [PubMed]
8. Cespedes, C.L.; Aqueveque, P.M.; Avila, J.G.; Alarcon, J.; Kubo, I. New advances in chemical defenses of plants: Researches in calceolariaceae. *Phytochem. Rev.* **2015**, *14*, 367–380. [CrossRef]
9. Muñoz, E.; Escalona, D.; Salazar, J.R.; Alarcon, J.; Céspedes, C.L. Insect growth regulatory effects by diterpenes from *Calceolaria talcana* Grau & Ehrhart (Calceolariaceae: Scrophulariaceae) against *Spodoptera frugiperda* and *Drosophila melanogaster*. *Ind. Crops Prod.* **2013**, *45*, 283–292. [CrossRef]
10. Muñoz, E.; Avila, J.G.; Alarcón, J.; Kubo, I.; Werner, E.; Céspedes, C.L. Tyrosinase inhibitors from *Calceolaria integrifolia* s.l.: *Calceolaria talcana* aerial parts. *J. Agric. Food Chem.* **2013**, *61*, 4336–4343. [CrossRef] [PubMed]
11. Wang, Y.; Liu, T.; Yang, Q.; Li, Z.; Qian, X. A Modeling Study for Structure Features of $\beta$-N-acetyl-D-hexosaminidase from *Ostrinia furnacalis* and its Novel Inhibitor Allosamidin: Species Selectivity and Multi-Target Characteristics. *Chem. Biol. Drug Des.* **2012**, *79*, 572–582. [CrossRef] [PubMed]
12. Speck-Planche, A.; Kleandrova, V.V.; Scotti, M.T. Fragment-based approach for the in silico discovery of multi-target insecticides. *Chemom. Intell. Lab. Syst.* **2012**, *111*, 39–45. [CrossRef]
13. Cavasotto, C.N.; Orry, A.J.W. Ligand docking and structure-based virtual screening in drug discovery. *Curr. Top. Med. Chem.* **2007**, *7*, 1006–1014. [CrossRef] [PubMed]
14. Tuccinardi, T. Docking-based virtual screening: Recent developments. *Comb. Chem. High Throughput Screen.* **2009**, *12*, 303–314. [CrossRef] [PubMed]
15. Cheng, T.; Li, Q.; Zhou, Z.; Wang, Y.; Bryant, S.H. Structure-Based Virtual Screening for Drug Discovery: A Problem-Centric Review. *AAPS J.* **2012**, *14*, 133–141. [CrossRef] [PubMed]
16. Kontoyianni, M. Docking and Virtual Screening in Drug Discovery. *Methods Mol. Biol.* **2017**, *1647*, 255–266. [PubMed]
17. Toledo Warshaviak, D.; Golan, G.; Borrelli, K.W.; Zhu, K.; Kalid, O. Structure-Based Virtual Screening Approach for Discovery of Covalently Bound Ligands. *J. Chem. Inf. Model.* **2014**, *54*, 1941–1950. [CrossRef] [PubMed]
18. Wang, L.; Gu, Q.; Zheng, X.; Ye, J.; Liu, Z.; Li, J.; Hu, X.; Hagler, A.; Xu, J. Discovery of New Selective Human Aldose Reductase Inhibitors through Virtual Screening Multiple Binding Pocket Conformations. *J. Chem. Inf. Model.* **2013**, *53*, 2409–2422. [CrossRef] [PubMed]
19. Ribeiro, F.F.; Mendonca Junior, F.J.B.; Ghasemi, J.B.; Ishiki, H.M.; Scotti, M.T.; Scotti, L. Docking of Natural Products against Neurodegenerative Diseases: General Concepts. *Comb. Chem. High Throughput Screen.* **2018**, *21*, 152–160. [CrossRef] [PubMed]
20. Saldivar-Gonzalez, F.; Gómez-García, A.; Sánchez-Cruz, N.; Ruiz-Rios, J.; Pilón-Jiménez, B.; Medina-Franco, J. Computational Approaches to Identify Natural Products as Inhibitors of DNA Methyltransferases. *Preprints* **2018**. [CrossRef]
21. Singh, P.; Bast, F. Multitargeted molecular docking study of plant-derived natural products on phosphoinositide-3 kinase pathway components. *Med. Chem. Res.* **2013**, *23*. [CrossRef]

22. Ambure, P.; Bhat, J.; Puzyn, T.; Roy, K. Identifying natural compounds as multi-target-directed ligands against Alzheimer's disease: An in silico approach. *J. Biomol. Struct. Dyn.* **2018**, *23*, 1–25. [CrossRef] [PubMed]
23. Lee, S.-H.; Ha, K.B.; Park, D.H.; Fang, Y.; Kim, J.H.; Park, M.G.; Woo, R.M.; Kim, W.J.; Park, I.-K.; Choi, J.Y.; et al. Plant-derived compounds regulate formation of the insect juvenile hormone receptor complex. *Pestic. Biochem. Physiol.* **2018**, *150*, 27–32. [CrossRef] [PubMed]
24. Jankowska, M.; Rogalska, J.; Wyszkowska, J.; Stankiewicz, M.; Jankowska, M.; Rogalska, J.; Wyszkowska, J.; Stankiewicz, M. Molecular Targets for Components of Essential Oils in the Insect Nervous System—A Review. *Molecules* **2017**, *23*, 34. [CrossRef] [PubMed]
25. Cespedes, C.L.; Muñoz, E.; Salazar, J.R.; Yamaguchi, L.; Werner, E.; Alarcon, J.; Kubo, I. Inhibition of cholinesterase activity by extracts, fractions and compounds from *Calceolaria talcana* and *C. integrifolia* (Calceolariaceae: Scrophulariaceae). *Food Chem. Toxicol.* **2013**, *62*, 919–926. [CrossRef] [PubMed]
26. Muñoz, E.; Lamilla, C.; Marin, J.C.; Alarcon, J.; Cespedes, C.L. Antifeedant, insect growth regulatory and insecticidal effects of *Calceolaria talcana* (Calceolariaceae) on *Drosophila melanogaster* and *Spodoptera frugiperda*. *Ind. Crops Prod.* **2013**, *42*, 137–144. [CrossRef]
27. Céspedes, C.L.; Salazar, J.R.; Alarcon, J. Chemistry and biological activities of *Calceolaria* spp. (Calceolariaceae: Scrophulariaceae). *Phytochem. Rev.* **2013**, *12*, 733–749. [CrossRef]
28. Thomsen, R.; Christensen, M.H. MolDock: A New Technique for High-Accuracy Molecular Docking. *J. Med. Chem.* **2006**, *49*, 3315–3321. [CrossRef] [PubMed]
29. Harel, M.; Kryger, G.; Rosenberry, T.; Mallender, W.; Lewis, T.; Fletcher, R.; Guss, J.; Silman, I.; Sussman, J.L. Three-Dimensional Structures of *Drosophila melanogaster* Acetylcholinesterase and of its Complexes with Two Potent Inhibitors. *Protein Sci.* **2000**, *9*, 1063–1072. [CrossRef] [PubMed]
30. Moras, D.; Billas, I.M.; Browning, C. Adaptability of the ecdysone receptor bound to synthetic ligands. [CrossRef]
31. Browning, C.; Martin, E.; Loch, C.; Wurtz, J.-M.; Moras, D.; Stote, R.H.; Dejaegere, A.P.; Billas, I.M.L. Critical role of desolvation in the binding of 20-hydroxyecdysone to the ecdysone receptor. *J. Biol. Chem.* **2007**, *282*, 32924–32934. [CrossRef] [PubMed]
32. Li, Y.; Wang, Y.; Jiang, H.; Deng, J. Crystal structure of *Manduca sexta* prophenoloxidase provides insights into the mechanism of type 3 copper enzymes. *Proc. Natl. Acad. Sci. USA* **2009**, *106*, 17002–17006. [CrossRef] [PubMed]
33. Cheung, J.; Rudolph, M.J.; Burshteyn, F.; Cassidy, M.S.; Gary, E.N.; Love, J.; Franklin, M.C.; Height, J.J. Structures of human acetylcholinesterase in complex with pharmacologically important ligands. *J. Med. Chem.* **2012**, *55*, 10282–10286. [CrossRef] [PubMed]
34. Cheung, J.; Gary, E.N.; Shiomi, K.; Rosenberry, T.L. Structures of Human Acetylcholinesterase Bound to Dihydrotanshinone I and Territrem B Show Peripheral Site Flexibility. *ACS Med. Chem. Lett.* **2013**, *4*, 1091–1096. [CrossRef] [PubMed]
35. Berman, H.M.; Westbrook, J.; Feng, Z.; Gilliland, G.; Bhat, T.N.; Weissig, H.; Shindyalov, I.N.; Bourne, P.E. The protein data bank. *Nucleic Acids Res.* **2000**, *28*, 235–242. [CrossRef] [PubMed]
36. Ogungbe, I.V.; Erwin, W.R.; Setzer, W.N. Antileishmanial phytochemical phenolics: Molecular docking to potential protein targets. *J. Mol. Graph. Model.* **2014**, *48*, 105–117. [CrossRef] [PubMed]
37. Loza-Mejía, M.A.; Salazar, J.R. Sterols and triterpenoids as potential anti-inflammatories: Molecular docking studies for binding to some enzymes involved in inflammatory pathways. *J. Mol. Graph. Model.* **2015**, *62*, 18–25. [CrossRef] [PubMed]
38. Krieger, E.; Vriend, G. YASARA View—Molecular graphics for all devices—From smartphones to workstations. *Bioinformatics* **2014**, *30*, 2981–2982. [CrossRef] [PubMed]
39. Yasara Dynamics. Available online: www.yasara.org (accessed on 23 October 2018).
40. Duan, Y.; Wu, C.; Chowdhury, S.; Lee, M.C.; Xiong, G.; Zhang, W.; Yang, R.; Cieplak, P.; Luo, R.; Lee, T.; et al. A point-charge force field for molecular mechanics simulations of proteins based on condensed-phase quantum mechanical calculations. *J. Comput. Chem.* **2003**, *24*, 1999–2012. [CrossRef] [PubMed]
41. Gan, R.; Zhao, L.; Sun, Q.; Tang, P.; Zhang, S.; Yang, H.; He, J.; Li, H. Binding behavior of trelagliptin and human serum albumin: Molecular docking, dynamical simulation, and multi-spectroscopy. *Spectrochim. Acta Part A Mol. Biomol. Spectrosc.* **2018**, *202*, 187–195. [CrossRef] [PubMed]

42. Ding, X.; Suo, Z.; Sun, Q.; Gan, R.; Tang, P.; Hou, Q.; Wu, D.; Li, H. Study of the interaction of broad-spectrum antimicrobial drug sitafloxacin with human serum albumin using spectroscopic methods, molecular docking, and molecular dynamics simulation. *J. Pharm. Biomed. Anal.* **2018**, *160*, 397–403. [CrossRef] [PubMed]

43. Kumar, A.; Srivastava, G.; Negi, A.S.; Sharma, A. Docking, molecular dynamics, binding energy-MM-PBSA studies of naphthofuran derivatives to identify potential dual inhibitors against BACE-1 and GSK-3β. *J. Biomol. Struct. Dyn.* **2018**, 1–16. [CrossRef] [PubMed]

44. Schwedes, C.; Tulsiani, S.; Carney, G.E. Ecdysone receptor expression and activity in adult *Drosophila melanogaster*. *J. Insect Physiol.* **2011**, *57*, 899–907. [CrossRef] [PubMed]

45. Li, Z.; Lazaridis, T. The Effect of Water Displacement on Binding Thermodynamics: Concanavalin A. *J. Phys. Chem. B* **2005**, *109*, 662–670. [CrossRef] [PubMed]

46. Whitehill, J.; Rigsby, C.; Cipollini, D.; Herms, D.A.; Bonello, P. Decreased emergence of emerald ash borer from ash treated with methyl jasmonate is associated with induction of general defense traits and the toxic phenolic compound verbascoside. *Oecologia* **2014**, *176*, 1047–1059. [CrossRef] [PubMed]

47. Harmatha, J.; Dinan, L. Biological activities of lignans and stilbenoids associated with plant-insect chemical interactions. *Phytochem. Rev.* **2003**, *2*, 321–330. [CrossRef]

48. Dinan, L.; Hormann, R.E. *Comprehensive Molecular Insect Science*; Elsevier: Amsterdam, The Netherlands, 2005; ISBN 9780444519245.

49. Jiang, H.; Wang, Y.; Kanost, M.R. Pro-phenol oxidase activating proteinase from an insect, *Manduca sexta*: A bacteria-inducible protein similar to *Drosophila* easter. *Proc. Natl. Acad. Sci. USA* **1998**, *95*, 12220–12225. [CrossRef] [PubMed]

50. Sugumaran, M.; Barek, H. Critical Analysis of the Melanogenic Pathway in Insects and Higher Animals. *Int. J. Mol. Sci.* **2016**, *17*, 1–24. [CrossRef] [PubMed]

51. Aloui, S.; Raboudi, F.; Ghazouani, T.; Salghi, R.; Hamdaoui, M.H.; Fattouch, S. Use of molecular and in silico bioinformatic tools to investigate pesticide binding to insect (Lepidoptera) phenoloxidases (PO): Insights to toxicological aspects. *J. Environ. Sci. Health B* **2014**, *49*, 654–660. [CrossRef] [PubMed]

52. Kanteev, M.; Goldfeder, M.; Fishman, A. Structure–function correlations in tyrosinases. *Protein Sci.* **2015**, *24*, 1360–1369. [CrossRef] [PubMed]

53. Karioti, A.; Protopappa, A.; Megoulas, N.; Skaltsa, H. Identification of tyrosinase inhibitors from *Marrubium velutinum* and *Marrubium cylleneum*. *Bioorg. Med. Chem.* **2007**, *15*, 2708–2714. [CrossRef] [PubMed]

54. Yoshimori, A.; Oyama, T.; Takahashi, S.; Abe, H.; Kamiya, T.; Abe, T.; Tanuma, S.I. Structure-activity relationships of the thujaplicins for inhibition of human tyrosinase. *Bioorg. Med. Chem.* **2014**, *22*, 6193–6200. [CrossRef] [PubMed]

55. Tan, X.; Song, Y.H.; Park, C.; Lee, K.W.; Kim, J.Y.; Kim, D.W.; Kim, K.D.; Lee, K.W.; Curtis-Long, M.J.; Park, K.H. Highly potent tyrosinase inhibitor, neorauflavane from *Campylotropis hirtella* and inhibitory mechanism with molecular docking. *Bioorg. Med. Chem.* **2016**, *24*, 153–159. [CrossRef] [PubMed]

56. Houghton, P.J.; Ren, Y.; Howes, M.-J. Acetylcholinesterase inhibitors from plants and fungi. *Nat. Prod. Rep.* **2006**, *23*, 181–199. [CrossRef] [PubMed]

57. Thapa, S.L.; Xu, H. Acetylcholinesterase: A Primary Target for Drugs and Insecticides. *Mini Rev. Med. Chem.* **2017**, *17*, 1665–1676. [CrossRef] [PubMed]

58. Kobayashi, H.; Suzuki, T.; Akahori, F.; Satoh, T. Acetylcholinesterase and Acetylcholine Receptors: Brain Regional Heterogeneity. *Anticholinesterase Pestic. Metab. Neurotox. Epidemiol.* **2011**, 3–18. [CrossRef]

59. Pang, Y.; Brimijoin, S.; Ragsdale, D.W.; Zhu, K.Y.; Suranyi, R.; Gormley, M.; Company, K. Novel and Viable Acetylcholinesterase Target Site for Developing Effective and Environmentally Safe Insecticides. *Curr. Drug Targets* **2012**, *13*, 471–482. [CrossRef] [PubMed]

60. Wiesner, J.; Kříž, Z.; Kuča, K.; Jun, D.; Koča, J. Acetylcholinesterases—The structural similarities and differences. *J. Enzyme Inhib. Med. Chem.* **2007**, *22*, 417–424. [CrossRef] [PubMed]

61. Katselou, M.G.; Matralis, A.N.; Kourounakis, A.P. Multi-target drug design approaches for multifactorial diseases: From neurodegenerative to cardiovascular applications. *Curr. Med. Chem.* **2014**, *21*, 2743–2787. [CrossRef] [PubMed]

62. Lu, J.J.; Pan, W.; Hu, Y.J.; Wang, Y.T. Multi-target drugs: The trend of drug research and development. *PLoS ONE* **2012**, *7*, 1–9. [CrossRef] [PubMed]

63. Lavecchia, A.; Cerchia, C. In silico methods to address polypharmacology: Current status, applications and future perspectives. *Drug Discov. Today* **2016**, *21*, 288–298. [CrossRef] [PubMed]

64. Prado-Prado, F.; García-Mera, X.; Abeijón, P.; Alonso, N.; Caamaño, O.; Yáñez, M.; Gárate, T.; Mezo, M.; González-Warleta, M.; Muiño, L.; et al. Using entropy of drug and protein graphs to predict FDA drug-target network: Theoretic-experimental study of MAO inhibitors and hemoglobin peptides from *Fasciola hepatica*. *Eur. J. Med. Chem.* **2011**, *46*, 1074–1094. [CrossRef] [PubMed]

65. Prado-Prado, F.J.; García, I.; García-Mera, X.; González-Díaz, H. Entropy multi-target QSAR model for prediction of antiviral drug complex networks. *Chemom. Intell. Lab. Syst.* **2011**, *107*, 227–233. [CrossRef]

66. Speck-Planche, A.; Kleandrova, V.; Scotti, M.; Cordeiro, M. 3D-QSAR Methodologies and Molecular Modeling in Bioinformatics for the Search of Novel Anti-HIV Therapies: Rational Design of Entry Inhibitors. *Curr. Bioinform.* **2013**, *8*, 452–464. [CrossRef]

67. Speck-Planche, A.; Kleandrova, V.; Luan, F.; Natalia, D.S.; Cordeiro, M. Multi-Target Inhibitors for Proteins Associated with Alzheimer: In Silico Discovery using Fragment-Based Descriptors. *Curr. Alzheimer Res.* **2013**, *10*, 117–124. [CrossRef] [PubMed]

68. Lackey, K.E. The Discovery of Lapatinib. In *Designing Multi-Target Drugs*; Morphy, J.R., Harris, J.C., Eds.; Royal Society of Chemistry: Cambridge, UK, 2012; pp. 181–205.

69. Alipieva, K.; Korkina, L.; Orhan, I.E.; Georgiev, M.I. Verbascoside—A review of its occurrence, (bio)synthesis and pharmacological significance. *Biotechnol. Adv.* **2014**, *32*, 1065–1076. [CrossRef] [PubMed]

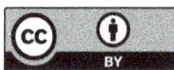

*biomolecules*

MDPI

*Article*

# BIOFACQUIM: A Mexican Compound Database of Natural Products

B. Angélica Pilón-Jiménez, Fernanda I. Saldívar-González, Bárbara I. Díaz-Eufracio and José L. Medina-Franco *

Department of Pharmacy, National Autonomous University of Mexico, Mexico City 04510, Mexico; angiepilon96@gmail.com (B.A.P.-J.); felilang12@gmail.com (F.I.S.-G.); debi_1223@hotmail.com (B.I.D.-E.)
* Correspondence: medinajl@unam.mx; Tel.: +5255-5622 3899

Received: 29 November 2018; Accepted: 15 January 2019; Published: 17 January 2019

**Abstract:** Compound databases of natural products have a major impact on drug discovery projects and other areas of research. The number of databases in the public domain with compounds with natural origins is increasing. Several countries, Brazil, France, Panama and, recently, Vietnam, have initiatives in place to construct and maintain compound databases that are representative of their diversity. In this proof-of-concept study, we discuss the first version of BIOFACQUIM, a novel compound database with natural products isolated and characterized in Mexico. We discuss its construction, curation, and a complete chemoinformatic characterization of the content and coverage in chemical space. The profile of physicochemical properties, scaffold content, and diversity, as well as structural diversity based on molecular fingerprints is reported. BIOFACQUIM is available for free.

**Keywords:** chemical space; chemical data set; chemoinformatics; consensus diversity plot; drug discovery; molecular diversity; visualization

---

## 1. Introduction

The significance of compound databases in drug discovery projects is continuously increasing. In fact, compound databases and chemical data sets are a centerpiece in pharmaceutical companies and other academic and government research centers [1]. In addition to their role in compound databases, natural products have been a major resource in drug discovery [2,3]. As reviewed elsewhere, there are several drugs recently approved for clinical use that are natural products or synthetic analogues of hit compounds initially identified from natural sources. A notable example is the fungi metabolite migalastat (Galafold®), approved in 2018 for the treatment of the Fabry disease [4]. Not unsurprisingly, natural product-based drug discovery is being coupled with other major drug discovery strategies such as high-throughput screening and virtual screening. Natural products are again gaining attention in the scientific community to address novel and/or difficult molecular endpoints, for instance, epigenetic targets [5,6].

Several compound databases of natural products have been constructed, curated and often maintained by academic and other not-for-profit research groups. Notable examples are the Universal Natural Product Database (UNPD) [7] and the Traditional Chinese Medicine (TCM) Database@Taiwan [8]. Of note, UNPD is no longer available online but represents the efforts of an academic group to assemble a large natural product database. Reference [4] confirms that there are other compound databases that collect natural products from specific geographical areas and countries, such as NuBBE_DB for natural products from Brazil [9] VIETHERB: A Database for Vietnamese Herbal Species was recently released to the public [10]. Other databases of natural products are discussed elsewhere [11–13]. Despite the fact that Mexico also has high levels of biodiversity, there are limited efforts to assemble a compound database of natural products. One example is UNIQUIM, recently reviewed by Medina-Franco [11].

The objective of this work is to introduce BIOFACQUIM as one of the first compound databases of natural products isolated and characterized in Mexico. In this proof-of-concept study, we discuss the assembly of the first version of this chemical data set along with a chemoinformatic characterization of molecular diversity, scaffold content and coverage in chemical space. The compound database is freely available via the web-interface BIOFACQUIM Explorer (https://biofacquim.herokuapp.com/), and is part of an initial effort towards building, updating and maintaining a compound database representative of the biodiversity of Mexico. Compounds in BIOFACQUIM are also available from ZINC15 at http://zinc15.docking.org/catalogs/biofacquimnp/

## 2. Materials and Methods

### 2.1. BIOFACQUIM Database

The database of natural products was assembled from a literature search. For the construction of the first version of BIOFACQUIM, the Scopus database (www.scopus.com) was searched using the keywords "natural products" and "School of Chemistry of the National Autonomous University of Mexico (FQ, UNAM)". This search led to a list of scientific papers and researchers that work with natural products. The eight journals that had contributed the most thus far were selected: *Journal of Ethnopharmacology*, *Natural Products Research*, *Journal of Agricultural and Food Chemistry*, *Journal of Natural Products*, *Planta Medica*, *Phytochemistry*, *Natural Product Letters*, and *Molecules*. As part of the search, three filters were used for the selection of the articles in each journal. The first filter was the search by institution (FQ, UNAM), the second was the search by publication year (2000–2018), and the last was the detailed analysis of the articles to identify if the procedure for the isolation, purification and characterization of the compounds from natural products was present. We want to emphasize that this is the first version of BIOFACQUIM; future versions will have natural products from more years, more peer-reviewed journals and more institutions, to achieve a database representative of the biodiversity of Mexico.

With the module 'Wash', from the molecular operating environment (MOE) program version 2018 [14], the database was curated. This was done to normalize and collect the most relevant information from the molecules. The data curation involved the elimination of salts, the adjustment of the protonation states, the optimization of the geometry by energy minimization and the elimination of the duplicated molecules. The default settings of the 'Wash' module were used.

### 2.2. Reference Data Sets

In order to characterize the diversity of BIOFACQUIM and to explore its coverage in chemical space, seven compound databases of broad interest in drug discovery were used as references. The structure files used in this work were taken from previous comparisons and chemoinformatic analyses of natural products [15]. The structures of the reference compounds were curated using the same procedure described to prepare BIOFACQUIM. Table 1 summarizes the reference databases and the number of compounds. Of note, the reference collections include seven data sets of natural products.

**Table 1.** Reference databases [15] compared for BIOFACQUIM.

| Database | Size [a] |
|---|---|
| Approved drugs | 1806 |
| Cyanobacteria metabolites | 473 |
| Fungi metabolites | 206 |
| Marine | 6253 |
| MEGx | 4103 |

**Table 1.** *Cont.*

| Database | Size [a] |
|---|---|
| Semi-synthetics (NATx) | 26,318 |
| NuBBE$_{DB}$ | 2214 |

[a] Number unique compounds after data curation.

*2.3. Molecular Properties of Pharmaceutical Relevance*

The curated BIOFACQUIM database was characterized by calculating six physicochemical properties of therapeutic interest, namely: molecular weight (MW), octanol/water partition coefficient (SlogP), topological surface area (TPSA), number of rotatable bonds (RB), number of H-bond donor atoms (HBD) and number of H-bond acceptor atoms (HBA). The statistical analysis was done, with the program DataWarrior [16], by calculating the mean, median and standard deviation of the calculated properties. Based on these statistics BIOFACQUIM was further compared with other natural products databases (NuBBE$_{DB}$, cyanobacteria, fungi, marine, and MEGx), approved drugs, and semisynthetic compounds (NATx) (Table 1).

*2.4. Scaffold Content*

Scaffold content analysis enabled us to identify the most frequent scaffolds in compound data sets and, in this work, to compare the scaffolds containing approved drugs with those containing natural products. The scaffold content analyses also enabled us to identify potential novel scaffolds. The most frequent core molecular scaffolds of BIOFACQUIM were computed using the definition described by Bemis and Murcko [17], in which the core scaffold is obtained by systematically removing the side chains of the compounds. The most frequent scaffolds in BIOFACQUIM were compared with data from the literature (vide infra).

*2.5. Visual Representation of Chemical Space*

In order to generate a visual representation of the chemical space of BIOFACQUIM, two visualization methods were used: principal component analysis (PCA) and *t*-distributed stochastic neighbor embedding (*t*-SNE). PCA reduces data dimensions by geometrically projecting them onto lower dimensions called principal components (PCs). The first PC is chosen to minimize the total distance between the data and its projection on the PC and to maximize the variance of the projected points.

*t*-SNE is a nonlinear dimension reduction in which Gaussian probability distributions over high-dimensional space are constructed and used to optimize a Student *t*-distribution in low-dimensional space. The low-dimensional space maintains the pairwise similarity to the high-dimensional space, leading to a clustering on the embedding space without any significant loss of structural information. Further details of each visualization method of the chemical space are discussed elsewhere [18,19]. In this work, for *t*-SNE, subsets of compounds were retrieved from large reference data sets (Table 1), namely: 40 % of the Marine, MEGx, and NuBBE$_{DB}$ data sets (2501, 1641, and 886 compounds, respectively). For NATx and approved drugs, 1000 molecules were used. For cyanobacteria metabolites and fungi data sets the entire databases were employed (473 and 206 compounds, respectively).

*2.6. Global Diversity: Consensus Diversity Analysis*

Since the chemical diversity strongly depends on the structure representation, it is practical to consider multiple representations for a complete, global assessment. To this end, consensus diversity (CD) plots have been proposed as simple two-dimensional graphs that enable the comparison of the diversity of compound data sets using four sets of structural representations [20]; these are typically the molecular fingerprints, scaffolds, molecular properties, and number of compounds. CD plots have been used to compare the diversity of natural products and other compound data sets [21]. Briefly, in a typical CD plot the scaffold and fingerprint diversity are represented along the *y*- and *x*-axes, respectively. The diversity based on whole molecular properties of pharmaceutical interest is represented by a continuous color scale and the number of compounds is mapped into the plot using different size data points. Further details are provided elsewhere [20]. To generate the CD plot of this work, for the *y*-axis we used the area under the cyclic system recovery curve [22]. For the *x*-axis, we employed the median of the fingerprint-based diversity computed with MACCS keys (166-bits) and the Tanimoto coefficient. Both are established and are representative metrics of the scaffold and fingerprint-based diversity. Subsets of the compounds were retrieved from large reference data sets (Table 1), considering the size of the databases. For NATx, Marine, MEGx, NuBBE$_{DB}$ and approved drugs, 2000, 1500, 1000, 800 and 700 molecules, respectively, were used. For cyanobacteria metabolites and fungi data sets, the entire databases were employed (473 and 206 compounds, respectively).

## 3. Results and Discussion

First, we present the results of the construction of the first proof-of-concept version of the BIOFACQUIM database followed by a first chemoinformatic characterization in terms of physicochemical properties, scaffold content, diversity and coverage in chemical space.

### 3.1. BIOFACQUIM Database

As described in the Materials and Methods section, after the first survey in Scopus with the researchers of the FQ, UNAM, three filters were applied to the eight selected journals. Each of the 92 scientific papers selected was analyzed individually to extract information about the natural products. Of note, in this manuscript we disclose the first version of BIOFACQUIM as a proof-of-concept collection in which current content may be biased by the type of compounds published by a research group (e.g., based on their expertise and/or the analytical techniques available to their groups) and the type of compounds and characteristics accepted for publication by a given journal (e.g., compounds with the biological activity of compounds with drug-like features). It is anticipated that these biases will be reduced as the content of BIOFACQUIM is updated in future releases, by increasing the number of research groups, number of journals and number of years covered (cf. the Conclusions section).

The current version of BIOFACQUIM contains the following information: identification number (ID), compound name, simplified molecular input line entry system (SMILES), reference (with the name of the journal, digital object identifier (DOI) number and publication year), kingdom (Plantae or Fungi), genus, species, and geographical location of the collection of the natural product. In addition, the biological activity, if it was reported in the publication, has been included. The current and first version of BIOFACQUIM has 423 compounds. It should be noted that 316 compounds were isolated from 49 different plant genera, 98 were isolated from 19 genera of fungi, and nine compounds were isolated from Mexican propolis (a sticky dark-colored hive product collected by bees from living plant sources). Figure 1 shows the distribution of compounds per year reported since the year 2000, as contained in the first version of the chemical data set. The compounds in the database that were published in 2018 are not included in Figure 1.

Figure 2 shows the chemical structures of representative compounds from the first version of BIOFACQUIM (discussed further below).

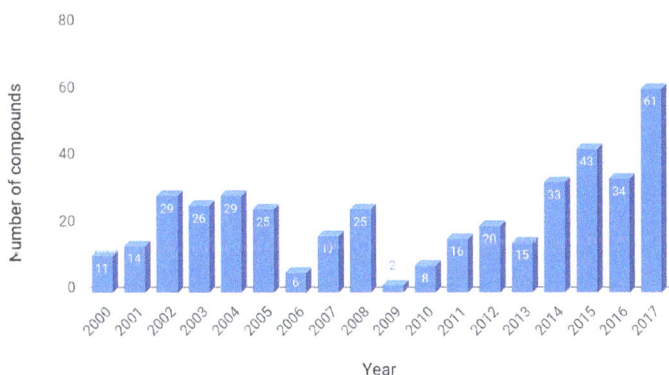

**Figure 1.** Distribution of compounds reported from 2000 to 2017, as contained in the first version of BIOFACQUIM. Compounds published in 2018 are not shown in this graph.

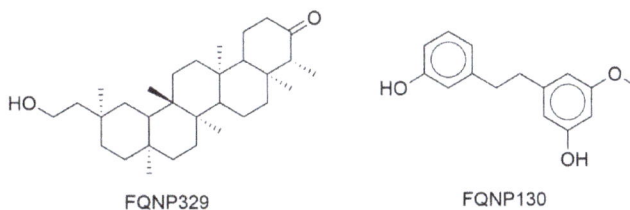

FQNP329                    FQNP130

**Figure 2.** Select compounds contained in BIOFACQUIM.

*3.2. Molecular Properties*

Figure 3 shows box plots of the distribution of the six calculated physicochemical properties (vide supra) calculated for BIOFACQUIM. For comparative purposes, the box plots also include the distribution of the same properties of the seven reference data sets that were retrieved from the literature [15]. The corresponding violin plots are shown in the Supplementary Figure S3. The three main molecular properties, size, flexibility, and molecular polarity, are described by MW, RB, and SlogP, TPSA, HBA, and HBD, respectively. In these plots, the boxes enclose the data points with values within the first and third quartile; the line that divides the box denotes the median of the distributions. The lines above and below indicate the upper and lower adjacent values. The red asterisks indicate the data points with values beyond the upper and lower adjacent values. Summary statistics are presented at the bottom of the box plots. The figure also includes a table below each box plot with the maximum, median, mean, standard deviation and minimum values for each property and each data set.

According to Figure 3 (and the violin plots in the Supplementary Material), based on the mean of RB, BIOFACQUIM compounds have comparable flexibility to approved drugs. The figure also shows that, except for cyanobacteria metabolites, all databases have a median of up to five rotatable bonds (including approved drugs). The median and mean MW of BIOFACQUIM are 340.5 and 412 g/mol, respectively. Notably, BIOFACQUIM and NuBBE_DB have the most similar MW profile compared to drugs. BIOFACQUIM has a median of 4 HBA, the same as that of the NuBBE_DB and Marine data sets. Furthermore, BIOFACQUIM has a very similar profile of HBA compared to MEGx. Comparing HBD, BIOFACQUIM, NuBBE_DB, NATx, and cyanobacteria have the same median values, with similar profiles to approved drugs and higher standard deviations than approved drugs. Regarding TPSA, the compounds in BIOFACQUIM are those that share the closest values to the approved drugs. It should be noted that the cyanobacteria metabolite set has the largest distribution and the highest mean values of TPSA, being the double of the mean of the approved drugs. The distribution of the SlogP values indicates that, overall, natural products are slightly more hydrophobic than approved drugs.

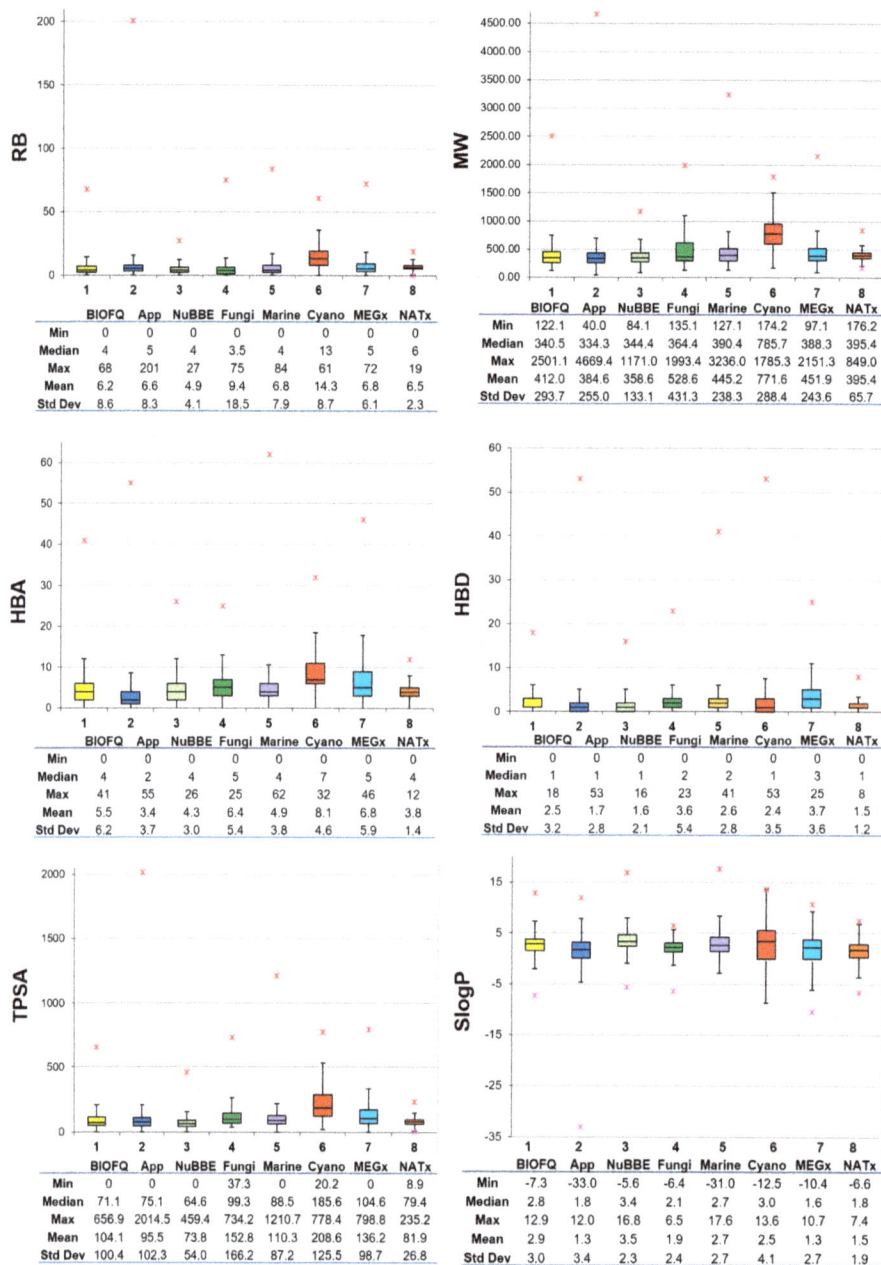

**Figure 3.** Box plots for the physicochemical properties of BIOFACQUIM (BIOFQ) and reference data sets (Table 1). The boxes enclose data points with values within the first and third quartile. The red asterisks indicate outliers. Summary statistics are included below each plot. RB: number of rotatable bonds; MW: molecular weight; HBA: number of H-bond acceptor atoms; HBD: number of H-bond donor atoms; TPSA: topological surface area; SlogP: octanol/water partition coefficient.

Taking together the results of the general profile of the properties, it can be concluded that the current version of BIOFACQUIM is, in general, most similar to the NuBBE$_{DB}$ and Fungi data sets. This outcome is in agreement with the findings that, while assembling BIOFACQUIM and analyzing the source papers in detail, the compounds were mostly isolated from plants and fungi.

### 3.3. Scaffold Content

Figure 4 shows the 27 most populated molecular scaffolds in BIOFACQUIM that included half (50.6 %) of the 423 compounds making up the database. Aside from benzene which is also frequent in several other compound databases [21], the second most frequent scaffold was a flavan-related scaffold (5 %), followed by 1,3-benzodioxole and dibenzyl core scaffolds (2.4 %). Interestingly, the last three frequent scaffolds in BIOFACQUIM are not the most frequent in other databases of natural products [15].

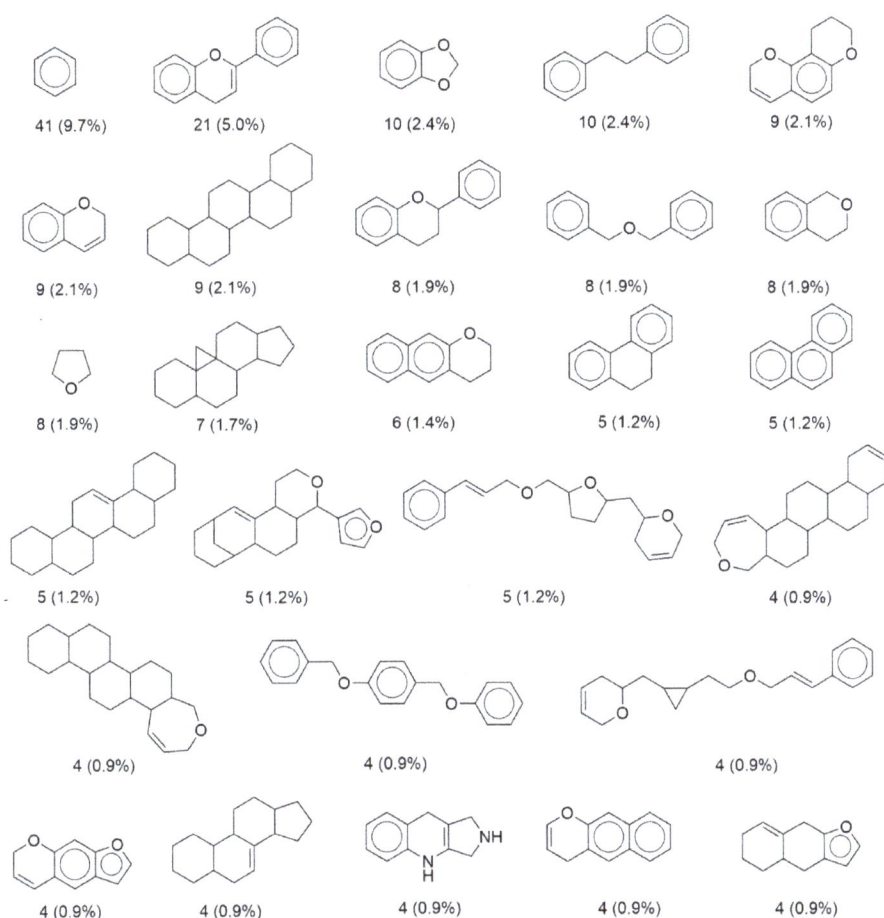

| 41 (9.7%) | 21 (5.0%) | 10 (2.4%) | 10 (2.4%) | 9 (2.1%) |
| 9 (2.1%) | 9 (2.1%) | 8 (1.9%) | 8 (1.9%) | 8 (1.9%) |
| 8 (1.9%) | 7 (1.7%) | 6 (1.4%) | 5 (1.2%) | 5 (1.2%) |
| 5 (1.2%) | 5 (1.2%) | 5 (1.2%) | | 4 (0.9%) |
| 4 (0.9%) | 4 (0.9%) | | 4 (0.9%) | |
| 4 (0.9%) | 4 (0.9%) | 4 (0.9%) | 4 (0.9%) | 4 (0.9%) |

**Figure 4.** Most frequent scaffolds in BIOFACQUIM. The frequency and percentage are shown. The 27 scaffolds shown in the figure contain half of the total compounds in the database (50.6%).

### 3.4. Chemical Space

As explained in the Materials and Methods section, a visual analysis of the chemical space of BIOFACQUIM was done with two visualization methods, PCA and *t*-SNE. The visual representation with PCA was based on the physicochemical properties while the visualization with *t*-SNE was based on the molecular topological fingerprints.

### 3.4.1. Visual Representation Based on Properties

Using the program KNIME [23], we did a visual comparison of the chemical space of BIOFACQUIM and the reference databases. We used the "Normalizer" node in KNIME which gives a linear transformation of all values, the minimum and maximum of each database. Then, PCA was applied to reduce the dimensionality of the six calculated physicochemical properties and to compare BIOFACQUIM with the reference collections (vide supra, Table 1).

Figure 5 shows a visual representation of the property-based chemical space. Table S1 in the Supplementary Material summarizes the corresponding loadings and eigenvalues for the first three PCs. The first two PCs capture 84% of the variance while the first three recover 92% of the variance. Table S1 shows that for the first PC, the larger loadings corresponded to SlogP, followed by RB, whereas for the second PC the largest loading corresponded to HBD.

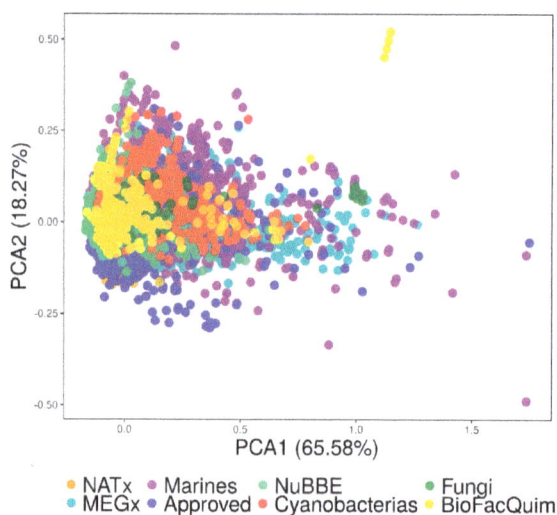

**Figure 5.** Visual representation of the chemical space based on the physicochemical properties of eight data sets. BIOFACQUIM (423 compounds, yellow); fungi metabolites (206 compounds, green); cyanobacteria metabolites (473 compounds, red); NuBBE$_{DB}$ (2214 compounds, light green); NATx (26318 compounds, orange); MEGx (4103 compounds, blue); marine metabolites (6253 compounds, lilac); US Food and Drug Administration (FDA)-approved drugs (1806 compounds, dark blue).

The visual representation of the chemical space in Figure 5 indicates that some of the natural product compounds occupy the same space as the already approved drugs. It also shows that there are molecules in BIOFACQUIM and the Marine set that cover neglected regions of the currently drug-like chemical space. Finally, Figure 5 suggests that BIOFACQUIM shares the chemical space of almost all Fungi and NuBBE$_{DB}$.

### 3.4.2. Visual Representation Based on Molecular Fingerprints

Figure 6 shows a visual representation of the chemical space of the current version of BIOFACQUIM based on topological fingerprints using *t*-SNE (see Materials and Methods). Figure 6a compares BIOFACQUIM with all other reference data sets. Figure 6b shows a comparison of BIOFACQUIM with approved drugs. Figure 6a shows three main groups or clusters in which all the databases have compounds. The clusters indicate that the visualization method and the fingerprints can distinguish three major core structures that would have detailed variations in the structure. Figure 6b indicates that there are compounds in BIOFACQUIM with high structural similarity to approved drugs. Notable examples are the compounds FQNP329 (chemical structure in Figure 2), similar to ethinylestradiol (App_75), and FQNP130, similar to choline (App_878). Other comparisons with *t*-SNE are shown in Figure S3 in the Supplementary Material.

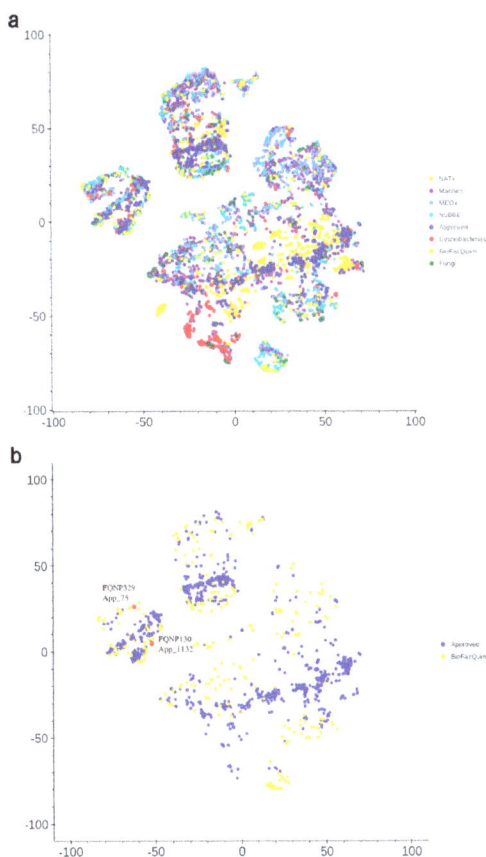

**Figure 6.** Visual representation of the chemical space of BIOFACQUIM compared with: (**a**) all reference data sets; and (**b**) approved drugs. The visualization was generated using *t*-distributed stochastic neighbor embedding (*t*-SNE) based on topological fingerprints. The red dots indicate the position of two representative compounds of BIOFACQUIM that are very similar to approved drugs.

Based on the assessment of the chemical space, in particular the position of BIOFACQUIM relative to other reference libraries in chemical space, it can be concluded that the compounds in BIOFACQUIM are very similar to drugs, based on their physicochemical properties (PCA) and structural fingerprints (*t*-SNE). Therefore, the chemical space analysis further supports the use of BIOFACQUIM in drug discovery projects.

*3.5. Global Diversity: Consensus Diversity Analysis*

As elaborated in the Materials and Methods section, a CD plot was used to compare the diversity of BIOFACQUIM with the diversity of the reference data sets, based on molecular fingerprints, scaffolds, and whole (physicochemical) properties. Figure 7 shows the CD plot, representing the

MACCS keys/Tanimoto similarity on the *x*-axis. Here, lower values indicate larger fingerprint-based diversity (further details of the fingerprint-based diversity assessment are presented in Figure S1 in the Supplementary Material). The *y*-axis of the CD plot represents the scaffold diversity where lower values (the area under the scaffold recovery curve—see Table S2 in the Supplementary Material) indicate higher scaffold diversity. The property-based diversity of BIOFACQUIM and each database was calculated as the Euclidean distance of the scaled properties. The values are represented on the color CD plot with data points on a continuous color scale. The darker color represents lower diversity while lighter colors represent higher diversity. Finally, the relative size of the databases is represented with different point sizes, where smaller data points indicate data sets with less number of molecules. The CD plot in Figure 7 shows that BIOFACQUIM and Cyanobacteria are found in the area representing low diversity of both scaffold and fingerprints. This may be attributed to the fact that this is the first version of the database. Regarding the diversity, based on physicochemical properties, the cyanobacteria metabolites were observed to have more diversity (e.g., lighter blue data point in Figure 7) than BIOFACQUIM. This is consistent with the analysis of the box plots discussed in Section 3.2. Figure 7 also indicates that approved drugs have high scaffold and fingerprint diversity that is consistent with previous reports [20,21].

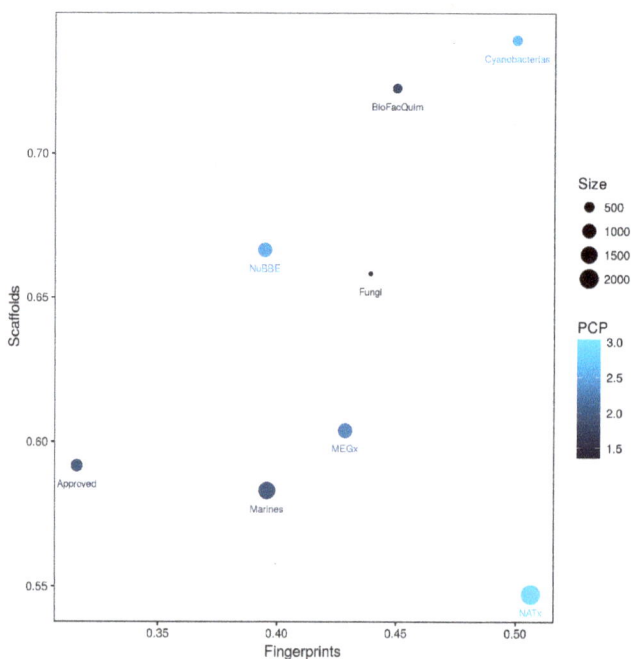

**Figure 7.** Consensus Diversity Plot comparing the global diversity of BIOFACQUIM with other natural product databases. The structural diversity (fingerprint diversity), calculated with the median Tanimoto coefficient of MACCS keys fingerprints, is plotted on the *x*-axis. The scaffold diversity of each database was defined as the area under the curve (AUC) of the respective scaffold recovery curves and is represented on the *y*-axis. The diversity, based on physicochemical properties (PCP), was calculated with the Euclidean distance of six scaled properties (SlogP, TPSA, MW, RB, HBD and HBA) and is shown on a color scale. The distance is represented with a continuous color scale from light blue (more diverse) to dark blue (less diverse). The relative size of the data set is represented with the size of the data point, smaller data points indicate compound data sets with fewer molecules.

## 4. Conclusions

BIOFACQUIM is a compound database of natural products from Mexico being constructed, curated and maintained by an academic group. The first and current version of BIOFACQUIM includes 423 compounds reported over the past 10 years at the School of Chemistry of the National Autonomous University of Mexico (UNAM). The compound database contains the chemical name, SMILES notation, reference (with name of the journal, year of publication and DOI number), kingdom (Plantae or Fungi), genus and species of the natural product, and geographical location of the collection. In addition, the biological activity, if it was reported in the publication, was included. The chemoinformatic characterization and analysis of the coverage and diversity of BIOFACQUIM in chemical space suggest broad coverage, overlapping with regions in the drug-like chemical space. The analysis also indicated that there are compounds in BIOFACQUIM with chemical structures very similar to drugs approved for clinical use that could, based on the similarity principle, be of pharmaceutical interest. Similar to other natural product databases, BIOFACQUIM can be used, via virtual screening, to identify potential lead compounds or starting points for additional optimization. The database is freely accessible through the website BIOFACQUIM Explorer, version 1.0 (https://biofacquim.herokuapp.com) and is part of the initiative D-TOOLS, described in detail elsewhere [24]. Compounds in BIOFACQUIM are also available from ZINC15 at http://zinc15.docking.org/catalogs/biofacquimnp/

One of the major objectives of this work, currently in progress, is to augment the size of BIOFACQUIM by expanding the search to other universities and research centers in Mexico, increasing the number of years and the number of scientific international peer-reviewed journals covered (with DOI number available). A second major objective of this work is to continue improving and maintaining the web-based interface BIOFACQUIM Explorer following general guidelines for the development and maintenance of public biological databases [25].

**Supplementary Materials:** The following are available online at http://www.mdpi.com/2218-273X/9/1/31/s1. Table S1. Loadings for the first three principal components of the property space of eight databases. Table S2. Statistics of the cyclic system recovery curves for BIOFACQUIM and the reference data sets. Figure S1. Distribution of the pairwise similarity values calculated for BIOFACQUIM and the reference data sets computed with MACCS keys (166-bits) and the Tanimoto coefficient. Figure S2. Visual representation of the chemical space of BIOFACQUIM generated with *t*-SNE. Figure S3. Violin plots for the physicochemical properties of BIOFACQUIM and reference data sets.

**Author Contributions:** Conceptualization, B.A.P.-J., F.I.S.-G., and J.L.M.-F.; methodology, B.A.P.-J., F.I.S.-G., and B.I.D.-E., formal analysis, B.A.P.-J. and B.I.D.-E.; writing and editing, B.A.P.-J. and J.L.M.-F.; funding acquisition, J.L.M.-F.

**Funding:** This research was supported by the Programa de Apoyo a la Investigación y el Posgrado (PAIP) grant 5000-9163, Facultad de Química, UNAM, and project PAPIME (DGAPA, UNAM) PE200118.

**Acknowledgments:** B.A.P.-J. is grateful for the support given by the subprogram 127 "Basic Training in Research" of the School of Chemistry, UNAM. F.I.S.-G. and B.I.D.-E. are thankful to Consejo Nacional de Ciencia y Tecnología, Mexico (CONACyT) for scholarships, numbers 629458 and 620289, respectively. Discussions with Oscar Palomino-Hernández to implement *t*-SNE are acknowledged. We also thank John Irwin and Khanh Tang for adding BIOFACQUIM in the database ZINC15.

**Conflicts of Interest:** The authors declare no conflicts of interest.

## References

1.  Miller, M.A. Chemical database techniques in drug discovery. *Nat. Rev. Drug Discov.* **2002**, *1*, 220–227. [CrossRef] [PubMed]
2.  Newman, D.J. From natural products to drugs. *Phys. Sci. Rev.* **2018**. [CrossRef]
3.  Newman, D.J.; Cragg, G.M. Natural products as sources of new drugs from 1981 to 2014. *J. Nat. Prod.* **2016**, *79*, 629–661. [CrossRef] [PubMed]
4.  Saldívar-González, F.I.; Pilón-Jiménez, B.A.; Medina-Franco, J.L. Chemical space of naturally occurring compounds. *Phys. Sci. Rev.* **2018**. [CrossRef]

5. Saldívar-González, F.I.; Gómez-García, A.; Chávez-Ponce de León, D.E.; Sánchez-Cruz, N.; Ruiz-Rios, J.; Pilón-Jiménez, B.A.; Medina-Franco, J.L. Inhibitors of DNA methyltransferases from natural sources: A computational perspective. *Front. Pharmacol.* **2018**, *9*, 1144. [CrossRef] [PubMed]
6. Thomford, N.; Senthebane, D.; Rowe, A.; Munro, D.; Seele, P.; Maroyi, A.; Dzobo, K. Natural products for drug discovery in the 21st century: Innovations for novel drug discovery. *Int. J. Mol. Sci.* **2018**, *19*, 1578. [CrossRef] [PubMed]
7. Gu, J.; Gui, Y.; Chen, L.; Yuan, G.; Lu, H.-Z.; Xu, X. Use of natural products as chemical library for drug discovery and network pharmacology. *PLoS ONE* **2013**, *8*, e62839. [CrossRef]
8. Chen, C.Y.-C. TCM database@Taiwan: The world's largest traditional chinese medicine database for drug screening in silico. *PLoS ONE* **2011**, *6*, e15939. [CrossRef]
9. Pilon, A.C.; Valli, M.; Dametto, A.C.; Pinto, M.E.F.; Freire, R.T.; Castro-Gamboa, I.; Andricopulo, A.D.; Bolzani, V.S. NuBBE$_{DB}$: An updated database to uncover chemical and biological information from brazilian biodiversity. *Sci Rep* **2017**, *7*, 7215. [CrossRef]
10. Nguyen-Vo, T.-H.; Le, T.Q.M.; Pham, D.T.; Nguyen, T.D.; Le, P.H.; Nguyen, A.D.T.; Nguyen, T.D.; Nguyen, T.-N.N.; Nguyen, V.A.; Do, H.T.; et al. VIETHERB: A database for vietnamese herbal species. *J. Chem. Inf. Model.* **2018**. [CrossRef]
11. Medina-Franco, J.L. Discovery and development of lead compounds from natural sources using computational approaches. In *Evidence-Based Validation of Herbal Medicine*; Mukherjee, P., Ed.; Elsevier: Amsterdam, The Netherlands, 2015; pp. 455–475.
12. Tung, C.-W. Public databases of plant natural products for computational drug discovery. *Curr. Comput. Aided Drug Des.* **2014**, *10*, 191–196. [CrossRef] [PubMed]
13. Chen, Y.; Garcia de Lomana, M.; Friedrich, N.-O.; Kirchmair, J. Characterization of the chemical space of known and readily obtainable natural products. *J. Chem. Inf. Model.* **2018**, *58*, 1518–1532. [CrossRef] [PubMed]
14. *Molecular Operating Environment (MOE)*, version 2018.08; Chemical Computing Group Inc.: Montreal, QC, Canada, 2018; Available online: http://www.chemcomp.com (accessed on 28 November 2018).
15. Saldívar-González, F.I.; Valli, M.; Andricopulo, A.D.; da Silva Bolzani, V.; Medina-Franco, J.L. Chemical diversity of NuBBE database: A chemoinformatic characterization. *J. Chem. Inf. Model.* **2019**. [CrossRef]
16. Sander, T.; Freyss, J.; von Korff, M.; Rufener, C. Datawarrior: An open-source program for chemistry aware data visualization and analysis. *J. Chem. Inf. Model.* **2015**, *55*, 460–473. [CrossRef] [PubMed]
17. Bemis, G.W.; Murcko, M.A. The properties of known drugs. 1. Molecular frameworks. *J. Med. Chem.* **1996**, *39*, 2887–2893. [CrossRef]
18. Van der Maaten, L.; Hinton, G. Visualizing data using t-SNE. *J. Mach. Learn Res.* **2008**, *9*, 2579–2605.
19. Osolodkin, D.I.; Radchenko, E.V.; Orlov, A.A.; Voronkov, A.E.; Palyulin, V.A.; Zefirov, N.S. Progress in visual representations of chemical space. *Exp. Opin. Drug Discov.* **2015**, *10*, 959–973. [CrossRef] [PubMed]
20. González-Medina, M.; Prieto-Martínez, F.D.; Medina-Franco, J.L. Consensus diversity plots: A global diversity analysis of chemical libraries. *J. Cheminf.* **2016**, *8*, 63. [CrossRef]
21. Naveja, J.; Rico-Hidalgo, M.; Medina-Franco, J. Analysis of a large food chemical database: Chemical space, diversity, and complexity. *F1000Research* **2018**, *7*, 993. [CrossRef]
22. Medina-Franco, J.L.; Martínez-Mayorga, K.; Bender, A.; Scior, T. Scaffold diversity analysis of compound data sets using an entropy-based measure. *QSAR Comb. Sci.* **2009**, *28*, 1551–1560. [CrossRef]
23. Berthold, M.R.; Cebron, N.; Dill, F.; Gabriel, T.R.; Kötter, T.; Meinl, T.; Ohl, P.; Sieb, C.; Thiel, K.; Wiswedel, B. Knime: The konstanz information miner. In *Data analysis, machine learning and applications: Proceedings of the 31st Annual Conference of the Gesellschaft für Klassifikation e.V., Albert-Ludwigs-Universität Freiburg, Freiburg im Breisgau, Germany, 7–9 March 2007*; Preisach, C., Burkhardt, H., Schmidt-Thieme, L., Decker, R., Eds.; Springer: Berlin/Heidelberg, Germany, 2008; pp. 319–326.
24. Naveja, J.J.; Oviedo-Osornio, C.I.; Trujillo-Minero, N.N.; Medina-Franco, J.L. Chemoinformatics: A perspective from an academic setting in Latin America. *Mol. Divers.* **2018**, *22*, 247–258. [CrossRef] [PubMed]
25. Helmy, M.; Crits-Christoph, A.; Bader, G.D. Ten simple rules for developing public biological databases. *PLoS Comput. Biol.* **2016**, *12*, e1005128. [CrossRef] [PubMed]

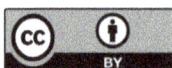

*biomolecules*

MDPI

*Article*

# A Marine Diterpenoid Modulates the Proteasome Activity in Murine Macrophages Stimulated with LPS

Yisett González [1], Deborah Doens [1], Héctor Cruz [1,2], Ricardo Santamaría [3], Marcelino Gutiérrez [3], Alejandro Llanes [1,*] and Patricia L. Fernández [1,*]

[1] Centro de Biología Celular y Molecular de Enfermedades, Instituto de Investigaciones Científicas y Servicios de Alta Tecnología (INDICASAT AIP),Edificio 219, Ciudad del Saber, 0801 Panamá, Panamá; ygonzalez@indicasat.org.pa (Y.G.); ddoens@gmail.com (D.D.); hector_cruz@outlook.com (H.C.)

[2] Facultad de Ciencias de la Salud Dr. William C. Gorgas, Universidad Latina de Panamá, 0801 Panamá, Panamá

[3] Centro de Biodiversidad y Descubrimiento de Drogas, INDICASAT AIP, Edificio 219, Ciudad del Saber, 0801 Panamá, Panamá; rsantamaria@indicasat.org.pa (R.S.); mgutierrez@indicasat.org.pa (M.G.)

* Correspondence: allanes@indicasat.org.pa (A.L.); pllanes@indicasat.org.pa (P.L.F.), Tel.: +507-517-0739

Received: 13 August 2018; Accepted: 1 October 2018; Published: 5 October 2018

**Abstract:** The proteasome is an intracellular complex that degrades damaged or unfolded proteins and participates in the regulation of several processes. The immunoproteasome is a specialized form that is expressed in response to proinflammatory signals and is particularly abundant in immune cells. In a previous work, we found an anti-inflammatory effect in a diterpenoid extracted from the octocoral *Pseudopterogorgia acerosa*, here called compound 1. This compound prevented the degradation of inhibitor κB α (IκBα) and the subsequent activation of nuclear factor κB (NFκB), suggesting that this effect might be due to inhibition of the ubiquitin-proteasome system. Here we show that compound 1 inhibits the proteasomal chymotrypsin-like activity (CTL) of murine macrophages in the presence of lipopolysaccharide (LPS) but not in its absence. This effect might be due to the capacity of this compound to inhibit the activity of purified immunoproteasome. The compound inhibits the cell surface expression of major histocompatibility complex (MHC)-I molecules and the production of proinflammatory cytokines induced by LPS in vitro and in vivo, respectively. Molecular docking simulations predicted that compound 1 selectively binds to the catalytic site of immunoproteasome subunits β1i and β5i, which are responsible for the CTL activity. Taken together these findings suggest that the compound could be a selective inhibitor of the immunoproteasome, and hence could pave the way for its future evaluation as a candidate for the treatment of inflammatory disorders and autoimmune diseases.

**Keywords:** marine diterpenoid; proteasome inhibitors; immunoproteasome

## 1. Introduction

The proteasome is an enzymatic complex found in the nucleus and cytoplasm of eukaryotic cells, archaea and certain bacteria. This complex is responsible for the degradation of intracellular proteins that are damaged or misfolded. It works in collaboration with the ubiquitin system, which tags proteins for proteasome processing. The proteasome plays an important role in the regulation of many cellular processes, such as the cell cycle, the defense against oxidative stress and inflammatory responses. The proteasome is composed of two types of domains: a core particle and one or two regulatory domains. The core particle is formed by four stacking rings, each of them consisting of seven α or β subunits. Central rings have three catalytic subunits, namely β1, β2 and β5, which have caspase-like, trypsin-like and chymotrypsin-like (CTL) activity, respectively. An alternative form of the proteasome, called immunoproteasome, is present in most animal cells but it is abundantly expressed in immune cells, where its primary role is to process proteins for antigen presentation by major histocompatibility complex (MHC) class I molecules [1,2]. Expression of the immunoproteasome is induced by interferon-γ (IFN-γ), tumor necrosis factor (TNF) and bacterial lipopolysaccharide (LPS) under inflammatory conditions, such as infections or autoimmune diseases [3–5]. In the presence of such stimuli, catalytic subunits of the constitutive form are respectively substituted by inducible subunits β1i (LPM2), β2i (MECL-1) and β5i (LMP7) to form the immunoproteasome. Unlike its constitutive counterparts, which have caspase-like activity, the β1i subunit also has CTL activity [6,7].

The proteasome has been implicated as a modulator of inflammatory responses by participating in the activation of nuclear factor κB (NFκB), a transcription factor that regulates the expression of many genes involved in inflammation [8]. Five NFκB family members have been described, namely RelA (p65), RelB, cRel, p50 and p52, respectively encoded by genes *rela, relb, crel, nfkb1* and *nfkb2*. After the stimulus, NFκB proteins form dimers, which bind to κB sites on target genes either as homodimers or heterodimers. In resting cells, NFκB is sequestered in the cytoplasm by inhibitor κB (IκB) proteins. Activation of NFκB is triggered by phosphorylation of IκB, followed by its ubiquitination and proteasomal degradation, thus releasing NFκB and promoting its translocation into the nucleus [9]. It has been demonstrated that the immunoproteasome subunit β1i is involved in the proteolytic processing of NFκB precursor proteins (p100/p105), as well as in the degradation of inhibitor κB α (IκBα) [10–12]. Later, it was observed that β1i-deficient retinal pigment epithelial cells exhibited diminished activation of NFκB in response to TNF [13]. However, the role of the immunoproteasome in NFκB activation and in the degradation of IκB proteins is still under debate [10,14–17]. Other studies have demonstrated that immunoproteasome subunits are not essential in the activation of NFκB either in cancer cell lines or in peritoneal macrophages stimulated with TNF [17,18].

Due to the role of the proteasome in many physiological processes, it has become a major target for the design of new drugs as a therapeutic for several diseases. Many proteasome inhibitors have been identified from natural and synthetic sources. Two of them, bortezomib and carfilzomib, are currently approved for the treatment of multiple myeloma. Although a number of second-generation proteasome inhibitors are in clinical trials [19], undesirable side effects have been associated to these molecules. The immunoproteasome has emerged as a therapeutic target and as a strategy to reduce the toxicity associated with the inhibition of the constitutive proteasome in cells [20,21]. These molecules are not only valuable as potential therapeutics but would also allow a better understanding of the physiological roles attributed to the immunoproteasome. Several highly selective immunoproteasome inhibitors have been recently described, including both peptidic [22] and nonpeptidic inhibitors [23].

In previous studies, we have shown a marked anti-inflammatory activity for a pseudopterane diterpene (compound 1) isolated from the octocoral *Pseudopterogorgia acerosa* [16]. Compound 1 inhibited the production and expression of proinflammatory mediators in macrophages stimulated with LPS, TNF and other toll-like receptor ligands. Our results showed that this anti-inflammatory effect is due to the inhibition of IκBα degradation and the subsequent activation of NFκB. We then analyzed if the effect of compound 1 might be influenced by a modulation of the ubiquitin-proteasome system, affecting the proteasomal degradation of phosphorylated IκBα. We show herein that compound 1 inhibits the CTL activity of the proteasome induced by LPS in vitro and reduces the expression of MHC class I in macrophages. This inhibitory effect might occur by a mechanism that involved the modulation of immunoproteasome activity, since a reduction in the CTL activity of the purified immunoproteasome was observed. In vivo, compound 1 reduces the production of proinflammatory mediators in the lung of animals treated by intranasal inoculation of LPS. Molecular docking simulations predicted that compound 1 preferentially interacts with the catalytic site of subunits β1i and β5i, suggesting that the effect of this compound might be dependent on immunoproteasome activity.

## 2. Materials and Methods

### 2.1. Mice

In vivo studies were carried out by using female C57Bl/6 mice with an age of eight weeks, obtained from Instituto de Investigaciones Científicas y Servicios de Alta Tecnología (INDICASAT)'s mouse facility. Mice were kept at 25 °C under a light/dark cycle of 12 h and had free access to food and water. All experiments were performed in accordance with guidelines from the Institutional Animal Welfare Committee and the Guide for the Care and Use of Laboratory Animals of the National Institutes of Health. The protocol was also approved by the Institutional Animal Care and Use Committee of INDICASAT AIP (IACUC-15-004).

### 2.2. Acute Pulmonary Inflammation

C57BL/6 mice ($n$ = 5) were anesthetized with Ketamine/Xylazine (93/6 mg/Kg) and then treated by intranasal inoculation with lipopolysaccharide (LPS) from *Escherichia coli* 0111:B4 (Sigma Aldrich, Saint Louis, MO, USA) (0.5 mg/Kg) or saline for control group. Compound 1 (5 mg/Kg) was administered by intraperitoneal (i.p.) injection 2 h before and 10 h after LPS administration. The control group was not treated with compound 1. Mice were euthanized 24 h after the challenge with LPS and the concentrations of tumor necrosis factor (TNF) and interleukin (IL)-6 were determined in lungs and in bronchoalveolar lavage (BAL) by the enzyme-linked immunosorbent assay (ELISA) method. The expression of proteasome and immunoproteasome subunits was determined by quantitative polymerase chain reaction (PCR) in whole lung homogenate of animals from LPS and control groups.

### 2.3. Cell Culture and Proteasome Activity Assay

Peritoneal macrophages from C57BL/6 mice were obtained five days after intraperitoneal instillation of 2 mL of thioglycollate 3%, by peritoneal washing with chilled Roswell Park Memorial Institute (RPMI) medium. Cells were seeded in RPMI with 10% fetal calf serum (FCS) at a density of $1 \times 10^6$/well in 24-well plates and cultured for 2 h at 37 °C in an atmosphere of 5% $CO_2$. Non-adherent cells were removed by washing and adherent cells were pre-incubated with compound 1 (25 μM) or isogorgiacerodiol (25 or 50 μM) for 2 h at 37 °C in an atmosphere of 5% $CO_2$. Then, cells were stimulated with bacterial LPS from *Escherichia coli* 0111:B4 (InvivoGen, San Diego, CA, USA) (1 μg/mL) for different periods of time (2, 4 or 8 h). Supernatants were discarded and cells were incubated with the fluorogenic peptide Suc-Leu-Leu-Val-Tyr-AMC to evaluate the proteasome CTL activity or Z-Leu-Leu-Glu-AMC to evaluate caspase-like activity as previously described [24,25]. After 2 h, supernatants were harvested and the fluorescence of free fluorophore 7-amino-4-methycoumarin (AMC) was measured by using FLx800 BioTek (Winooski, VT, USA) at wavelength/band pass 360/40 for excitation and 460/40 for emission.

### 2.4. Western Blot Analysis

Western blot analysis was performed as previously described by González et al. [16]. Briefly, peritoneal macrophages were stimulated with 1 μg/mL of LPS with or without 25 μM of compound 1. Cells were further lysed and 20 μg of total extracts were diluted in loading buffer, boiled and applied to a sodium dodecyl sulfate (SDS) polyacrilamide gel (12%) under reducing conditions. Protein bands were transferred to a polyvinylidene difluoride (PVDF) membrane and further incubated overnight with a monoclonal antiubiquitin antibody specific for Lys48 [26]. For Western blot image densitometry, ImageJ v. 1.50i [27] was used as recommended by the software developer.

### 2.5. Major Histocompatibility Complex Class I Flow Cytometry Analysis

The experiments of cell surface quantification of MHC-I expression were performed in bone marrow-derived macrophages (BMDM), since these cells have lower levels of basal MHC-I expression than elicited peritoneal macrophages. The BMDM were extracted and cultured as previously described by González et al. [16]. Cultured cells were stimulated with LPS at a concentration of 1 µg/mL in the presence or absence of compound 1 (25 µM). After 24 h, expression of MHC-I was evaluated by flow cytometry.

After 24 h of stimulus, cells were collected, washed with phosphate-buffered saline (PBS) and blocked for 15 min with 200 µL bovine serum albumin (BSA) 1% in PBS. Cells were then washed and incubated for 30 min at 4 °C with antimouse CD11b fluorescein isothiocyanate (FITC) (5 µg/mL) and/or phycoerythrin (PE) antimouse H-2Ld/H-2Db clone 28-14-8 (Biolegend, San Diego, CA, USA) diluted in PBS BSA 1%. After several washes, cells were resuspended in PBS and analyzed by flow cytometry. Event acquisition was performed with a Partec CyFlow® cytometer and the data were analyzed using FlowMax software (PARTEC, Münster, Germany) and FCS Express 4 Flow Cytometry (De Novo software, Los Angeles, CA, USA).

*2.6. Quantitative Real Time Polymerase Chain Reaction*

Elicited peritoneal macrophages were stimulated with LPS (10 ng/mL) for 2, 4 and 8 h or preincubated for 1 h with compound 1 (25 µM), PR-957 (200 nM) or Polymyxin B (15 µg/mL) and then stimulated with LPS (10 ng/mL) for 8 h. After the stimuli, total RNA was extracted using TRIzol (Life Technology Corporation: Invitrogen and Applied Biosystems, Foster City, CA, USA). The cDNA was obtained by using a High-Capacity cDNA Reverse Transcription Kit (Life Technology Corporation: Invitrogen and Applied Biosystems). The ABI 7500 (Applied Biosystems) was used to perform the quantitative real-time PCR analysis using SYBR Green master mix (Applied Biosystems). Amplification conditions were: 95 °C (10 min), 40 cycles of 95 °C (15 s), and 59 °C (60 s). The data were normalized to the hypoxanthine phosphoribosyltransferase (HPRT) expression and were represented as the difference relative to the control level. The $2^{-\Delta\Delta CT}$ method was used to analyze the relative gene expression. The following forward/reverse primer pairs were used: 5'-TGACCAAGGACGAATGTCTG-3'/5'-GATTTGGTCTCCCAAAAGCA-3' for β1; 5'-GTGAATCAGCACGGGTTTT-3'/5'-AATCCGCTGCAACAATGACT-3' for β5; 5'-CATCATGGCAGTGGAGTTTGAC-3'/5'-ACCTGAGAGGGCACAGAAGATG-3' for β1i; 5'-ACCACACTCGCCTTCAAGTTC-3'/5'-GCCAAGCAGGTAAGGGTTAATC-3' for β5i and 5'-GCTGGTGAAAAGGACCTCT-3'/5'-CACAGGACTAGAACACCTGC-3' for HPRT.

*2.7. Purified Proteasome Activity Assay*

The assay was performed by using the Proteasome-Glo™ Assay Systems (Promega, Madiscon, WI, USA) following the manufacturer's instructions. Briefly, 2 nM of mouse 20S proteasome or immunoproteasome (Boston Biochem, Cambridge, MA, USA) were added to a white 96-well plate in a volume of 50 µL. Then, 50 µL of compound 1 was added at different concentrations (50, 25 and 12.5 µM) and the plate was incubated for 1 h at 37 °C. Following, 50 µL of the Proteasome-Glo™ reagent containing the luciferin detection reagent and the substrates (Suc-LLVY for Chymotrypsin-like or Z-nLPnLD for Caspase-like) were added. The plate was mixed at 300–500 rpm for 30 s and incubated at room temperature for 30 min. Luminescence was measured by using a plate reader Synergy HT from BioTek.

*2.8. Cytokine Measurements*

Animals were euthanized and the BAL was obtained by injecting 1 mL of PBS into the trachea and collecting again. The BAL was centrifuged and the supernatants were harvested. The whole lung homogenate was obtained by homogenization of the tissue in 1X PBS containing 0.1% of Triton100 and protease inhibitors. Homogenates were centrifuged and the supernatants were stored. The concentrations of TNF and IL-6 in lungs and BAL were determined by ELISA (DuoSet kit, R&D System, Minneapolis, MN, USA), according to the manufacturer's protocol.

*2.9. Molecular Docking Simulation*

ACD/ChemSketch v. 12 (ACD/Labs, Toronto, Canada) was used to draw the 2D structures of compound 1 and isogorgiacerodiol, and to convert them into 3D structural data. Avogadro v.1.1.1 [28] was used to optimize the geometry of both molecules. Antechamber v.1.27 [29] was used for an additional energy minimization step before docking. For preparation of the receptor protein, we isolated the dimer formed by chains K and L from the murine constitutive proteasome (Protein Data Bank (PDB) accession code 3UNB) and immunoproteasome (PDB accession code 3UNF), corresponding to subunits β5/β5i and β6, respectively. All ligands and water molecules were removed before docking. The co-crystallized ligand in both structures was used to define the position of the binding site of subunits β5/β5i and to set grid parameters for docking. Docking simulations per se were performed with Dock v. 6.7 [30] by using grid score and Hawkings GB/SA as primary and secondary energy scoring functions, respectively. The program was set to output the best 10 docking poses and those with the lowest energy were selected for further analyses in each experiment. Prediction of hydrogen bonds and other noncovalent interactions were done with Chimera v.1.11 [31] and LigPlot+ [32].

*2.10. Statistical Analysis*

Data are presented as means + standard error of the mean (SEM) or mean + standard deviation (SD). Results were analyzed using a statistical software package (GraphPad Prism 6). Statistical analyses were performed by unpaired *t* test, Mann-Whitney test, Kruskal-Wallis multiple comparisons test. A difference between groups was considered to be significant if $p < 0.05$ (* $p < 0.05$; ** $p < 0.01$; *** $p < 0.001$). The half maximal inhibitory concentration ($IC_{50}$) was calculated adjusting a sigmoidal dose−response curve following GraphPad Prism 6 procedure.

## 3. Results

*3.1. Compound 1 Inhibits the Activity of the Proteasome with the Consequent Accumulation of Ubiquitinated Proteins*

We have previously demonstrated that compound 1 (Figure 1a) inhibits the degradation of IκBα, leading to the prevention of NFκB activation and the subsequent transcription of genes encoding pro-inflammatory mediators [16]. Considering the effect of compound 1 on the degradation of IκB, we determined if it interferes with the ubiquitin-proteasome system. We first analyzed if compound 1 modulates the proteasome CTL and caspase-like activities, which have been largely implicated in the regulation of immune responses [33]. Macrophages were treated with LPS and compound 1 for different time points and then incubated with the fluorogenic peptides Suc-Leu-Leu-Val-Tyr-AMC or Z-Leu-Leu-Glu-AMC, substrates for CTL and caspase-like activities respectively. Treatment with LPS induced an increase in CTL activity after 4 h of stimulus that was maintained until 8 h. Compound 1 considerably reduced CTL activity 2 and 4 h after treatment (Figure 1b). Compound 1 also inhibited the caspase-like activity at 8 h of stimulus (Figure 1c). Although the compound has no apparent effect on the CTL activity in the absence of stimulus with LPS, it significantly inhibits caspase-like activity (Figure S5). The inhibitory effect of compound 1 is not due to cell death since we have previously demonstrated that compound 1 is not cytotoxic [16]. The effect of compound 1 on proteasome activity was also evidenced by the accumulation of polyubiquitinated (poly-Ub) proteins in macrophages stimulated with LPS (Figure 1d). The accumulation of poly-Ub proteins was detected by immunoblotting in macrophage extracts obtained from cells stimulated with LPS in the presence or absence of compound 1. Western blot analysis shows a notably higher accumulation of poly-Ub proteins in the presence of compound 1 than in its absence (Figure 1d,e). These results suggest that compound 1 might have an effect on proteasome activity.

(a)  (b)  (c)

(d)  (e)

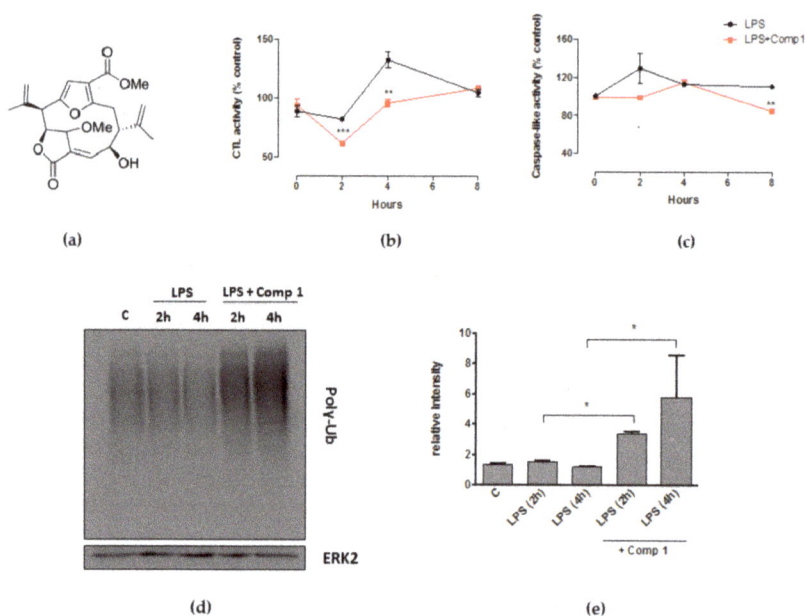

**Figure 1.** Compound 1 inhibits proteasome activity in the presence of lipopolysaccharide (LPS). (a) Schematic representation of compound 1. Macrophages were stimulated with LPS (1 μg/mL) in the presence or absence of compound 1 (25 μM) for 2, 4 or 8 h. Hydrolysis of fluorogenic peptides Suc-Leu-Leu-Val-Tyr-AMC (b) or Z-Leu-Leu-Glu-AMC (c) was measured in cell supernatants by detection of free 7-amino-4-methycoumarin (AMC). Results were normalized with DMSO-treated controls. Results represent mean ± standard error of the mean (SEM) from treatments performed in triplicates and are representative of two different experiments. (d) Immunoblotting for poly-Ub detection in macrophage extracts obtained from cells stimulated with LPS in the presence or absence of compound 1. The Anti-Ubiquitin Lys48 antibody was used to detect poly-Ub. Detection of ERK2 was used as a loading control. The figure is representative of two different experiments with similar results. (e) Relative intensity calculated by the ratio of area under the curve from poly-Ub/area under the curve for total. Results represent mean + SEM from two different experiments * $p < 0.05$; ** $p < 0.01$; *** $p < 0.001$ compared to LPS alone. CTL: chemotrypsin-like.

### 3.2. Compound 1 did not Affect the Expression of β1i and β5i Subunits in Peritoneal Macrophages Stimulated with Lypopolisaccharide

It has been previously demonstrated that LPS induces the expression of immunoproteasome subunits [5]. Then, we evaluated, in our experimental conditions, the capacity of LPS to induce the expression of the subunits involved in the CTL activity of the immunoproteasome, β1i and β5i, and their counterparts in the constitutive proteasome, β1 and β5. We stimulated peritoneal macrophages with LPS at different time points and the expression of the subunits was evaluated by quantitative PCR. The LPS treatment significantly increased the expression of β1i and β5i 4 and 8 h after the stimuli (Figure S6). We did not find statistically significant differences in the level of expression of both subunits induced by LPS (Figure S6). Although there is a slight increase in the expression of the constitutive subunits β1 and β5 induced by LPS, compared to nonstimulated controls, the levels of expression of these subunits were fivefold less than the expression of β1i and β5i (Figure S6).

We then analyzed if compound 1 interferes with the expression of proteasome subunits. Macrophages were treated with LPS for 8 h in the presence or absence of compound 1. The expression of the subunits induced by LPS was not affected by the treatment with compound 1 (Figure 2a,b).

A known inhibitor of the immunoproteasome, PR-957, did not interfere with the expression of β1i and β5i either. As expected, the pretreatment of cells with polymyxin B, which binds to lipid A and interferes with the binding of LPS to TLR4, completely abrogated the increase of β1i and β5i expression induced by LPS (Figure 2a,b). The expression of β1 and β5 was not affected by the treatment of cells with compound 1 (data not shown).

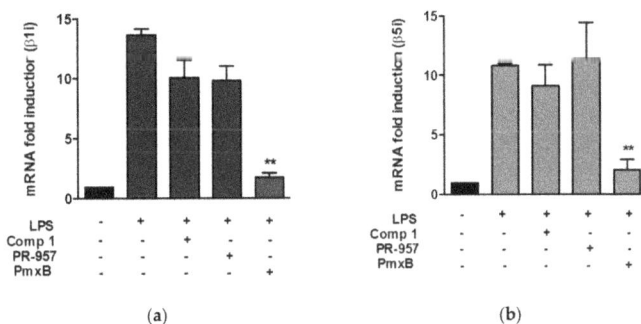

(a)                  (b)

**Figure 2.** Compound 1 does not appear to interfere with the expression of immunoproteasome subunits. Peritoneal macrophages were pre-treated with compound 1 (25 µM), PR-957 (200 nM) or Polimixin B (PmxB) (15 µg/mL) and then stimulated with LPS (1 ng/mL) for 8 h. Total RNA was isolated and the amount of mRNA was determined for β1i (a) or β5i (b). Values were normalized by using hypoxanthine phosphoribosyltransferase (HPRT) expression and are shown as fold induction of mRNA expression with respect to control samples. Results represent means + SEM from two independent experiments performed in duplicates, ** $p < 0.005$.

### 3.3. Compound 1 Inhibits the Chemotrypsin-like Activity of Purified Proteasomes

In order to rule out the possibility of an unspecific effect of compound 1 on proteasome activity, we evaluated if the compound inhibits the activity of purified constitutive proteasome and immunoproteasome. Purified proteasomes were incubated with compound 1 at different concentrations and the CTL activity was determined after the addition of Suc-LLVY substrate. Compound 1 significantly reduced the activity of the immunoproteasome even at a concentration of 12.5 µM (Figure 3a), with an $IC_{50}$ value of 9.767 µM (Figure S7). The compound also reduced the CTL activity of the constitutive proteasome at the concentration of 50 µM (Figure 3b). We did not observe any effect of compound 1 on the caspase-like activity of the constitutive proteasome (data not shown).

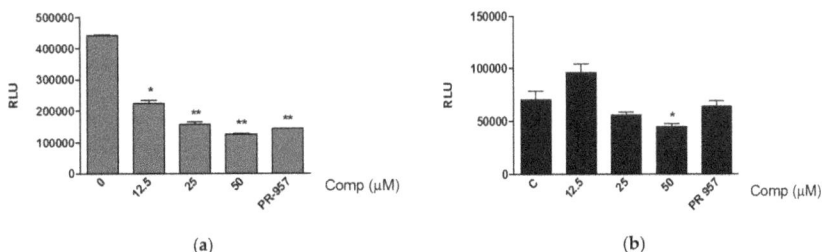

(a)                  (b)

**Figure 3.** Compound 1 inhibits the activity of immunoproteasome at low concentration. Purified immunoproteasome (a) and constitutive proteasome (b) (2 nM) were incubated with different concentrations of compound 1 (12.5, 25 and 50 µM) or PR-957 (200 nM) at 37 °C. After 1 h the substrate Suc-LLVY was added and the luminescence was reported as relative light units (RLU). Results represent mean + standard deviation (SD) from treatments performed in triplicates.

*3.4. Compound 1 Inhibits the Expression of MHC-I In Vitro and the Production of Pro-Inflammatory Mediators In Vivo*

Immunoproteasome has been implicated in the presentation of certain classes of peptides by the MHC class I. The expression of MHC class I is also modulated by the immunoproteasome [2]. As we believe that compound 1 might be affecting immunoproteasome activity, we then analyzed if the compound interferes with the expression of MHC class I induced by LPS in macrophages. We stimulated bone marrow-derived macrophages with LPS and treated with compound 1. The levels of MHC-I on cell surface were analyzed by flow cytometry after 24 h of treatments. The histogram shows that LPS induced an increase in the levels of MHC-I expressed on macrophages surface, and this effect was reverted by the treatment of cells with compound 1 (Figure 4). The inhibition of MHC-I expression might be due to immunoproteasome modulation induced by compound 1.

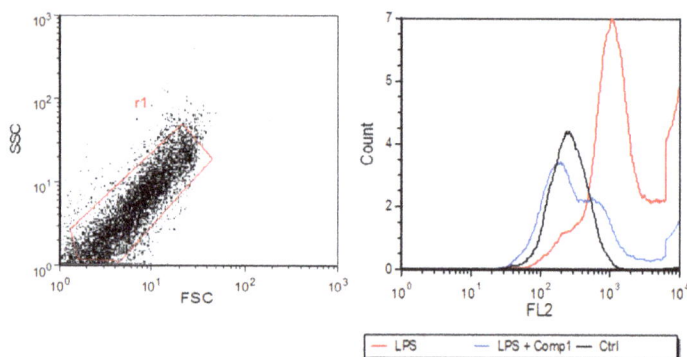

**Figure 4.** Expression of major histocompatibility complex (MHC)-I induced by LPS in macrophages appears to be inhibited by compound 1. LPS (1 µg/mL) was used to stimulate bone marrow-derived macrophages in the presence or absence of compound 1 (25 µM). Expression of MHC-I (H-2Ld/H-2Db) was measured on CD11b+ cells after 24 h. Figure shows a histogram of MHC-I expression representative of two different experiments. Control (Ctrl) corresponds to non-stimulated cells.

It has been observed that the selective inhibition of the immunoproteasome downregulates the expression of proinflammatory mediators in a variety of immune pathologies [34]. Hence, we determined whether compound 1 has an effect on the inflammatory response induced by LPS in vivo. Mice were treated with compound 1 by intraperitoneal (i.p.) administration 2 h before and 10 h later after intranasal inoculation of LPS. We first evaluated the expression of immunoproteasome subunits induced by LPS and we observed higher levels of β1i and β5i in the animals treated with LPS, compared with the control group (Figure S8). These levels were correlated with increased production of inflammatory mediators in lungs and BAL (Figure 5). Compound 1 significantly reduced the production of TNF in the lungs of animals treated with LPS (Figure 5a,b). Although the reduction of IL-6 in lungs was not statistically significant, we have observed a conserved trend in the experiments. The suppression of TNF and IL-6 in the presence of compound 1 was also observed in the bronchoalveolar lavage of treated animals (Figure 5c,d). LPS treatment did not increase the expression of β1 and β5 subunits from the constitutive proteasome (Figure S8). Thus, the effect of compound 1 in the inflammatory response in vivo could occur, at least in part, by means of the modulation of immunoproteasome activity.

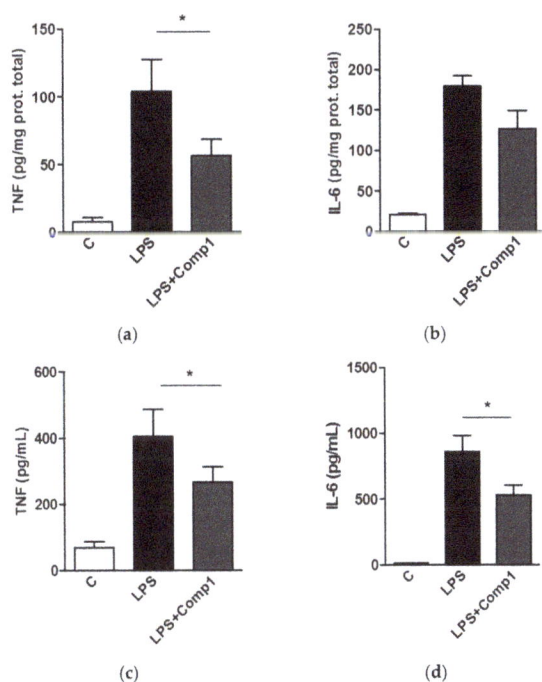

**Figure 5.** Compound 1 inhibits the production of pro-inflammatory mediators in vivo. C57BL/6 mice were injected intraperitoneal (i.p.) with compound 1 (5 mg/Kg), 2 h before and 10 h later after LPS (0.5 mg/Kg) inoculation. After 24 h of LPS treatment, protein levels of tumor necrosis factor (TNF) and interleukin (IL)-6 were quantified in lung tissue (**a**,**b**) and bronchoalveolar lavage (**c**,**d**). Results represent mean + SEM from two different experiments *, $p < 0.05$.

### 3.5. Compound 1 Appears to Bind to the Catalytic Pocket of β5i Subunit of the Immunoproteasome

We used molecular docking simulation to further study the binding of compound 1 to the catalytic site of β5i subunit of the murine proteasomes. It has been previously shown that neighboring subunits contribute to interactions within the binding sites of proteasomal catalytic subunits [35]. Hence, we also included subunit β6 when performing the docking simulation for binding sites of subunits β5 and β5i. Compound 1 was predicted to bind to subunits β5 and β5i with energy estimates of −97.03 and −104.72 kJ/mol, respectively. Although energy values are relatively similar for both subunits, there are notable differences in the sites where the compound is predicted to bind (Figure 6).

Compound 1 was predicted to be oriented towards the catalytic site of subunit β5i of the immunoproteasome (Figure 6a), almost fully inserted in the corresponding S1 specificity pocket (Figure 6c). The S1 pocket has been found to be critical in determining selective binding of ligands to subunits β5 and β5i. This pocket also contains an N-terminal Thr1 residue that is essential for the catalytic activity of the subunits [36]. Compound 1 appears to form two hydrogen bonds with residues from the β5i subunit, one between the carbonyl group at C-16 and the Thr1 residue, and another one between the methoxyl group at C-9 and the Gly23 residue (Figure 6a). Conversely, in the subunits of the constitutive proteasome, compound 1 is predicted to bind towards the neighboring β6 subunit, relatively away from the catalytic site of subunit β5 and its S1 pocket (Figure 6b,d). In this case, compound 1 also appears to form a hydrogen bond with Gly23, but involves a carbonyl group at C-20 rather than the methoxyl group at C-9.

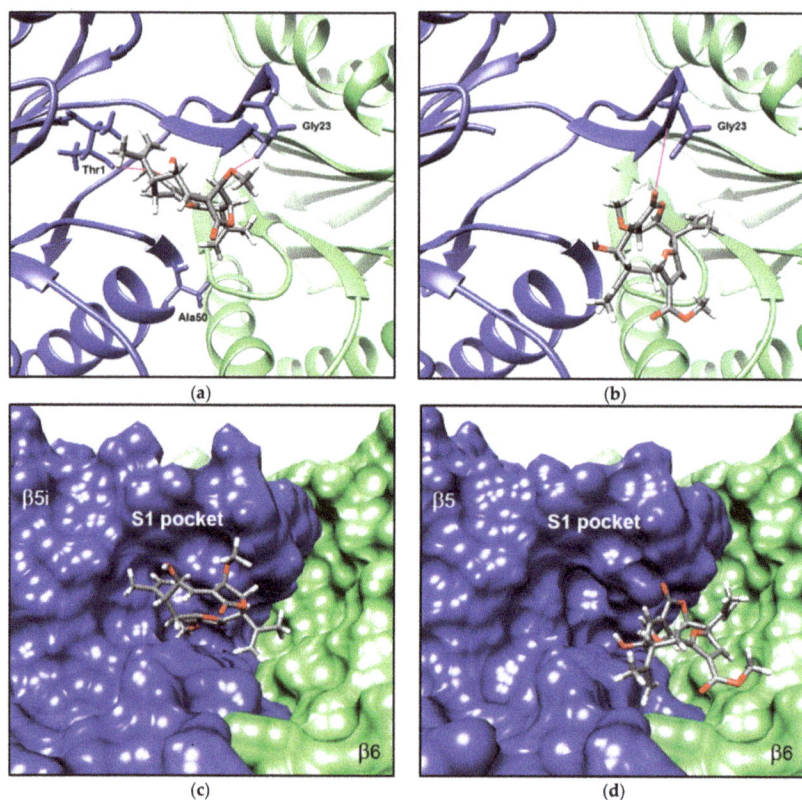

**Figure 6.** Molecular docking simulation predicted specific binding of compound 1 to the catalytic site of subunit β5i of the murine immunoproteasome. Lowest-energy pose predicted for the interaction of compound 1 with subunits β5i-β6 of the immunoproteasome (**a**) and with subunits β5-β6 of the constitutive form (**b**). Orientation of compound 1 within the S1 pocket of subunits β5i (**c**) and β5 (**d**) is also shown. Subunits β5/β5i are colored blue and β6 subunits are colored green. Purple lines indicate predicted hydrogen bonds between the ligand and amino acid residues from the subunits.

Further prediction of noncovalent interactions with LigPlot+ revealed that binding of compound 1 to the S1 pocket of the β5i subunit is also facilitated by hydrophobic contacts with several amino acid residues from the pocket (Figure 7a). Among those residues are Ala20 and Ala49, which in turn are involved in the CTL activity of the subunit [36]. Although hydrophobic interactions with residues from the β5 subunit also appear to be relevant for binding of compound 1 to the constitutive proteasome, these involve additional contacts with residues from the neighboring β6 subunit (Figure 7b). These results suggest that compound 1 might modulate the β5i subunit activity due to its specific interaction with amino acids involved in the catalytic activity of the subunit.

We also analyzed the interaction of compound 1 with β1i subunit and with the corresponding β1 subunit of the constitutive proteasome. Compound 1 was predicted to bind to the catalytic site of subunit β1i, while binding to a different but relatively closer site in subunit β1 (Figure S9). Predicted energy values were −102.09 and −106.69 kJ/mol, for the β1 and β1i subunits respectively.

In order to determine the functional groups that could be involved in the interaction of compound 1 to the β5i subunit, we performed docking simulations for the structurally related compound isogorgiacerodiol, which presents a weaker anti-inflammatory activity [16]. This compound differs from compound 1 only in the substitution of the methoxyl group at C-9 by a hydroxyl group

(Figure S1–S4). The compound was predicted to bind outside the catalytic site of subunits β5 and β5i (Figure S10). In the immunoproteasome, this compound appears to form a hydrogen bond with its hydroxyl group at C-20 and residue Ala50 of the β5i subunit, which is close to the interface between subunits β5i and β6. Furthermore, orientation of this compound is favored by a pattern of hydrophobic interactions involving residues Asp125 and Pro126 from the β6 subunit. Isogorgiacerodiol does not inhibit the CTL activity in vitro (Figure S10). These results indicate that the methoxyl group at C-9 of compound 1, which is not present in isogorgiacerodiol, may be critical for the orientation that facilitates its binding to the catalytic site of the β5i subunit.

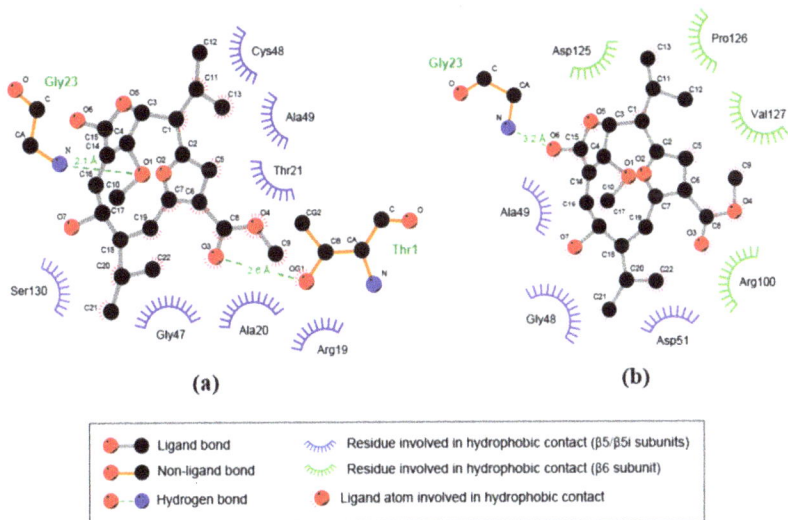

**Figure 7.** A different pattern of noncovalent interactions is involved in binding of compound 1 to β5 and β5i subunits. Two-dimensional representation of ligand–protein interactions for compound 1 and the β5/β5i-β6 subunits of the murine immunoproteasome (**a**) and the constitutive proteasome (**b**). Atoms are represented by their chemical symbol. For side chains of amino acids, CA, CB and CG indicate the α, β, and γ carbon atoms, respectively.

## 4. Discussion

We have previously shown that compound 1 inhibits the inflammatory response induced in macrophages after LPS challenge by a mechanism involving the reduction of IκBα degradation [16]. Since the proteasome is critical for IκBα degradation and activation of NFκB, we suspected that the compound might be interfering with the activity of the proteasome. Here, we found accumulation of polyubiquitinated proteins in murine macrophages stimulated with LPS and treated with compound 1, which correlates with a reduced proteasomal CTL and caspase-like activities. Analyses on purified proteasomes revealed that compound 1 inhibits the CTL activity of immunoproteasome. We also showed that compound 1 reduces the LPS-induced surface expression of MHC class I molecules in vitro and the production of proinflammatory mediators in vivo. Docking simulations have predicted a selective interaction of compound 1 with the β5i subunit. Thus, the anti-inflammatory effect of this compound might be dependent, at least in part, on the modulation of immunoproteasome activity.

It has been previously shown that LPS induces proteasomal activation in immune cells and that a proteasome inhibitor, lactacystin, blocks the expression of multiple genes involved in the response of macrophages to LPS [4]. Hence, we determined the effect of compound 1 on the proteasome activity in LPS-stimulated macrophages. Considering the relevance of chymotrypsin-like activity of proteasomes in the inflammatory response of macrophages [37,38], we evaluated the effect of compound 1 on β1i and β5i immunoproteasome subunits and their counterparts in the constitutive proteasome. We showed herein that compound 1 inhibits the CTL activity of the proteasome, thus resulting in the accumulation of polyubiquitinated proteins. This effect of compound 1 on CTL activity did not occur in the absence of LPS, suggesting that the compound might be modulating the immunoproteasome activity. Compound 1 also inhibited the caspase-like activity of the proteasome; however, this effect did not exclusively occur in the presence of LPS. The inhibition of constitutive proteasomal CTL activity has been previously reported for different plant-derived terpenoids, and this effect is associated with anti-inflammatory and/or anti-cancer properties of these compounds [39,40].

The effect of compound 1 on purified immunoproteasome and constitutive proteasome was further evaluated. While compound 1 inhibited the CTL activity of immunoproteasome at the three concentrations analyzed, the inhibition of the constitutive proteasome only occurred at a higher compound concentration. Previous reports have shown that in RAW 264.7 cells early TNF production induced by LPS is not regulated by the immunoproteasome and that the inhibition of β2 and β5 constitutive proteasome subunits is required for a decrease in the production of this cytokine [5]. However, we have previously demonstrated that compound 1 inhibits the expression and secretion of inflammatory mediators, including TNF, in peritoneal macrophages stimulated with LPS as early as 3 h of stimulus [16]. Differences in the kinetic expression of immunoproteasome subunits induced by LPS in cell lines and primary macrophages might explain these discrepancies.

In immune cells, pro-inflammatory stimuli induce the replacement of the constitutive proteasome by the immunoproteasome, which increases MHC class I antigen processing and regulates inflammatory responses. Stimulation of cells with IFN-γ and TNF leads to the expression of immunoproteasome subunits [26,41]. It has been reported that the expression of LPS-induced immunoproteasome subunits is implicated in the production of certain inflammatory mediators [5]. We have shown that LPS preferentially increased mRNA expression of β1i and β5i compared to β1 and β5 in murine peritoneal macrophages that were not affected by treatment with compound 1. No expression of mRNA for proteasome subunits was observed in control cells without stimulus. However, β5i protein has been detected in the cytoplasm of nonstimulated peritoneal macrophages [17]. Although we have not found differences in mRNA expression between β1i and β5i in LPS-stimulated macrophages, other authors have reported higher protein levels of β1i than those of β5i after stimulation with IFN-γ [17]. Previous reports of the occurrence of mixed-subunit proteasomes, involving one or two inducible subunits coupled with constitutive ones, may support these findings [12,42]. Further studies are necessary to characterize the proteasome composition influenced by LPS stimulus.

Immunoproteasome has been largely implicated in the processing of MHC class I-restricted peptides [43]. Activation of cytotoxic T lymphocytes depends on the recognition of peptides presented by MHC-I molecules. Immunoproteasome generates peptides for MHC-I presentation more efficiently than the constitutive proteasome, probably by means of the substitution of the caspase-like activity of β1 subunit by the CTL activity of β1i [44]. Proinflammatory stimuli such as IFN-γ, TNF and LPS upregulate the cell surface expression of MHC-I molecules [45,46]. Our results show that LPS induces an increment in the levels of MHC-I in cell surface, an effect that was avoided by compound 1. These results are congruent with the idea that compound 1 might be interfering with immunoproteasome activity, affecting MHC-I expression. Our data are consistent with previous findings in which the inhibition of immunoproteasome subunits by using PR-957 reduces cell surface expression of MHC-I in splenocytes and cytokine production in monocytes [47]. Deficiency of β5i in mice generates a reduction in MHC-I cell surface expression levels compared to wild type mice [2], which was not observed in the absence of β1i [48]. These results point out a role of β5i in MHC class I expression.

In vivo, inhibition of immunoproteasome modulates immune responses and disease progression in several models. Treatment of animals with PR-957 reduces signs of experimental arthritis, which is associated with a reduction in joint expression of proinflammatory mediators [47]. This inhibitor also attenuated the progression of experimental autoimmune encephalomyelitis and prevented the expression of pro-inflammatory mediators in the brain and spinal cord of animals [49]. A mouse colitis model has revealed that the blockage of β5i subunit reduced the pathological sings of the disease and cytokine production in the colon [34]. Immunoproteasome subunits are rapidly induced in lungs after viral infection of mice [50]. Here we have shown that compound 1 inhibited the production of proinflammatory mediators in the lungs and in the bronchoalveolar lavage of mice treated with LPS. This effect could be at least partially dependent on the inhibition of immunoproteasome subunits, since LPS significantly upregulated the expression of β1i and β5i in lungs. Further studies are necessary to demonstrate the interaction of compound 1 with immunoproteasome in vivo.

Molecular docking simulations supported the notion that compound 1 inhibits CTL activity of the immunoproteasome. The compound was predicted to bind to the catalytic site of the β5i subunit, oriented towards its S1 specificity pocket. The compound forms at least two hydrogen bonds with residues from the subunit, one between a methoxyl group and residue Gly23, and another between a carbonyl group and the N-terminal Thr1 residue. Thr1 is actively involved in the catalytic mechanism of the subunit [51,52] and was recently shown to participate in the activation of proteolytic activity during biogenesis of the proteasome [53]. Furthermore, several well-studied proteasome inhibitors, such as PR-957, interact with this residue [36].

Conversely, in the subunits of the constitutive proteasome, compound 1 was predicted to bind towards a small cavity of the neighboring β6 subunit, leaving the S1 pocket empty. The compound also appears to form a hydrogen bond with residue Gly23, but involves a carbonyl group at C-20 rather than a methoxyl group. Taken together with the experimental evidence, these predictions suggest that compound 1 might selectively inhibit the CTL activity of the immunoproteasome, by binding to the β5i subunit. Docking of the structurally-related compound isogorgiacerodiol, which presents a substitution of the methoxyl by a hydroxyl group at C-9, was predicted to bind outside the catalytic site of the β5i subunit, oriented towards the neighboring β6 subunit. These results point out the methoxyl group of compound 1 as critical for the orientation that facilitates its binding to the catalytic site of the β5i subunit.

Since it has been demonstrated that the β1i subunit of the immunoproteasome has CTL activity, we also evaluated the interaction of compound 1 with this subunit. The compound was also predicted to bind to the catalytic site of the β1i subunit, with binding energy estimates similar to those for the β5i subunit. Results suggest that the effect of the compound on the CTL activity of the immunoproteasome could be the consequence of binding to two subunits with similar activity. This finding is consistent with reported evidence that inhibition of multiple proteolytic sites is needed for a marked reduction of proteasome-mediated proteolysis [54].

Different contributions to inflammatory responses and other functions related to the immune system have been attributed to different proteasome subunits. Deficiency in the β1i subunit induced a reduction of cytokine production by murine B cells stimulated with LPS, through a mechanism partially dependent on NFκB inhibition [12]. Altered NFκB activity in nonobese diabetic mice has been attributed to a defect in proteasome function due to a lack of β1i subunit expression [10]. Selective inhibition of the β5i subunit leads to partial reduction of TNF and IL-6 production induced by LPS in vitro, which is completely abrogated if β1i and β2i are also inhibited [47]. The in vitro and in vivo identification of heterogeneous proteasome populations that differ in their enzymatic features [55] may explain the role attributed to individual proteasome subunits in pathological conditions.

Proteasome inhibitors are promising candidates for the treatment of inflammatory diseases and cancer. Currently, there are three proteasome inhibitors approved by the United States Food and Drug Administration (FDA) for clinical use in humans, namely, bortezomib, carfilzomib and ixazomib. The immunoproteasome is overexpressed in malignant cells and in cells involved in autoimmune disorders [20,56]. Selective inhibitors of the immunoproteasome have the advantage of being effective as a treatment for such conditions, while preventing the onset of undesirable side effects associated with the inhibition of the constitutive proteasome [40]. Here we propose a natural compound as a potential specific inhibitor of the CTL activity of the immunoproteasome, opening a path for further studies to characterize this compound as a new agent for the treatment of inflammatory and autoimmune diseases.

## 5. Conclusions

We have shown here a diterpenoid as a potential inhibitor of CTL activity of the proteasome. This compound inhibited the expression of MHC class I molecules in vitro and reduced the levels of pro-inflammatory cytokines in response to LPS in vivo. Molecular docking has predicted that the compound selectively interacts with the S1 pocket of the β5i subunit of the immunoproteasome, a common feature among immunoproteasome inhibitors. The immunoproteasome has been implicated in the induction and maintenance of inflammation and a more efficient generation of peptides for MHC-I presentation. The immunoproteasome has been proposed as a potential therapeutic target, since it is associated with several pathological conditions including cancer and inflammation. This work suggests that this compound might be a selective inhibitor of the immunoproteasome, hence pointing it out as a candidate in the search for new drugs for the treatment of inflammatory disorders and autoimmune diseases.

**Supplementary Materials:** The following are available online at http://www.mdpi.com/2218-273X/8/4/109/s1, Figure S1: $^1$H-NMR and $^{13}$C-NMR spectra and structure of compound **1**, Figure S2: $^1$H-NMR and $^{13}$C-NMR spectra and structure of isogorgiacerodiol, Figure S3: HRAPCI-MS spectra and structure of compound **1**, Figure S4: HRAPCI-MS spectra and structure of isogorgiacerodiol, Figure S5: Compound **1** inhibits caspase-like activity but not CTL activity in the absence of LPS, Figure S6: LPS induces the expression of immunoproteasome subunits, Figure S7: IC50 sigmoidal curve of the effect of compound 1 on CTL activity of the immunoproteasome, Figure S8: LPS selectively induces the expression of immunoproteasome subunits in vivo, Figure S9: Predicted orientation of compound **1** within the catalytic sites of subunits β1 and β1i of the murine constitutive and immunoproteasome, respectively, Figure S10: Effect of isogorgiacerodiol on proteasome CTL activity.

**Author Contributions:** Conceptualization, A.L. and P.L.F.; Funding acquisition, P.L.F.; Methodology, Y.G., D.D., H.C., R.S., A.L. and P.L.F.; Resources, M.G. and P.L.F.; Writing—original draft, Y.G., D.D., H.C., M.G., A.L. and P.L.F.

**Funding:** This research was funded by Secretaría Nacional de Ciencia Tecnología e Innovación (SENACYT) of the Republic of Panama (grant numbers FID11-082 and FID14-024) and the Sistema Nacional de Investigación (SNI) (grant number SNI163-2016). Héctor Cruz was supported by funds from Deveaux Foundation.

**Acknowledgments:** Financial support by SENACYT and SNI is gratefully acknowledged. We thank Ricardo Lleonart for densitometry analysis and Gabrielle Britton for critical review of the manuscript.

**Conflicts of Interest:** The authors declare no conflict of interest. The funders had no role in the design of the study; in the collection, analyses, or interpretation of data; in the writing of the manuscript, and in the decision to publish the results.

## References

1. Brown, M.G.; Driscoll, J.; Monaco, J.J. Structural and serological similarity of MHC-linked LMP and proteasome (multicatalytic proteinase) complexes. *Nature* **1991**, *353*, 355–357. [CrossRef] [PubMed]
2. Fehling, H.J.; Swat, W.; Laplace, C.; Kühn, R.; Rajewsky, K.; Müller, U.; von Boehmer, H. MHC class I expression in mice lacking the proteasome subunit LMP-7. *Science* **1994**, *265*, 1234–1237. [CrossRef] [PubMed]
3. Griffin, T.A.; Nandi, D.; Cruz, M.; Fehling, H.J.; Kaer, L. V; Monaco, J.J.; Colbert, R.A. Immunoproteasome assembly: cooperative incorporation of interferon gamma (IFN-γ)-inducible subunits. *J. Exp. Med.* **1998**, *187*, 97–104. [CrossRef] [PubMed]
4. Qureshi, N.; Perera, P.; Shen, J.; Zhang, G.; Lenschat, A.; Splitter, G.; Morrison, D.C.; Vogel, S.N. The proteasome as a lipopolysaccharide-binding protein in macrophages: differential effects of proteasome inhibition on lipopolysaccharide-induced signaling events. *J. Immunol.* **2003**, *171*, 1515–1525. [CrossRef] [PubMed]

5.  Reis, J.; Guan, X.Q.; Kisselev, A.F.; Papasian, C.J.; Qureshi, A.A.; Morrison, D.C.; van Way, C.W.; Vogel, S.N.; Qureshi, N. LPS-Induced Formation of Immunoproteasomes: TNF-α and Nitric Oxide Production are Regulated by Altered Composition of Proteasome-Active Sites. *Cell. Biochem. Biophys.* **2011**, *60*, 77–88. [CrossRef] [PubMed]

6.  Reidlinger, J.; Pike, A.M.; Savory, P.J.; Murray, R.Z.; Rivett, A.J. Catalytic properties of 26 S and 20 S proteasomes and radiolabeling of MB1, LMP7, and C7 subunits associated with trypsin-like and chymotrypsin-like activities. *J. Biol. Chem.* **1997**, *272*, 24899–24905. [CrossRef] [PubMed]

7.  Ho, Y.K.; Bargagna-Mohan, P.; Wehenkel, M.; Mohan, R.; Kim, K.B. LMP2-Specific Inhibitors: Chemical Genetic Tools for Proteasome Biology. *Chem. Biol.* **2007**, *14*, 419–430. [CrossRef] [PubMed]

8.  Palombella, V.J.; Rando, O.J.; Goldberg, A.L.; Maniatis, T. The ubiquitin-proteasome pathway is required for processing the NF-κB1 precursor protein and the activation of NF-κB. *Cell.* **1994**, *78*, 773–785. [CrossRef]

9.  Karin, M.; Ben-Neriah, Y. Phosphorylation Meets Ubiquitination: The Control of NF-κB Activity. *Annu. Rev. Immunol.* **2000**, *18*, 621–663. [CrossRef] [PubMed]

10. Hayashi, T.; Faustman, D. NOD mice are defective in proteasome production and activation of NF-κB. *Mol. Cell. Biol.* **1999**, *19*, 8646. [CrossRef] [PubMed]

11. Hayashi, T.; Faustman, D. Essential role of human leukocyte antigen-encoded proteasome subunits in NF-κB activation and prevention of tumor necrosis factor-α-induced apoptosis. *J. Biol. Chem.* **2000**, *275*, 5238–5247. [CrossRef] [PubMed]

12. Hensley, S.E.; Zanker, D.; Dolan, B.P.; David, A.; Hickman, H.D.; Embry, A.C.; Skon, C.N.; Grebe, K.M.; Griffin, T. a; Chen, W.; Bennink, J.R.; Yewdell, J.W. Unexpected role for the immunoproteasome subunit LMP2 in antiviral humoral and innate immune responses. *J. Immunol.* **2010**, *184*, 4115–4122. [CrossRef] [PubMed]

13. Maldonado, M.; Kapphahn, R.J.; Terluk, M.R.; Heuss, N.D.; Yuan, C.; Gregerson, D.S.; Ferrington, D.A. Immunoproteasome Deficiency Modifies the Alternative Pathway of NFκB Signaling. *PLoS ONE* **2013**, *8*. [CrossRef] [PubMed]

14. Kessler, B.M.; Lennon-Duménil, A.M.; Shinohara, M.L.; Lipes, M.A.; Ploegh, H.L. LMP2 expression and proteasome activity in NOD mice. *Nat. Med.* **2000**, *6*, 1064. [CrossRef] [PubMed]

15. Visekruna, A.; Joeris, T.; Seidel, D.; Kroesen, A.; Loddenkemper, C.; Zeitz, M.; Kaufmann, S.H.E.; Schmidt-Ullrich, R.; Steinhoff, U. Proteasome-mediated degradation of IκBα and processing of p105 in Crohn disease and ulcerative colitis. *J. Clin. Invest.* **2006**, *116*, 3195–3203. [CrossRef] [PubMed]

16. González, Y.; Doens, D.; Santamaría, R.; Ramos, M.; Restrepo, C.M.; Barros De Arruda, L.; Lleonart, R.; Gutiérrez, M.; Fernández, P.L. A pseudopterane diterpene isolated from the octocoral Pseudopterogorgia acerosa inhibits the inflammatory response mediated by TLR-ligands and TNF-α in macrophages. *PLoS ONE* **2013**, *8*, e84107. [CrossRef] [PubMed]

17. Bitzer, A.; Basler, M.; Krappmann, D.; Groettrup, M. Immunoproteasome subunit deficiency has no influence on the canonical pathway of NF-κB activation. *Mol. Immunol.* **2017**, *83*, 147–153. [CrossRef] [PubMed]

18. Jang, E.R.; Lee, N.-R.; Han, S.; Wu, Y.; Sharma, L.K.; Carmony, K.C.; Marks, J.; Lee, D.-M.; Ban, J.-O.; Wehenkel, M.; et al. Revisiting the role of the immunoproteasome in the activation of the canonical NF-κB pathway. *Mol. Biosyst.* **2012**, *8*, 2295–2302. [CrossRef] [PubMed]

19. Teicher, B.A.; Tomaszewski, J.E. Proteasome inhibitors. *Biochem. Pharmacol.* **2015**, *96*, 1–9. [CrossRef] [PubMed]

20. Lee, W.; Kim, K.B. The immunoproteasome: an emerging therapeutic target. *Curr. Top. Med. Chem.* **2011**, *11*, 2923–2930. [CrossRef] [PubMed]

21. Miller, Z.; Ao, L.; Kim, K.B.; Lee, W. Inhibitors of the immunoproteasome: current status and future directions. *Curr. Pharm. Des.* **2013**, *19*, 4140–4151. [CrossRef] [PubMed]

22. Sula Karreci, E.; Fan, H.; Uehara, M.; Mihali, A.B.; Singh, P.K.; Kurdi, A.T.; Solhjou, Z.; Riella, L.V.; Ghobrial, I.; Laragione, T.; et al. Brief treatment with a highly selective immunoproteasome inhibitor promotes long-term cardiac allograft acceptance in mice. *Proc. Natl. Acad. Sci.* **2016**. [CrossRef] [PubMed]

23. Sosič, I.; Gobec, M.; Brus, B.; Knez, D.; Živec, M.; Konc, J.; Lešnik, S.; Ogrizek, M.; Obreza, A.; Žigon, D. Nonpeptidic Selective Inhibitors of the Chymotrypsin-Like (β5 i) Subunit of the Immunoproteasome. *Angew. Chemie.* **2016**. [CrossRef]

24. Nam, S.; Smith, D.M.; Dou, Q.P. Ester Bond-containing Tea Polyphenols Potently Inhibit Proteasome Activity in Vitro and in Vivo. *J Biol Chem.* **2001**, *20*. [CrossRef]

25. Cheng, X.; Shi, W.; Zhao, C.; Zhang, D.; Liang, P.; Wang, G.; Lu, L. Triptolide sensitizes human breast cancer cells to tumor necrosis factor-α-induced apoptosis by inhibiting activation of the nuclear factor-κB pathway. *Mol. Med. Rep.* **2016**. [CrossRef] [PubMed]

26. Akiyama, K.; Yokota, K.; Kagawa, S.; Shimbara, N.; Tamura, T.; Akioka, H.; Nothwang, H.G.; Noda, C.; Tanaka, K.; Ichihara, A. cDNA cloning and interferon gamma down-regulation of proteasomal subunits X and Y. *Science* **1994**, *265*, 1231–1234. [CrossRef] [PubMed]

27. Schneider, C.A.; Rasband, W.S.; Eliceiri, K.W. NIH Image to ImageJ: 25 years of image analysis. *Nat. Methods* **2012**, *9*, 671–675. [CrossRef] [PubMed]

28. Hanwell, M.D.; Curtis, D.E.; Lonie, D.C.; Vandermeerschd, T.; Zurek, E.; Hutchison, G.R. Avogadro: An advanced semantic chemical editor, visualization, and analysis platform. *J. Cheminform.* **2012**, *4*. [CrossRef] [PubMed]

29. Wang, J.; Wang, W.; Kollmann, P.; Case, D. Antechamber, An Accessory Software Package For Molecular Mechanical Calculation. *J. Comput. Chem.* **2005**, *25*, 1157–1174. [CrossRef] [PubMed]

30. Allen, W.J.; Balius, T.E.; Mukherjee, S.; Brozell, S.R.; Moustakas, D.T.; Lang, P.T.; Case, D.A.; Kuntz, I.D.; Rizzo, R.C. DOCK 6: Impact of new features and current docking performance. *J. Comput. Chem.* **2015**, *36*, 1132–1156. [CrossRef] [PubMed]

31. Pettersen, E.F.; Goddard, T.D.; Huang, C.C.; Couch, G.S.; Greenblatt, D.M.; Meng, E.C.; Ferrin, T.E. UCSF Chimera—A Visualization System for Exploratory Research and Analysis. *J. Comput. Chem* **2004**, *25*, 1605–1612. [CrossRef] [PubMed]

32. Laskowski, R.A.; Swindells, M.B. LigPlot+: Multiple ligand-protein interaction diagrams for drug discovery. *J. Chem. Inf. Model.* **2011**, *51*, 2778–2786. [CrossRef] [PubMed]

33. Groettrup, M.; Kirk, C.J.; Basler, M. Proteasomes in immune cells: More than peptide producers? *Nat. Rev. Immunol.* **2010**, *10*, 73–78. [CrossRef] [PubMed]

34. Basler, M.; Dajee, M.; Moll, C.; Groettrup, M.; Kirk, C.J. Prevention of experimental colitis by a selective inhibitor of the immunoproteasome. *J. Immunol.* **2010**, *185*, 634–641. [CrossRef] [PubMed]

35. Lei, B.; Abdul Hameed, M.; Hamza, A.; Wehenkel, M.; Muzyka, J.L.; Yao, X.J.; Kim, K.B.; Zhan, C.G. Molecular basis of the selectivity of the immunoproteasome catalytic subunit LMP2-specific inhibitor revealed by molecular modeling and dynamics simulations. *J. Phys. Chem. B* **2010**, *114*, 12333–12339. [CrossRef] [PubMed]

36. Huber, E.M.; Basler, M.; Schwab, R.; Heinemeyer, W.; Kirk, C.J.; Groettrup, M.; Groll, M. Immuno- and constitutive proteasome crystal structures reveal differences in substrate and inhibitor specificity. *Cell.* **2012**, *148*, 727–738. [CrossRef] [PubMed]

37. Shen, J.; Reis, J.; Morrison, D.C.; Papasian, C.; Raghavakaimal, S.; Kolbert, C.; Qureshi, A.A.; Vogel, S.N.; Qureshi, N. Key inflammatory signaling pathways are regulated by the proteasome. *Shock* **2006**, *25*, 472–484. [CrossRef] [PubMed]

38. Shen, J.; Gao, J.J.; Zhang, G.; Tan, X.; Morrison, D.C.; Papasian, C.; Vogel, S.N.; Qureshi, N. Proteasome-mediated regulation of CpG DNA- and peptidoglycan-induced cytokines, inflammatory genes, and mitogen-activated protein kinase activation. *Shock* **2006**, *25*, 594–599. [CrossRef] [PubMed]

39. Yang, H.; Chen, D.; Qiuzhi, C.C.; Yuan, X.; Dou, Q.P. Celastrol, a triterpene extracted from the Chinese "Thunder of God Vine," is a potent proteasome inhibitor and suppresses human prostate cancer growth in nude mice. *Cancer Res.* **2006**, *66*, 4758–4765. [CrossRef] [PubMed]

40. Lu, L.; Kanwar, J.; Schmitt, S.; Cui, Q.C.; Zhang, C.; Zhao, C.; Dou, Q.P. Inhibition of tumor cellular proteasome activity by triptolide extracted from the Chinese medicinal plant "thunder god vine". *Anticancer Res.* **2011**, *31*, 1–10. [PubMed]

41. Boes, B.; Hengel, H.; Ruppert, T.; Multhaup, G.; Koszinowski, U.H.; Kloetzel, P.M. Interferon γ stimulation modulates the proteolytic activity and cleavage site preference of 20S mouse proteasomes. *J. Exp. Med.* **1994**, *179*, 901–909. [CrossRef] [PubMed]

42. Guillaume, B.; Chapiro, J.; Stroobant, V.; Colau, D.; Van Holle, B.; Parvizi, G.; Bousquet-Dubouch, M.-P.; Théate, I.; Parmentier, N.; Van den Eynde, B.J. Two abundant proteasome subtypes that uniquely process some antigens presented by HLA class I molecules. *Proc. Natl. Acad. Sci. U.S.A.* **2010**, *107*, 18599–18604. [CrossRef] [PubMed]

43. Kloetzel, P.M. Antigen processing by the proteasome. *Nat. Rev. Mol. Cell. Biol.* **2001**, *2*, 179–187. [CrossRef] [PubMed]

44. Groettrup, M.; van den Broek, M.; Schwarz, K.; Macagno, A.; Khan, S.; de Giuli, R.; Schmidtke, G. Structural plasticity of the proteasome and its function in antigen processing. *Crit. Rev. Immunol.* **2001**, *21*, 339–358. [CrossRef] [PubMed]

45. MacAry, P.A.; Lindsay, M.; Scott, M.A.; Craig, J.I.; Luzio, J.P.; Lehner, P.J. Mobilization of MHC class I molecules from late endosomes to the cell surface following activation of CD34-derived human Langerhans cells. *Proc. Natl. Acad. Sci. USA* **2001**, *98*, 3982–3987. [CrossRef] [PubMed]

46. Boehm, U.; Klamp, T.; Groot, M.; Howard, J.C. Cellular responses to interferon-γ. *Annu. Rev. Immunol.* **1997**, *15*, 749–795. [CrossRef] [PubMed]

47. Muchamuel, T.; Basler, M.; Aujay, M.; Suzuki, E.; Kalim, K.W.; Lauer, C.; Sylvain, C.; Ring, E.R.; Shields, J.; Jiang, J.; et al. A selective inhibitor of the immunoproteasome subunit LMP7 blocks cytokine production and attenuates progression of experimental arthritis. *Nat. Med.* **2009**, *15*, 781–787. [CrossRef] [PubMed]

48. Van Kaer, L.; Ashton-Rickardt, P.G.; Eichelberger, M.; Gaczynska, M.; Nagashima, K.; Rock, K.L.; Goldberg, A.L.; Doherty, P.C.; Tonegawa, S. Altered peptidase and viral-specific T cell response in LMP2 mutant mice. *Immunity* **1994**, *1*, 533–541. [CrossRef]

49. Basler, M.; Mundt, S.; Muchamuel, T.; Moll, C.; Jiang, J.; Groettrup, M.; Kirk, C.J. Inhibition of the immunoproteasome ameliorates experimental autoimmune encephalomyelitis. *EMBO Mol. Med.* **2014**, *6*, 226–238. [CrossRef] [PubMed]

50. Keller, I.E.; Vosyka, O.; Takenaka, S.; Kloß, A.; Dahlmann, B.; Willems, L.I.; Verdoes, M.; Overkleeft, H.S.; Marcos, E.; Adnot, S.; et al. Regulation of Immunoproteasome Function in the Lung. *Sci. Rep.* **2015**, *5*, 10230. [CrossRef] [PubMed]

51. Löwe, J.; Stock, D.; Jap, B.; Zwickl, P.; Baumeister, W.; Huber, R. Crystal structure of the 20S proteasome from the archaeon T. acidophilum at 3.4 A resolution. *Science* **1995**, *268*, 533–539. [CrossRef] [PubMed]

52. Groll, M.; Ditzel, L.; Löwe, J.; Stock, D.; Bochtler, M.; Bartunik, H.D.; Huber, R. Structure of 20S proteasome from yeast at 2.4 A resolution. *Nature* **1997**, *386*, 463–471. [CrossRef] [PubMed]

53. Huber, E.M.; Heinemeyer, W.; Li, X.; Arendt, C.S.; Hochstrasser, M.; Groll, M. A unified mechanism for proteolysis and autocatalytic activation in the 20S proteasome. *Nat. Commun.* **2016**, *7*, 10900. [CrossRef] [PubMed]

54. Kisselev, A.F.; Callard, A.; Goldberg, A.L. Importance of the different proteolytic sites of the proteasome and the efficacy of inhibitors varies with the protein substrate. *J. Biol. Chem.* **2006**, *281*, 8582–8590. [CrossRef] [PubMed]

55. Dahlmann, B.; Ruppert, T.; Kuehn, L.; Merforth, S.; Kloetzel, P.M. Different proteasome subtypes in a single tissue exhibit different enzymatic properties. *J. Mol. Biol.* **2000**, *303*, 643–653. [CrossRef] [PubMed]

56. Yewdell, J.W. Immunoproteasomes: Regulating the regulator. *Proc. Natl. Acad. Sci.* **2005**, *102*, 9089–9090. [CrossRef] [PubMed]

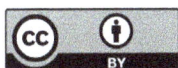

*biomolecules*

MDPI

*Article*

# Analysis of Flavonoids Bioactivity for Cholestatic Liver Disease: Systematic Literature Search and Experimental Approaches

Juan Carlos Sánchez-Salgado [1,2,*], Samuel Estrada-Soto [2,*], Sara García-Jiménez [2], Sergio Montes [3], Jaime Gómez-Zamudio [4] and Rafael Villalobos-Molina [5,6]

1   Instituto de Medicina Molecular y Ciencias Avanzadas, Mexico City 01900, Mexico
2   Facultad de Farmacia, Universidad Autónoma del Estado de Morelos, Cuernavaca, MOR 62209, Mexico; saragarcia@uaem.mx
3   Instituto Nacional de Neurología y Neurocirugía, Mexico City 14269, Mexico; montesergio@yahoo.com
4   Unidad de Investigación Médica en Bioquímica, Hospital de Especialidades, Centro Médico Nacional Siglo XXI, IMSS, México City 06720, Mexico; jaime_gomez_zamudio@hotmail.com
5   Unidad de Biomedicina, Facultad de Estudios Superiores-Iztacala, Universidad Nacional Autónoma de México, Tlalnepantla 54090, Mexico; villalobos@campus.iztacala.unam.mx
6   Departamento de Bioquímica, Facultad de Medicina, Universidad Nacional Autónoma de México, Ciudad de México 04510, México
*   Correspondence: juanc.sanchez@immca.com.mx (J.C.S.-S.); enoch@uaem.mx (S.E.-S.); Tel.: +52-777-329-7089 (S.E.-S)

Received: 2 December 2018; Accepted: 7 March 2019; Published: 14 March 2019

**Abstract:** Flavonoids are naturally occurring compounds that show health benefits on the liver. However, there is little investigation about identification and evaluation of new flavonoid-containing drugs for cholestatic liver disease, one of the most common liver illnesses. We aimed to a systematic search regarding efficacy of flavonoids for treatment of cholestatic liver disease, and then evaluate naringenin (NG) as representative flavonoid in an obstructive cholestasis model. We searched for information of experimental and clinical studies in four major databases without time and language limits. Intervention was defined as any flavonoid derivate compared with other flavonoid, placebo, or without comparator. In addition, we evaluated NG on a bile duct-ligated model in order to contribute evidence of its actions. Eleven experimental reports that support the efficacy of flavonoids in cholestatic liver disease were identified. However, there was no homogeneity in efficacy endpoints evaluated and methodology. On the other hand, NG showed beneficial effects by improving specific metabolic (cholesterol and lipoproteins) and liver damage (bilirubin and alkaline phosphatase) biomarkers. The review lacks homogeneous evidence about efficacy of flavonoids in experimental settings, and is susceptible to risk for bias. NG only showed improvements in specific disease biomarkers. More investigation is still needed to determine its potential for drug development.

**Keywords:** flavonoids; systematic review; cholestasis

## 1. Introduction

Liver disease is a prominent health problem with an important epidemiological and economic burden worldwide, accounting for 25% of prevalence [1,2]. However, this estimation is inconsistent since there is no reliable and applicable diagnostic test yet [2].

Cholestasis is an impaired bile flow from liver to duodenum that triggers unspecific cellular damage, which initiates inflammatory and fibro-genic processes in the liver, as well as cirrhosis and hepatocellular cancer in advanced stages [3]. This alteration might be provoked by an impaired export of bile acids to bile canaliculi (intrahepatic cholestasis), or by physical obstruction of bile flow due to gall stones, parasites, or biliary tumor growth (extrahepatic cholestasis) [4].

The most accepted and well established experimental model that reproduces pathobiochemical alterations is the bile duct-ligated (BDL) rodent model [3,5]. The surgical bile duct ligation induces an obstructive cholestatic damage, which results in typical phenotype as in human cholestasis [3,5,6]. In this context, there are exhaustive efforts to found new therapeutic agents able to decrease pathological severity and progression of cholestatic liver diseases. Despite this, there are limited approved drug interventions for the treatment of this disease, i.e., ursodeoxycholic acid (UDCA) is the only approved oral drug for cholestatic liver diseases, such as primary biliary cirrhosis and obstructive cholestasis [7,8]. Additionally, silymarin, a mixture of flavolignans from Silybum marianum (milk thistle), has been proposed as an alternative for primary biliary cirrhosis due to its antioxidant and hepatoprotective properties [9–11].

Systematic reviews and meta-analysis have become increasingly important in decision making for drug discovery. In fact, this technique is a powerful evidence-based strategy to ensure there is justification for further research on bioactive molecules or re-planning research objectives [12]. A little investigation has been carried out on flavonoid efficacy in disease. Only a systematic review summarizes biological activities of prenylated flavonoids and suggests the structural implications for their bioactivities [13]. However, there is no information about efficacy of these compounds on cholestatic liver disease despite previous evidence for silymarin.

Previously we reported the beneficial effects of flavonoid-rich extract of *Cochlospermum vitifolium* bark for improvement of liver enzymes activity in BDL rat [14]. Then, HPLC analysis showed that one of its main bioactive compounds was naringenin (NG), a widely spread flavonoid in nature [15]. Recently, a chemical analysis revealed the presence of other flavonoids in the bark extract of this species [16].

This work summarizes and compares the efficacy endpoints reported for flavonoids in cholestatic liver disease, taking into account clinical and experimental settings, by systematic literature search in four major databases. Moreover, we evaluated the efficacy of NG in a BDL Wistar rat model in order to compare retrieved information from literature. To the best of our knowledge, this is the first systematic search of flavonoids as candidates for cholestasis therapy, as well as to show the biological effects of NG on the BDL rat.

## 2. Materials and Methods

### 2.1. Systematic Review

#### 2.1.1. Sources

We conducted a systematic search for peer-reviewed articles in four major databases: Pubmed (Medline), Cochrane Library, Trip Database, and Lilacs. PRISMA statement was followed in order to establish the evidence-based minimum set of items for reporting on systematic reviews.

#### 2.1.2. Eligibility Criteria

A PICO strategy was developed as described in Table S1. Briefly, the databases were searched using combinations of the following terms: flavonoid, cholestasis, and bile duct ligated. A species filter for human or animal was applied to identify clinical trials or experimental assays, respectively. Simple literature reviews, case reports, editorial letters, comments, as well as duplicated or no abstract articles were excluded. The searching did not consider time and language limits.

#### 2.1.3. Studies Selection

The inclusion criteria for the selection of manuscripts were: all articles containing keywords in title, abstract or full-text, as well as those reporting clinical trials or experimental studies of isolated flavonoids for the treatment of cholestatic liver diseases (primary biliary cirrhosis, primary sclerosing cholangitis, biliary atresia, or Alagille syndrome). Only with BDL were selected in order to compare our experimental data. The selection was conducted by two independent reviewers, who analyzed the articles for discrepancies.

### 2.1.4. Meta-Analysis

A meta-analysis of the retrieved data could not be carried out due to methodological heterogeneity such as dosing, mode of administration, animal species, and time of exposure.

### 2.1.5. Risk of Bias Assessment

In order to assess the risk of biases of the animal studies reported in this systematic review, we applied a modified version of Cochrane's RoB tool denominated Systematic Review Centre for Laboratory animal Experimentation (SYRCLE). This tool considers six types of biases: Selection, performance, detection, attrition, reporting, and other biases, comprised of 10 items [17].

## 2.2. Experimental Studies

### 2.2.1. Reagents and Materials

Naringenin ~95% were purchased from Sigma-Aldrich Co. (St. Louis, MO, USA). Other reagents and surgical supplies were purchased from local sources.

### 2.2.2. Sample Preparation

Briefly, test samples were dissolved using a 10% aqueous solution of dimethylsulfoxide (DMSO). Dose of NG used was 50 mg/kg/day; the control group received 2 mL of vehicle.

### 2.2.3. Animal Model

Male Wistar rats (250–300 g, b.w.) were used under laboratory conditions with standard rodent diet and water ad libitum. All of the protocols were conducted as established by Federal Regulations for Animal Experimentation and Care (NOM-062-ZOO-1999, SAGARPA) and approved by Scientific and Bioethics Committee of Facultad de Farmacia (UAEM).

All animals were anesthetized by intraperitoneal injection of sodium pentobarbital (35 mg/kg), shaved and sanitized using a surgical disinfecting solution. A 1 cm incision below xiphoid process was made to extract gastrohepatic epiplon and locate duodenum segment. Once bile duct was cleaned for connective tissue, a triple ligation was made on bile duct using non-absorbable monofilament nylon suture (Farmacéutica Internacional S.A. de C.V., Mexico City, Mexico), and cut in two segments. Unconscious animals were gently sutured and allocated in warmed room until recovery. Sham animals (surgery control group) were subjected to the same protocol, but without ligation.

After 24 h post-surgery, animals were randomly allocated in three experimental groups ($n = 10$ animals per group) and began to receive the treatment. The experimental groups were: Sham + vehicle, BDL + vehicle, and BDL + NG. Aseptic cleaning was made along experiments using povidone-iodine 10% solution as palliative care. After 10 days of treatment all animals were sacrificed by dislocation and blood samples extracted by cardiac puncture. ARRIVE guidelines were followed for reporting this assay.

### 2.2.4. Biomarkers Quantification

Fresh collected blood samples were centrifuged at 3000 g for 10 min. Serum was separated from cell fraction and stored at $-20$ °C until analysis. Non-specific cholestasis biomarkers alanine transaminase (ALT), aspartate transaminase (AST), alkaline phosphatase (AP), and $\gamma$-glutamyltranspeptidase (GGT) activities) were determined as described by Rivera-Macías et al. [18].

Additionally, metabolic biomarkers were determined such as glucose, total cholesterol, triglycerides, very low-density lipoprotein (VLDL), high-density lipoprotein (HDL), and low-density lipoprotein (LDL). Quantitative enzymatic spectrophotometry was carried out using commercial kits (Wiener Labs, Mexico City, Mexico).

### 2.2.5. Data Analysis and Statistics

Data shown are expressed as mean $\pm$ standard error of the mean (SEM) obtained from three independent experiments. Plots were constructed with Microcal™ Origin 6.0 software (Microcal Software Inc., Northampton, MA, USA). Statistical analysis was done with IBM® SPSS® software (IBM Corporation, Somer, NY, USA) by Student's t-test and One-way ANOVA. Statistical significance was established when $p < 0.05$. Bonferroni post-hoc analysis was used for ANOVA.

## 3. Results

### 3.1. Systematic Review

Of all ninety articles identified in the primary search (Pubmed = 76, Trip Database = 5, Lilacs = 9, Cochrane Library = 0), we selected 12 of the experimental studies and one clinical trial (a pilot study on primary biliary cirrhosis). After full-text revision, we selected 11 articles for data discussion (Figure 1). All of them were on experimental studies on BDL rodents, as described in Table 1. Despite use of synonyms terms to retrieve a larger number of articles, we did not have more available information. Meta-analysis was not possible because of different animal species, route of administration, time of exposure, or methodology.

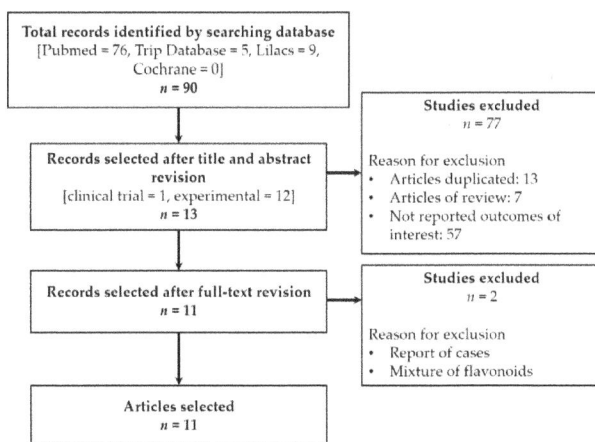

**Figure 1.** Flowchart showing the selection process for included studies on this systematic review.

Table 1. Efficacy endpoints studied on selected articles of systematic review.

| No | Chemical Structure | Compound Name | Dose Applied | Species | Liver Function | Fibrosis | Oxidative Stress | Inflammation | Reference |
|----|---|---|---|---|---|---|---|---|---|
| 1 | | Diosmin | 100 mg/kg/day, p.o. for 28 days | Wistar rat | X | X | X | X | Ali et al 2018 |
| 2 | | | 30 mg/kg/day p.o. for 28 days | Wistar rat | X | X | X | | Kabirifar et al 2017 |
| 3 | | Quercetin | 25 mg/kg/day p.o. for 28 days * | Sprague Dawley rat | X | X | X | X | Lin et al 2014 |
| 4 | | | 75, 150, 300 µmol/kg/day i.p. for 28 days | Wistar rat | X | X | X | | Peres et al 2000 |
| 5 | | Rutin | 25mg/kg/day p.o. for 28 days * | Sprague Dawley rat | X | X | X | X | Pan et al 2014 |
| 6 | | Genistein | 5 µg/rat/day p.o. for 56 days | Wistar rat | X | X | | | Salas et al 2007 |
| 7 | | Silybin/ Silibinin | 0.4g/kg ad libitum p.o. for 28 days | Wistar rat | | | X | | Serviddio et al 2014 |
| 8 | | | Dose not determined for 28 days | Wistar rat | | | | X | Stanca et al 2013 |
| 9 | | Epigallo- catechin 3-gallate | 30mg/kg/day i.p. for 14 days ** | C57BL/6 mice | | X | X | X | Shen et al 2015 |
| 10 | | | 25 mg/kg/day p.o. for 14 days | Sprague Dawley rat | X | X | | X | Yu et al 2015 |
| 11 | | Baicalin | 50 mg/kg/day i.p. for 14 days ** | C57BL/6 mice | X | X | | X | Shen et al 2017 |

* Compound administration began 1 week before surgery and 3 weeks postoperative. ** Compound administration began 2 h before surgery and 14 days postoperative.

The major flavonoids identified from this search were diosmin, bacailin, quercetin, epigallocatechin 3-gallate, silybin or silibinin (major active component of silymarin), rutin (quercetin-3-O-rutinoside), and genistein (Table 1). Interestingly, no evidence was found about NG, one of the most naturally occurring flavonoid studied due of its health benefits on metabolic and cardiovascular diseases (Figure 2). This no evidence scenario encouraged us to evaluate NG as candidate for drug discovery, and contribute to experimental pharmacological data of flavonoids.

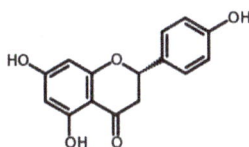

**Figure 2.** Chemical structure of naringenin (NG).

The biological processes altered on obstructive cholestasis are liver function, extracellular matrix components processing, redox status, and inflammation balance [3]. In this context, only diosmin, quercetin and rutin were evaluated for all these components (Table 1). Lin et al. showed that quercetin supplementation produced alleviation of liver histological integrity, serum biomarkers stabilization, reduction of fibrotic and inflammatory processes, and resolution of oxidative stress probably by modulation of bile duct proliferation and ductal reaction, blockade of mitogenic and fibrogenic signaling, and antioxidant effect [19]. Additionally, they evaluated rutin (quercetin-3-O-rutinoside), the O-glycoside compound that combine quercetin and disaccharide rutinose, on the same model and evaluated the same endpoints. The evidence showed that rutin had similar effects taking into account that it is converted to quercetin during metabolism [20].

On the other hand, Ali et al. reported data on efficacy of diosmin alone or in combination with sildenafil (erectile dysfunction approved drug with antioxidant and anti-inflammatory properties [21,22]) on the same model. Interestingly, diosmin alone was able to restore redox homeostasis by regulation of antioxidant enzymes GSR and SOD, a putative mechanism proposed for this molecule [23].

In order to compare parameters of the liver function and metabolic status on BDL-treated animals, we show tables of percentage change of each parameter vs. untreated cholestatic rats (Tables 2 and 3). It should be noticed that only one study reported mortality as valid endpoint for evaluation of experimental efficacy [23]. Additionally, ductal enzymes AP and GGT were missing on several studies despite these biomarkers are pivotal for cholestasis diagnostic [24].

**Table 2.** Percentage changes of liver function parameters induced by flavonoids on BDL model.

| No | Reference | Compound | Change % | | | | | |
|----|-----------|----------|------|------|------|------|--------------------|-----------|
| | | | ALT | AST | AP | GGT | Total Bilirubin | Mortality |
| 1 | Ali et al 2018 | Diosmin | 48.77 | 48.32 | 50.53 | 46.37 | 56.77 | 20% |
| 2 | Kabirifar et al 2017 | Quercetin | 32.89 | 34.32 | 44.44 | ND | ND | ND |
| 3 | Lin et al 2014 | Quercetin | 30.05 | 35.98 | ND | 55.87 | 36.26 | ND |
| 4 | Peres et al 2000 * | Quercetin | 55.81 | 78.57 | 49.86 | ND | ND | ND |
| 5 | Pan et al 2014 | Rutin | 37.16 | 44.55 | ND | 63.49 | 40.66 | ND |
| 6 | Salas et al 2007 | Genistein | 51.53 | ND | 59.88 | 73.68 | 68.97 | ND |
| 7 | Serviddio et al 2014 | Silybin/Silibinin | ND | ND | ND | ND | ND | ND |
| 8 | Stanca et al 2013 | Silybin/Silibinin | 30.76 | 23.68 | 27.78 | ND | 39.76 | ND |
| 9 | Shen et al 2015 | Epigallocatechin 3-Gallate | ND | ND | ND | ND | ND | ND |
| 10 | Yu et al 2015 | Epigallocatechin 3-Gallate | −29.77 | 3.66 | ND | ND | -4.64 | ND |
| 11 | Shen et al 2017 | Baicalin | ND | ND | ND | ND | ND | ND |
| 12 | Current article | NG | −6.79 | −40.02 | 19.78 | −7.82 | 38.91 | 30% |

ND, not determined; NG, Naringenin; ALT, alanine transaminase; AST, aspartate transaminase; AP, alkaline phosphatase; GGT, gamma glutamyltranspeptidase. * Only was considered dose 150 µg/mL for this analysis since this dose was administered for 28 days. Negative values means an augmentation of the parameter in comparison with untreated cholestatic animals.

**Table 3.** Percentage changes of metabolic parameters induced by flavonoids on BDL model.

| No | Reference | Compound | Change % | | | | | | |
|---|---|---|---|---|---|---|---|---|---|
| | | | Glucose | Cholesterol | Triglycerides | Insulin | VLDL | LDL | HDL |
| 3 | Lin et al 2014 | Quercetin | ND | 14.78 | 26.47 | ND | ND | ND | ND |
| 5 | Pan et al 2014 | Rutin | ND | 19.13 | 25.00 | ND | ND | ND | ND |
| 10 | Yu et al 2015 | Epigallocatechin 3-Gallate | ND | 0.69 | ND | ND | ND | 0.74 | −18.52 |
| 12 | Current article | NG | −2.51 | 36.33 | 29.43 | 44.44 | 29.43 | 58.44 | −48.50 |

ND, not determined; NG, naringenin; VLDL, very low density lipoprotein; LDL, low density lipoprotein; HDL, high density lipoprotein. Negative values means an augmentation of the parameter in comparison with untreated cholestatic animals.

Flavonoids showed a good performance in hepatoprotection since almost all compounds showed a marked serum decrease of the liver and ductal enzymes (about 50% on average). In accordance with these data, it seems that genistein (5 µg/rat/day, p.o.) and quercetin (150 µmol/kg/day, i.p.) had a better performance than other flavonoids; however, intraperitoneal high dose (about 45 mg daily), and a confusing mode of administration (it began four weeks before biliary obstruction and was continued for a further four weeks) were inconclusive [25,26].

It is important to mention that quantification of metabolic biomarkers such as cholesterol, depicts indirect improvements on bile acid synthesis; however, metabolites such as glucose, triglycerides, and lipoproteins might determine a correct function of the liver, since this organ plays a central role in lipid and carbohydrate metabolism [24]. As seen above, few investigations consider metabolic parameters as pivotal endpoints for the evaluation of efficacy. Only three studies measured serum cholesterol, two measured triglycerides, and one measured lipoprotein content (LDL and HDL) (Table 3).

Further, it was remarkable to consider that risk of bias assessment show that the majority of studies assessed had a high risk for selection, performance, and detection biases (Figure S1). This evidence exposes an unmet need to improve the quality of the experimental protocols for most confident information in drug discovery. This was another reason for not including a meta-analysis in this investigation.

### 3.2. Experimental Study

#### 3.2.1. Signature of Obstructive Cholestasis in the Rat

As reported, bile duct obstruction produced significant alterations in serum biomarkers concentration compared with sham-operated rats. Major alterations were decrease of glucose (Figure 3a) and HDL (Figure 3d), as well as increase of total cholesterol (Figure 3b), LDL (Figure 3d), and bilirrubin (Figure 4d) in comparison with the sham group. Triglycerides and VLDL concentrations were unaltered similar to the report by Stedman et al. [27]. Increase of liver enzymes ALT and AST, and bile ductal enzymes GGT and AP were determinant for cholestatic liver disease signature in BDL (Figure 4), due to hepatocellular damage produced by high concentrations of toxic bile acids [28].

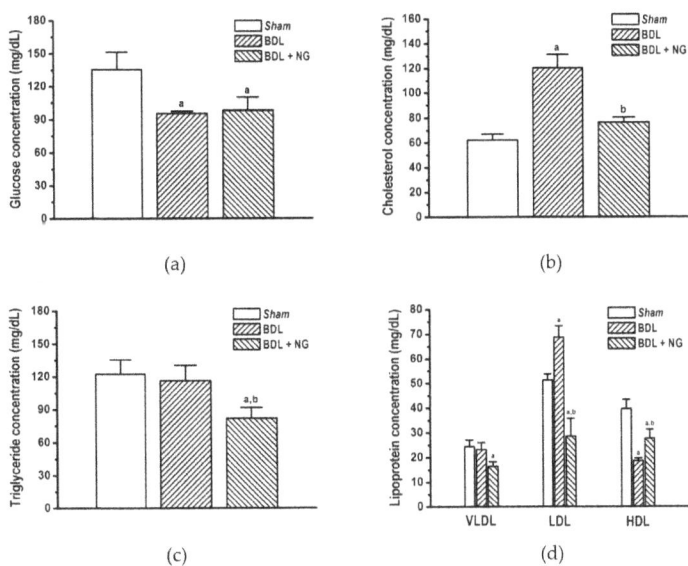

**Figure 3.** Metabolic biomarkers quantified on bile duct-ligated (BDL) model after administration of naringenin (NG, 50 mg/kg/day) for 10 days. (**a**) Glucose, (**b**) total cholesterol, (**c**) triglycerides, (**d**) lipoprotein (very low-density lipoprotein (VLDL), low-density lipoprotein (LDL), and high-density lipoprotein (HDL)). Data are expressed as means ± SEM ($n$ = 8–10). a: Significantly different from sham control group at $p < 0.05$, and b: Significantly different from BDL group at $p < 0.05$.

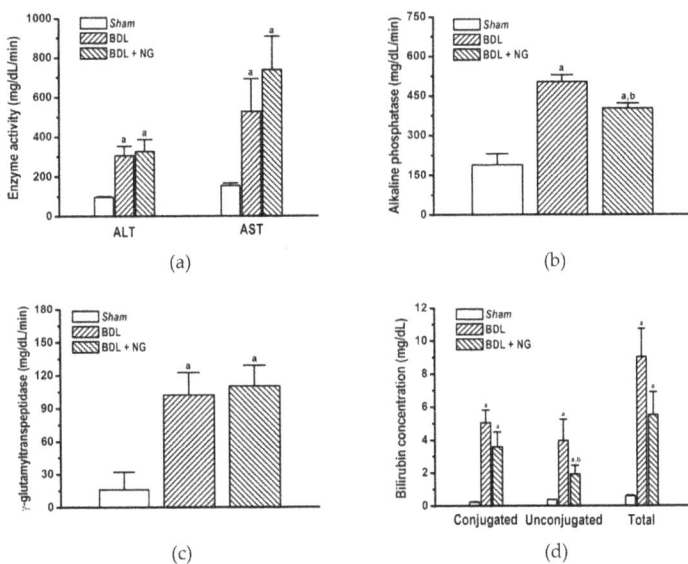

**Figure 4.** Liver function and cholestasis biomarkers quantified on bile duct-ligated (BDL) model after administration of naringenin (NG, 50 mg/kg/day) for 10 days. (**a**) Transaminases (ALT and AST), (**b**) alkaline phosphatase, (**c**) γ-glutamyltranspeptidase (**d**), and bilirubin were expressed from each group. Data are expressed as means ± SEM ($n$ = 8–10). a: Significantly different from sham control group at $p < 0.05$, and b: Significantly different from BDL group at $p < 0.05$.

### 3.2.2. Efficacy of NG in Obstructive Cholestasis

Naringenin significantly improved serum cholesterol (Figure 4b) and low and high-density lipoproteins (Figure 4d) in the BDL model. Interestingly, despite triglycerides and VLDL were not modified on cholestatic damage, this flavonoid decreased both parameters. Additionally, significant decrease in bilirubin (Figure 4d) and AP activity (Figure 4b) suggests an improvement of liver and bile duct damage.

Finally, biochemical improvements attributed to NG allowed reduced mortality. By contrast, body weight changes along time had no modification. In fact, treated BDL rats suffered more weight loss than the BDL group (Figure 5).

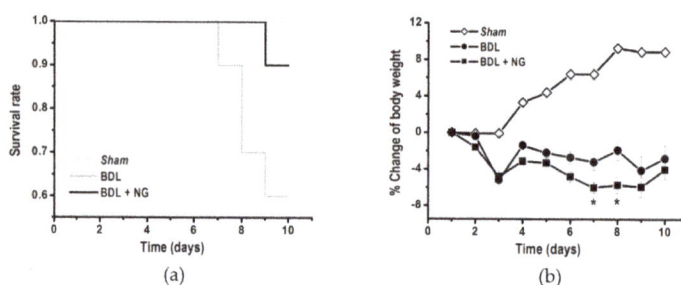

**Figure 5.** Survival rate (**a**), and percentage change of body weight (**b**) measured after administration of naringenin (NG, 50 mg/kg/day) for 10 days. *Significantly different from bile duct-ligated (BDL) group at $p < 0.05$ ($n = 10$ animals/group).

## 4. Discussion

Flavonoids are naturally occurring compounds with beneficial health effects in chronic diseases, being cardiovascular and metabolic diseases that are better characterized. Further, higher intake of these compounds has been associated with lower mortality rates from specific vascular diseases and cancer [29]. The importance of flavonoid-rich foods consumption in preventing cholestasis mortality remains uncertain. For this reason, we aimed to show the state-of-the-art of flavonoids for the drug design of new anti-cholestatic agents through a systematic review.

Currently, some articles have applied systematic searching in order to analyze proficiency of natural products on specific illnesses (e.g. triterpenes on wound healing) [30]. Recently, Chen et al. reviewed phenylated flavonoids and their biological effects; this investigation focused on structural properties of the phenylated flavonoids and the implication in biological activity. However, no evidence was found on cholestatic liver disease or liver disease related abnormalities [13]. For this reason, the anti-cholestatic effect of flavonoids remains an outstanding issue in drug discovery.

Silymarin has been the most studied flavonoid for liver disease. This extract has been characterized as a potent antioxidant, immunomodulatory, and anti-fibrotic agent indicated as adjuvant treatment for all-causes liver disorders [11]. Our analysis shows that one major component of this extract, silibinin or silybin, improved serum transaminase, AP, and bilirubin in BDL model; which is possible by a decrease of pro-inflammatory lipids (platelet-activating factor, PAF), and improved activity and expression of both lysophosphatidylcholine acyltransferase LPCAT1 and LPCAT2, key enzymes in PAF remodeling [31]. Despite evidence, there is no more investigation about flavonoid-based therapeutic interventions for the treatment of cholestasis. This situation suggests an opportunity for medicinal chemists, computer-aided designers, or organic chemists to evaluate flavonoid as a potential scaffold for new lead compounds.

Our database search shows no evidence for evaluation of flavonoids efficacy and safety in a clinical setting. Only a pilot study ($n = 27$) was found where oral silymarin was assessed in UDCA non-responsive primary biliary cirrhosis (PBC) patients. Despite UDCA therapy for 52.6 ± 10.4

months, elevation of AP activity (2 times above normal) was persistent, neither adjuvant therapy with silymarin improved clinical endpoints [11]. In this context, diosmin, quercetin, or genistein should be good options since these flavonoids decreased AP activity 40–50% (Table 2). However, more clinical investigation is still needed to assess this potential.

On the other hand, eleven reports were retrieved from systematic search. The analysis showed a variety of administration and time framework, i.e., some reported pre-operative (one week) and post-operative (three weeks) administration [19,20]. This approach might bias in the therapeutic effect assessment, since it began one week before a cholestatic pattern is established. Additionally, animal species were different and possibly crucial for biological behavior. The most used is the Wistar rat (six studies) followed by Sprague Dawley (three studies). Despite Sprague Dawley was developed from Wistar strain, data show that Wistar strain is prone for metabolic impairments [32]. This should be relevant in taking into account the metabolic component of cholestasis [33,34].

As mentioned, metabolic impairment is a pivotal alteration on obstructive cholestasis. Alterations in glucose, cholesterol, LDL, and HDL were observed in the BDL group (Figure 4). Modification of cholesterol and lipoprotein on cholestasis by bile duct ligation surgery is known [35]; also, high concentration of plasma insulin [36,37] and low concentration of glucose [38] have been reported for this model. In contrast, other studies reported contradictory values suggesting a wide metabolic disparity between species, rodent strain, and time of damage exposure [38,39]. In addition, it has been established that intrahepatic cholestasis of pregnancy (ICP) and PBC are associated with impaired metabolic profile, including glucose intolerance and dyslipidemia [33,34]. Our analysis showed few data on metabolic parameters for BDL (Table 3).

This is the first time that NG is evaluated in a BDL model, despite that a simple review about beneficial effects of this flavonoid in ethanol- and carbon tetrachloride-induced liver diseases and its putative mechanisms was published with no evidence about obstructive cholestasis [40]. Mulvihill and colleagues reported similar effects in their studies using LDL receptor-null ($LDL^{-/-}$) mice fed with a Western high caloric diet, which expressed metabolic impairments as dyslipidemia (increased VLDL and LDL), hyperinsulinemia, and weight gain vs. wild-type littermates. Treatment with NG 1% or 3% (wt/wt) improved triglyceride, total cholesterol, and lipoprotein concentrations after four weeks. In contrast, HDL was unaltered in animals with the Western diet, and NG did not modify this condition [41]. Our findings contribute for the beneficial metabolic effects induced by this flavonoid, taking into account that cholestasis have a distinct etiology and target organ than the diet-induced dyslipidemia.

Finally, the precise mechanism by which flavonoids exert their hepatoprotective effects is unclear yet. However, there is evidence suggesting that flavonoids might improve imbalance in oxidant/antioxidant status. For example, Kabirifar et al. reported that quercetin might improve the antioxidant capacity of the liver tissue by decreasing the activity of NADPH oxidase 1 (NOX1), a major intracellular producer of reactive oxygen species [42], and the expression of its activator Rac1. Further, an increase of the antioxidant enzymes catalase and glutathione superoxide dismutase (SOD) was reported [43]. Lin et al. showed similar evidences where an elevated mRNA expression of Mn-SOD, Cu/Zn-SOD, and catalase was observed. [19] On the other hand, it has been reported that flavonoids exert a regulation of inflammatory response and deposition of extracellular matrix by the decrease of mitogenic IL-1β and fibrogenic TGF-β1 expression and down-regulated BDL-induced hepatic Smad2/3 phosphorylation. [19] More investigation must be encouraged to promote comprehensive studies that describe the beneficial effects of flavonoids and its mechanism.

## 5. Conclusions

Flavonoids comprise a group of natural products with promising efficacy for the management of cholestatic liver disease. More clinical and experimental investigation should be driven to promote the drug design of flavonoid-based pharmaceuticals for the treatment of these pathologies with the lowest risk of bias. Naringenin is a flavonoid with specific beneficial effects on liver function and metabolic flow altered in cholestasis. Further investigation needs is required to characterize its pharmacological mechanism and applicability in a clinical setting.

**Supplementary Materials:** The following are available online at http://www.mdpi.com/2218-273X/9/3/102/s1, Figure S1: SYRCLE's tool for assessing risk of bias of the selected studies, Table S1: PICO strategy developed for systematic review.

**Author Contributions:** J.C.S.-S.; methodology, data curacy, writing first draft, S.E.-S; validation, supervision, administration of the project, S.G.-J; methodology, S.M.; methodology, J.G.-Z; methodology, and R.V.-M.; supervision, verification.

**Funding:** This study was financed by a grant from CONACYT (SEP-2003-C02-43440/280) and PROMEP-SEP. J.C.S.-S. is a CONACYT fellow (reference number: 198277).

**Acknowledgments:** Juan Carlos Sánchez-Salgado and Samuel Estrada-Soto belong to Red Nacional de Investigación Preclínica de Productos Naturales.

**Conflicts of Interest:** All authors declare do not have some conflict of interest.

## References

1. Williams, R. Global challenges in liver disease. *Hepatology* **2006**, *44*, 521–526. [CrossRef]
2. Araújo, A.R.; Rosso, N.; Bedogni, G.; Tiribelli, C.; Bellentani, S. Global epidemiology of non-alcoholic fatty liver disease/non-alcoholic steatohepatitis: What we need in the future. *Liver Int.* **2018**, *38*, 47–51. [CrossRef]
3. Abshagen, K.; König, M.; Hoppe, A.; Müller, I.; Ebert, M.; Weng, H.; Holzhütter, H.-G.; Zanger, U.M.; Bode, J.; Vollmar, B.; et al. Pathobiochemical signatures of cholestatic liver disease in bile duct ligated mice. *BMC Syst. Biol.* **2015**, *9*, 83. [CrossRef] [PubMed]
4. Heathcote, E.J. Diagnosis and management of cholestatic liver disease. *Clin. Gastroenterol. Hepatol.* **2007**, *5*, 776–782. [CrossRef] [PubMed]
5. Bosoi, C.R.; Oliveira, M.M.; Ochoa-Sanchez, R.; Tremblay, M.; Ten Have, G.A.; Deutz, N.E.; Rose, C.F.; Bemeur, C. The bile duct ligated rat: A relevant model to study muscle mass loss in cirrhosis. *Metab. Brain Dis.* **2017**, *32*, 513–518. [CrossRef] [PubMed]
6. Wang, H.; Vohra, B.P.S.; Zhang, Y.; Heuckeroth, R.O. Transcriptional profiling after bile duct ligation identifies PAI-1 as a contributor to cholestatic injury in mice. *Hepatology* **2005**, *42*, 1099–1108. [CrossRef] [PubMed]
7. Rudic, J.S.; Poropat, G.; Krstic, M.N.; Bjelakovic, G.; Gluud, C. Ursodeoxycholic acid for primary biliary cirrhosis. *Cochrane Database Syst. Rev.* **2012**, *12*, CD000551. [CrossRef] [PubMed]
8. Thompson, J.N.; Cohen, J.; Blenkharn, J.I.; McConnell, J.S.; Barr, J.; Blumgart, L.H. A randomized clinical trial of oral ursodeoxycholic acid in obstructive jaundice. *Br. J. Surg.* **1986**, *73*, 634–636. [CrossRef]
9. Federico, A.; Dallio, M.; Loguercio, C. Silymarin/Silybin and Chronic Liver Disease: A Marriage of Many Years. *Molecules* **2017**, *22*, 191. [CrossRef] [PubMed]
10. Crocenzi, F.A.; Roma, M.G. Silymarin as a new hepatoprotective agent in experimental cholestasis: New possibilities for an ancient medication. *Curr. Med. Chem.* **2006**, *13*, 1055–1074. [CrossRef]
11. Angulo, P.; Patel, T.; Jorgensen, R.A.; Therneau, T.M.; Lindor, K.D. Silymarin in the treatment of patients with primary biliary cirrhosis with a suboptimal response to ursodeoxycholic acid. *Hepatology* **2000**, *32*, 897–900. [CrossRef] [PubMed]
12. Schuler, J.; Hudson, M.L.; Schwartz, D.; Samudrala, R. A Systematic Review of Computational Drug Discovery, Development, and Repurposing for Ebola Virus Disease Treatment. *Molecules* **2017**, *22*, 177. [CrossRef] [PubMed]
13. Chen, X.; Mukwaya, E.; Wong, M.-S.; Zhang, Y. A systematic review on biological activities of prenylated flavonoids. *Pharm. Biol.* **2014**, *52*, 655–660. [CrossRef]
14. Sánchez-Salgado, J.C.; Ortiz-Andrade, R.R.; Aguirre-Crespo, F.; Vergara-Galicia, J.; León-Rivera, I.; Montes, S.; Villalobos-Molina, R.; Estrada-Soto, S. Hypoglycemic, vasorelaxant and hepatoprotective effects of Cochlospermum vitifolium (Willd) Sprengel: A potential agent for the treatment of metabolic syndrome. *J. Ethnopharmacol.* **2007**, *109*, 400–405.
15. Sánchez-Salgado, J.C.; Castillo-España, P.; Ibarra-Barajas, M.; Villalobos-Molina, R.; Estrada-Soto, S. Cochlospermum vitifolium induces vasorelaxant and antihypertensive effects mainly by activation of NO/cGMP signaling pathway. *J. Ethnopharmacol.* **2010**, *130*, 477–484. [CrossRef] [PubMed]

16. Aguilar-Guadarrama, A.B.; Rios, M.Y. Flavonoids, Sterols and Lignans from Cochlospermum vitifolium and Their Relationship with Its Liver Activity. *Molecules* **2018**, *23*, 1952. [CrossRef] [PubMed]

17. Hooijmans, C.R.; Rovers, M.M.; de Vries, R.B.M.; Leenaars, M.; Ritskes-Hoitinga, M.; Langendam, M.W. SYRCLE's risk of bias tool for animal studies. *BMC Med. Res. Methodol.* **2014**, *14*, 43. [CrossRef]

18. Rivera-Mancía, S.; Montes, S.; Méndez-Armenta, M.; Muriel, P.; Ríos, C. Morphological changes of rat astrocytes induced by liver damage but not by manganese chloride exposure. *Metab. Brain. Dis.* **2009**, *24*, 243–255. [CrossRef]

19. Lin, S.-Y.; Wang, Y.-Y.; Chen, W.-Y.; Chuang, Y.-H.; Pan, P.-H.; Chen, C.-J. Beneficial effect of quercetin on cholestatic liver injury. *J. Nutr. Biochem.* **2014**, *25*, 1183–1195. [CrossRef]

20. Pan, P.-H.; Lin, S.-Y.; Wang, Y.-Y.; Chen, W.-Y.; Chuang, Y.-H.; Wu, C.-C.; Chen, C.-J. Protective effects of rutin on liver injury induced by biliary obstruction in rats. *Free Radic. Biol. Med.* **2014**, *73*, 106–116. [CrossRef]

21. Zahran, M.H.; Hussein, A.M.; Barakat, N.; Awadalla, A.; Khater, S.; Harraz, A.; Shokeir, A.A. Sildenafil activates antioxidant and antiapoptotic genes and inhibits proinflammatory cytokine genes in a rat model of renal ischemia/reperfusion injury. *Int. Urol. Nephrol.* **2015**, *47*, 1907–1915. [CrossRef] [PubMed]

22. Kaur, M.; Singh, A.; Kumar, B.; Singh, S.K.; Bhatia, A.; Gulati, M.; Prakash, T.; Bawa, P.; Malik, A.H. Protective effect of co-administration of curcumin and sildenafil in alcohol induced neuropathy in rats. *Eur. J. Pharmacol.* **2017**, *805*, 58–66. [CrossRef]

23. Ali, F.E.M.; Azouz, A.A.; Bakr, A.G.; Abo-Youssef, A.M.; Hemeida, R.A.M. Hepatoprotective effects of diosmin and/or sildenafil against cholestatic liver cirrhosis: The role of Keap-1/Nrf-2 and P38-MAPK/NF-κB/iNOS signaling pathway. *Food Chem. Toxicol.* **2018**, *120*, 294–304. [CrossRef] [PubMed]

24. Lawrence, Y.A.; Steiner, J.M. Laboratory Evaluation of the Liver. *Vet. Clin. North Am. Small Anim. Pract.* **2017**, *47*, 539–553. [CrossRef] [PubMed]

25. Salas, A.L.; Ocampo, G.; Fariña, G.G.; Reyes-Esparza, J.; Rodríguez-Fragoso, L. Genistein decreases liver fibrosis and cholestasis induced by prolonged biliary obstruction in the rat. *Ann. Hepatol.* **2007**, *6*, 41–47.

26. Peres, W.; Tuñón, M.J.; Collado, P.S.; Herrmann, S.; Marroni, N.; González-Gallego, J. The flavonoid quercetin ameliorates liver damage in rats with biliary obstruction. *J. Hepatol.* **2000**, *33*, 742–750. [CrossRef]

27. Stedman, C.; Liddle, C.; Coulter, S.; Sonoda, J.; Alvarez, J.G.; Evans, R.M.; Downes, M. Benefit of farnesoid X receptor inhibition in obstructive cholestasis. *Proc. Natl. Acad. Sci. USA* **2006**, *103*, 11323–11328. [CrossRef]

28. Higuchi, H.; Gores, G.J. Bile acid regulation of hepatic physiology: IV. Bile acids and death receptors. *Am. J. Physiol. Gastrointest. Liver Physiol.* **2003**, *284*, G734–G738.

29. Ivey, K.L.; Jensen, M.K.; Hodgson, J.M.; Eliassen, A.H.; Cassidy, A.; Rimm, E.B. Association of flavonoid-rich foods and flavonoids with risk of all-cause mortality. *Br. J. Nutr.* **2017**, *117*, 1470–1477. [CrossRef]

30. Agra, L.C.; Ferro, J.N.S.; Barbosa, F.T.; Barreto, E. Triterpenes with healing activity: A systematic review. *J. Dermatolog. Treat.* **2015**, *26*, 465–470. [CrossRef]

31. Stanca, E.; Serviddio, G.; Bellanti, F.; Vendemiale, G.; Siculella, L.; Giudetti, A.M. Down-regulation of LPCAT expression increases platelet-activating factor level in cirrhotic rat liver: potential antiinflammatory effect of silybin. *Biochim. Biophys. Acta.* **2013**, *1832*, 2019–2026. [CrossRef] [PubMed]

32. Marques, C.; Meireles, M.; Norberto, S.; Leite, J.; Freitas, J.; Pestana, D.; Faria, A.; Calhau, C. High-fat diet-induced obesity Rat model: A comparison between Wistar and Sprague-Dawley Rat. *Adipocyte* **2015**, *5*, 11–21. [CrossRef] [PubMed]

33. Menżyk, T.; Bator, M.; Derra, A.; Kierach, R.; Kukla, M. The role of metabolic disorders in the pathogenesis of intrahepatic cholestasis of pregnancy. *Clin. Exp. Hepatol.* **2018**, *4*, 217–223. [CrossRef] [PubMed]

34. Vignoli, A.; Orlandini, B.; Tenori, L.; Biagini, M.R.; Milani, S.; Renzi, D.; Luchinat, C.; Calabrò, A.S. The metabolic signature of Primary Biliary Cholangitis and its comparison with Coeliac Disease. *J. Proteome Res.* **2018**, *18*, 1228–1236. [CrossRef] [PubMed]

35. Bauer, J.E.; Meyer, D.J.; Campbell, M.; McMurphy, R. Serum lipid and lipoprotein changes in ponies with experimentally induced liver disease. *Am. J. Vet. Res.* **1990**, *51*, 1380–1384.

36. Jessen, N.; Buhl, E.S.; Schmitz, O.; Lund, S. Impaired insulin action despite upregulation of proximal insulin signaling: novel insights into skeletal muscle insulin resistance in liver cirrhosis. *J. Hepatol.* **2006**, *45*, 797–804. [CrossRef] [PubMed]

37. Lin, S.-Y.; Sheu, W.H.-H.; Chen, W.-Y.; Lee, F.-Y.; Huang, C.-J. Stimulated resistin expression in white adipose of rats with bile duct ligation-induced liver cirrhosis: relationship to cirrhotic hyperinsulinemia and increased tumor necrosis factor-alpha. *Mol. Cell. Endocrinol.* **2005**, *232*, 1–8. [CrossRef]

38. Enochsson, L.; Isaksson, B.; Strömmer, L.; Erlanson-Albertsson, C.; Permert, J. Bile duct obstruction is associated with early postoperative upregulation of liver uncoupling protein-2 and reduced circulating glucose concentration in the rat. *Nutrition* **2010**, *26*, 405–410. [CrossRef]
39. Catala, J.; Daumas, M.; Chanh, A.P.; Lasserre, B.; Hollande, E. Insulin and glucagon impairments in relation with islet cells morphological modifications following long term pancreatic duct ligation in the rabbit–a model of non-insulin-dependent diabetes. *Int. J. Exp. Diabetes Res.* **2001**, *2*, 101–112. [CrossRef]
40. Hernández-Aquino, E.; Muriel, P. Beneficial effects of naringenin in liver diseases: Molecular mechanisms. *World J. Gastroenterol.* **2018**, *24*, 1679–1707. [CrossRef]
41. Mulvihill, E.E.; Allister, E.M.; Sutherland, B.G.; Telford, D.E.; Sawyez, C.G.; Edwards, J.Y.; Markle, J.M.; Hegele, R.A.; Huff, M.W. Naringenin prevents dyslipidemia, apolipoprotein B overproduction, and hyperinsulinemia in LDL receptor-null mice with diet-induced insulin resistance. *Diabetes* **2009**, *58*, 2198–2210. [CrossRef] [PubMed]
42. Choi, S.S.; Sicklick, J.K.; Ma, Q.; Yang, L.; Huang, J.; Qi, Y.; Chen, W.; Li, Y.-X.; Goldschmidt-Clermont, P.J.; Diehl, A.M. Sustained activation of Rac1 in hepatic stellate cells promotes liver injury and fibrosis in mice. *Hepatology* **2006**, *44*, 1267–1277. [CrossRef] [PubMed]
43. Kabirifar, R.; Ghoreshi, Z.-A.-S.; Safari, F.; Karimollah, A.; Moradi, A.; Eskandari-Nasab, E. Quercetin protects liver injury induced by bile duct ligation via attenuation of Rac1 and NADPH oxidase1 expression in rats. *HBPD INT* **2017**, *16*, 88–95. [CrossRef]

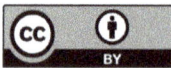

*biomolecules*

MDPI

*Article*

# Synthesis of a Novel α-Glucosyl Ginsenoside F1 by Cyclodextrin Glucanotransferase and Its In Vitro Cosmetic Applications

Seong Soo Moon [1,†], Hye Jin Lee [1,†], Ramya Mathiyalagan [2], Yu Jin Kim [1], Dong Uk Yang [1,3], Dae Young Lee [4], Jin Woo Min [1], Zuly Jimenez [2] and Deok Chun Yang [1,2,*]

[1]   Department of Oriental Medicinal Biotechnology, College of Life Science, Kyung Hee University, 1 Seocheon-dong, Giheung-gu, Yongin-si, Gyeonggi-do 17104, Korea; ssm8656@hanmail.net (S.S.M.); serendipity27@nate.com (H.J.L.); yujinkim@khu.ac.kr (Y.J.K.); rudckfeo23@naver.com (D.U.Y.); hero304@khu.ac.kr (J.W.M.)

[2]   Graduate School of Biotechnology, College of Life Science, Kyung Hee University, 1 Seocheon-dong, Giheung-gu, Yongin-si, Gyeonggi-do 17104, Korea; ramyabinfo@gmail.com (R.M.); zejp78@gmail.com (Z.J.)

[3]   K-gen (corp), 218, Gajeong-ro, Yuseong-gu, Daejeon 34129, Korea

[4]   Department of Herbal Crop Research, National Institute of Horticultural and Herbal Science, RDA, Eumseong 27709, Korea; dylee0809@gmail.com

*   Correspondence: dcyang@khu.ac.kr; Tel.: +82-31-201-2100; Fax: +82-31-205-2688

†   These authors contributed equally to this work.

Received: 28 August 2018; Accepted: 30 October 2018; Published: 10 November 2018

**Abstract:** Ginsenosides from *Panax ginseng* (Korean ginseng) are unique triterpenoidal saponins that are considered to be responsible for most of the pharmacological activities of *P. ginseng*. However, the various linkage positions cause different pharmacological activities. In this context, we aimed to synthesize new derivatives of ginsenosides with unusual linkages that show enhanced pharmacological activities. Novel α-glycosylated derivatives of ginsenoside F1 were synthesized from transglycosylation reactions of dextrin (sugar donor) and ginsenoside F1 (acceptor) by the successive actions of Toruzyme®3.0L, a cyclodextrin glucanotransferase. One of the resultant products was isolated and identified as (20S)-3β,6α,12β-trihydroxydammar-24ene-(20-O-β-D-glucopyranosyl-(1→2)-α-D-glucopyranoside) by various spectroscopic characterization techniques of fast atom bombardment-mass spectrometry (FAB-MS), infrared spectroscopy (IR), proton-nuclear magnetic resonance ($^1$H-NMR), $^{13}$C-NMR, gradient heteronuclear single quantum coherence (gHSQC), and gradient heteronuclear multiple bond coherence (gHMBC). As expected, the novel α-glycosylated ginsenoside F1 (G1-F1) exhibited increased solubility, lower cytotoxicity toward human dermal fibroblast cells (HDF), and higher tyrosinase activity and ultraviolet A (UVA)-induced inhibitory activity against matrix metalloproteinase-1 (MMP-1) than ginsenoside F1. Since F1 has been reported as an antiaging and antioxidant agent, the enhanced efficacies of the novel α-glycosylated ginsenoside F1 suggest that it might be useful in cosmetic applications after screening.

**Keywords:** cyclodextrin glycosyltransferase; cyclodextrin glycosyltransferase (CGTase); ginsenoside F1; α-glucosyl ginsenoside F1

## 1. Introduction

Ginseng saponins, referred to as ginsenosides, are one of the major bioactive substances of *Panax ginseng* Meyer, a commonly used traditional herbal medicine in Korea, China, and Japan. Ginsenosides have been reported to have antifatigue and antioxidant activities, improve brain function, enhance stamina, and regulate blood circulation with approval from the Korea Food and Drug Administration (KFDA), in addition to various other pharmacological activities including anticancer [1,2],

*Biomolecules* **2018**, *8*, 142

anti-inflammation [3], and antidiabetes [1,4] functions. These various pharmacological activities of ginsenosides typically depend on the types of sugar moieties and the position and linkage of their attachment [4,5]. More than 289 distinct saponins had been identified from different *Panax* sp. up to 2012 [6], and these compounds show different biological activities based on structural differences [3].

Ginsenosides are mainly classified as protopanaxadiol-type (PPD), protopanaxatriol-type (PPT), and oleanane-type saponins and further grouped into major and minor saponins based on the position and linkages of sugar moieties. The minor saponins, which are ginsenoside metabolites, are responsible for most of the pharmacological activities of ginseng which include ginsenoside F1, Rh1, compound K, and Rh2 [7]. These ginsenosides are mainly absorbed into systemic circulation [8]. Ginsenoside F1 is a minor saponin from the leaf of *P. ginseng* that was reported to have skin whitening activity [9], modulate skin diseases [10], and function as an antiaging and antioxidant agent [11], suggesting that it might be a candidate for cosmetic applications.

Synthesis of novel and diversified compounds is a way to extend the efficacy of natural products. Such diversity can be generated by biosynthetic reactions such as glucosylation [12,13]. Especially, enzymatic glycosylation provides more regioselectiveness than conventional chemical synthesis [14]. A number of reports have suggested that transglycosylation by enzymes can be used to improve physiochemical functions such as taste, solubility in water, and oxidative stability of numerous active substances [15,16]. Among these enzymes, cyclodextrin glycosyltransferase (CGTase), 1,4-α-D-glucan: 1,4-α-D-glycopyranosyltransferase, cyclizing, EC 2.4.1.19) [17] has been reported to accelerate reactions between natural products and starch hydrolysate or β-cyclodextrin to produce glucosylated modifications of natural compounds such as hesperidin, glycosylglycerol [14,16] rutin [18], and steroidal saponins [19].

Although the beta isomer was prominent, the alpha isomer has attracted much attention in recent years. The increased solubility of hesperidin [16,18] and decreased bitterness of glycosylated stevioside [15] by CGTase was reported. Other studies reported the mild sweet taste with no odor, no tongue-pricking, and increased stability of O-α-glucosylthiamin compared with thiamin hydrochloride [20] and the powerful skin whitening activity of alpha arbutin [21] compared with beta arbutin [22] as a result of glycosylation by CGTase.

In this study, we aimed to synthesize the unusual alpha glycosylated ginsenoside F1 by a reaction involving ginsenoside F1, dextrin, and CGTase. One of the resultant novel compounds was purified, and the structure was elucidated by various nuclear magnetic resonance (NMR) spectra and Fourier-transform infrared spectroscopy (FTIR). We also evaluated the cytotoxicity and protective effect of α-glycosylated ginsenoside F1 against ultraviolet (UV) damage by measuring matrix metalloproteinase-1 (MMP-1) expression in human dermal fibroblast cells. In addition, the in vitro antityrosinase activity of α-glycosylated ginsenoside F1 was evaluated against mushroom tyrosinase.

## 2. Materials and Methods

### 2.1. Materials

Ginsenosides compound K (CK), Rh2, Rh1, F1, aglycone PPD (aPPD), and aglycone PPT (aPPT) were obtained from the laboratory of Hanbangbio, Kyung Hee University, South Korea. Toruzyme 3.0L (the crude enzyme of CGTase) obtained from Novozymes, China, was extracted from *Thermoanaerobacter* sp. Dextrin was supplied by Fluka Chemie AG (Buchs, Switzerland), and all the other chemicals used were of analytical grade and from commercial sources.

### 2.2. Biotransformation

The preliminary screening of glycosylation was carried out as the method of Wang et al., 2010 [19]. Different ginsenosides, CK (1.6 mM, 1 eq), Rh2 (1.6 mM, 1 eq), Rh1 (1.56 mM,1 eq), F1 (1.56 mM, 1 eq), aPPD (2.17 mM), and aPPT (2.09 mM) together with the sugar donor dextrin (9.9mM, 6 eq, 10–15 units of glucose) were dissolved in 20 mM sodium phosphate buffer (1 mL, pH 7.0). Next, 25 µL of Toruzyme® 3.0L with initial activity of 3.0 KNU (kilo novo units)/g [17] was added to the reaction mixture and reacted at 50 °C for 2 h. and kept in boiling water for 5 min to inactivate the enzyme. The mixture was extracted three times with an equal volume of *n*-butanol, and the *n*-butanol layer was washed twice with distilled water to remove excess dextrin, dried in a rotary evaporator under vacuum [19], and dissolved in methanol for thin-layer chromatography (TLC).

## 2.3. Glycosylation of Ginsenoside F1

For further experimental analysis, F1 was used as a substrate. The effects of different concentrations of dextrin (0–7 mg) and Toruzyme® (5–30 μL) and different reaction durations (0.5–3 h) on specificity of F1 glycosylation were examined using the procedure described above. For purification of glycosylated F1, F1 (500 mg, 1.56 mM, 1 eq) and dextrin (2g, 7.92 mM, 5 eq) were dissolved in 500 mL of 20 mM sodium phosphate buffer and then treated with 15 mL of Toruzyme® 3.0 L.

## 2.4. Identification of Glycosylated Ginsenoside F1

Semiqualitative screening of the glycosylated products was carried out by TLC and high-performance liquid chromatography (HPLC) was carried out by Ramya et al., 2015 and Quan et al., 2012 [13,23] with slight modifications. TLC was performed with silica gel plates (60 F254, Merck, Darmstadt, Germany) using the developing solvent $CHCl_3$:$CH_3OH$:$H_2O$ (65:35:10, *v/v*, lower phase). The TLC plates were dried, dipped in 10% $H_2SO_4$, and air dried with heating at 110 to 120 °C. The HPLC analysis was carried out on an Agilent 1260 series with a $C_{18}$ (250 × 4.6 mm, ID 5 μm) column using distilled water as solvent A and acetonitrile as solvent B mobile phases. The following gradient was used: A:B ratios of 80.5:19.5 for 0–29 min, 70:30 for 29–36 min, 68:32 for 36–45 min, 66:34 for 45–47 min, 64.5:35.5 for 47–49 min, 0:100 for 49–61 min, and 80.5:19.5 for 61–66 min with a flow rate of 1.6 mL/min. The sample was detected at a wavelength of 203 nm.

## 2.5. Nuclear Magnetic Resonance Analysis

Structural elucidation of the new compound by NMR spectra ($^1$H NMR, $^{13}$C NMR, gHSQC (heteronuclear single quantum correlation) and heteronuclear multiple bond correlation (gHMBC)) were performed using a Varian Unity INOVA AS 400 FT-NMR spectrometer (Varian, Palo Alto, CA, USA), and chemical shifts were expressed in δ (ppm), with tetramethylsilane (TMS) used as an internal standard. The dimethyl sulfoxide-$d_6$ (DMSO-$d_6$) was used as a solvent. Melting points were obtained using a Fisher-John's melting point apparatus. Optical rotations were measured on a JASCO P-1010 digital polarimeter. Infrared spectra were obtained on a Perkin Elmer Spectrum One FTIR spectrometer (Perkin-Elmer, Walthanm, MA, USA). High resolution fast-atom bombardment mass spectrometry (HR-FAB/MS) were recorded using a JEOL JMS-700 (JEOL, Tokyo, Japan) mass spectrometer.

## 2.6. Cell Lines and Cell Culture

Human dermal fibroblasts (HDF) were purchased from the Korean Cell Line Bank (Seoul, Korea). The cells were grown in Dulbecco's modified essential media (DMEM) supplemented with 10% fetal bovine serum (FBS) and 1% penicillin–streptomycin at 37 °C in a humidified atmosphere containing 95% air and 5% $CO_2$.

### 2.6.1. Ultraviolet Irradiation and Sample Treatment

A high-pressure metal halide lamp (UVASUN 3000, Mutzhas, Munich, Germany) emitting wavelengths in the range of 340 to 450 nm was used as a UV source. Human dermal fibroblasts cells were seeded at 4 × 10 cell/dish in 60-mm culture dishes for 24 h. Prior to UV irradiation, cells were washed twice with phosphate buffer saline (PBS), and the medium was replaced with 1 mL of PBS. The incident dose at the surface of the cells was 66 mW/s. The spectral distribution of the

UVASUN 3000 source was determined with a Beckman UV 5270 spectrophotometer (Beckman, Munich, Germany, FRG).

### 2.6.2. Cytotoxicity Assay

Human dermal fibroblasts cells were cultured at a density of $1 \times 10^4$ cells/well in 96-well flat-bottomed plates in a 5% $CO_2$ humidified atmosphere at 37 °C. After 24 h of culture, the medium was exchanged with medium containing different concentrations of ginsenoside F1 (F1) and α-glycosylated ginsenoside F1 (Glycosylated F1), and the cells were incubated for a further 24 h. Cell viability was determined by the 3-(4,5-dimethylthiazol-2-yl)-2,5-diphenyltetrazolium bromide (MTT) assay [24] with slight modification. Briefly, 10 μL of MTT solution (5 mg/mL) was added to each well and incubated for 4 h. After removal of MTT, the cells were lysed with 100 μL DMSO, and absorbance was measured at 570 nm using a microplate reader (Bio-Tek Instruments, Winooski, VT, USA).

### 2.6.3. In Vitro Tyrosinase Inhibition Activity

Tyrosinase from *Agricus bisporus* (mushroom) was purchased from Sigma Chemicals Co. (St Louis, MO, USA). Inhibition of tyrosinase activity was measured as previously described [22]. L-DOPA (3-(3,4-dihydroxyphenyl)-L-alanine, 0.83 or 3.3 mM) was used as the substrate, and 600 units of tyrosinase was added in the presence or absence of F1, glycosylated F1, or arbutin. The absorbance was measured at 475 nm in a microplate reader (Bio-Tek Instruments, Winooski, VT, USA).

### 2.6.4. Assay for Inhibition of Matrix Metalloproteinase-1 Expression

Matrix metalloproteinase-1 (MMP-1) level was quantified using a sandwich ELISA Quantikine total human MMP-1 kit (R&D Systems Inc., Minneapolis, MN, USA) After UV irradiation, HDF cells were cultured in DMEM with F1, and glycosylated F1, or ((−)-*cis*-3,3′,4′,5,5′,7-hexahydroxy-flavane-3-gallate) (EGCG) as a positive control. The culture supernatants were harvested, and MMP-1 was measured according to the manufacturer's instructions. Absorbance was measured at 490 nm in a microplate reader microplate reader (Bio-Tek Instruments, Winooski, VT, USA).

## 3. Results and Discussion

### 3.1. Biotransformation of Minor Ginsenosides by Cyclodextrin glycosyltransferase (CGTase)

Among the major ginsenosides, Rb1, Rc, Re, and Rg1 have already been used as substrates for the synthesis of series of new α-glycosylginsenosides through transglycosylation [13,25,26]. However, after oral administration, the major ginsenosides were converted into minor ginsenosides by intestinal microflora. Therefore, we used minor ginsenosides CK, Rh2, F1, Rh1, aPPD, and aPPT as acceptors with dextrin as a sugar donor during CGTase enzyme transglycosylation. As a result, CK, Rh2, F1, and Rh1 yielded new transglycosylated compounds with different retention factor ($R_f$) values compared with known ginsenoside standards (Figure S1). Among these, PPT type ginsenosides Rh1 and F1 showed more glycosylated products, possibly due to the glucose attached to α-OH at C-6 and another –OH at C-20 of the dammerendiol steroidal aglycone. We chose F1 for further studies because of the distinct separation of glycosylated products in addition to its previous reported application in cosmetics and skin care. PPD and PPT aglycone did not generate glycosylated products, indicating that sugar molecules are primarily involved in transglycosylation.

### 3.2. Specificity of Transglycosylation of Ginsenoside F1

Even though the effects of various factors on transglycosylation by Toruzyme were already reported [19,27], this should be validated for the effective synthesis of new compounds. Therefore, the effects of different concentrations of dextrin and CGTase (Toruzyme) on the degree of glycosylation were investigated by HPLC. As shown in Figure S2a, the 5:1 $w/w$ ratio of dextrin: F1 showed the highest yield. There was no significant difference for greater than five volumes, and it was difficult to separate saponin after biotransformation due to the combined extraction of sugar with saponin in the recovery process. In addition, increasing the amount of enzyme rapidly increased the yield up to 20 μL of enzyme with 1 mg of F1 and 5 mg of dextrin, as determined by HPLC (Figure S2b).

### 3.3. Transglycosylation Analysis of Ginsenoside F1

The glycosylation of F1 with dextrin and CGTase for different time durations yielded several new spots that appeared below F1 on TLC (Figure S3). The reaction products were washed several times with water to remove the unreacted excess sugar molecules. The six new spots (G1–F1, G2–F1, G3–F1, G4–F1, G5–F1, and G6–F1) under ginsenoside F1 on TLC (Figure 1a) and the corresponding peaks (G1–F1, G2–F1, G3–F1, G4–F1, G5–F1, and G6–F1), other than ginsenoside F1 on HPLC analysis (Figure 1b), were considered new glycosylated products from F1. G1–F1 ($R_f$ = 0.53) on TLC was isolated as a pure form by silica gel chromatography and elution with $CHCl_3/CH_3OH$ (9:1). The yield of compound G1–F1 was 12% (74 mg) and the structure was identified by ${}^1$H-NMR, ${}^{13}$C-NMR, and two-dimensional (2D) NMR and by correlations with the HSQC and HMBC spectra. The low percentage of yield is due to the formation of other products (G2–F1, G3F1, G4–F1, G5–F1, and G6–F1).

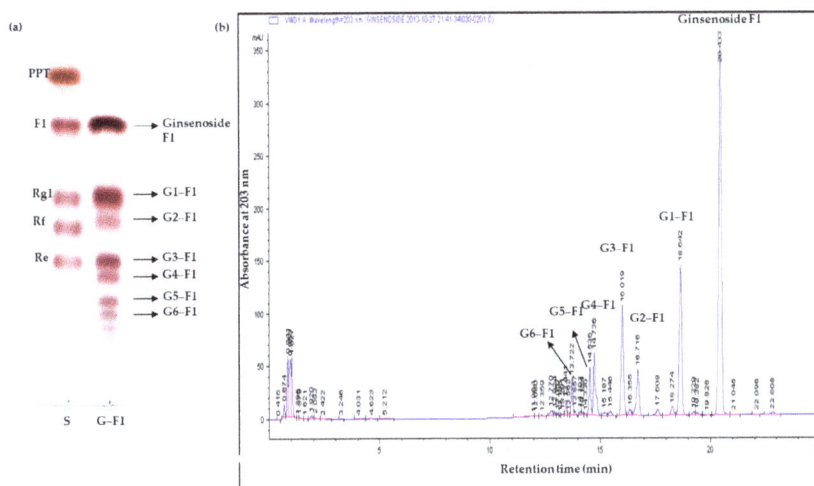

**Figure 1.** (a) Thin layer chromatography of new F1 glycosylated products after removal of excess sugar. (b) High-performance liquid chromatography (HPLC) analysis of F1 and various glycosylated products after reaction. G1–F1, compound **1**; G2–F1, compound **2**; G3–F1, compound **3**; G4–F1, compound **4**; G5–F1, compound **5**; G6–F1, compound **6**.

Compound **1** (G1–F1) was obtained as a white powder. The molecular formula of G1–F1 was determined to be $C_{42}H_{72}O_{14}$ from the pseudomolecule ion peak *m/z* 799.4843 [M-H]$^-$ in negative high-resolution fast atom bombardment-mass spectrometry (FAB-MS). The infrared spectrum showed strong absorbance from hydroxyl groups (3366 cm$^{-1}$) and a double bond (1650 cm$^{-1}$) in G1–F1 (Figure S4). In the ${}^1$H NMR spectrum, proton signals of one olefin methine ($\delta_H$ 5.30, dd, *J* = 6.0, 6.4 Hz, H-24), three oxygenated methines ($\delta_H$ 3.48, H-3; 4.10, H-12; 4.38, H-6), and eight singlet methyls ($\delta_H$ 1.98 (H-28), 1.58 (H-26), 1.56 (H-27), 1.55 (H-21), 1.45 (H-29), 1.08 (H-18), 1.01 (H-19), 0.98 (H-30)) were observed, indicating that G1–F1 has a protopanaxatriol-type triterpene moiety. Proton signals due to the sugar moiety, two anomeric proton signals at $\delta_H$ 5.81 (d, *J* = 3.6 Hz, H-1″) and 5.04 (d, *J* = 8.0 Hz, H-1′), and several oxygenated methines and methylene proton signals at $\delta_H$ 3.72~4.56 were observed (Figure S5a). The ${}^{13}$C NMR spectrum of G1–F1 (Figure S5b) exhibited 42 carbon signals due to a triterpene with two hexoses. An olefin quaternary carbon signal at $\delta_C$ 131.0 (C-25), one olefin methine carbon signal at $\delta_C$ 125.9 (C-24), one oxygenated quaternary carbon signal at 83.5 (C-20), three oxygenated methine carbon signals ($\delta_C$ 78.6 (C-3), 67.8 (C-6), 70.2 (C-12)), and eight methyl carbon signals ($\delta_C$ 32.0 (C-28), 25.7 (C-26), 22.3 (C-21), 17.8 (C-18), 17.6 (C-19), 17.5 (C-27, 30), 16.3 (C-29)) were observed for the protopanaxatriol-type aglycone moiety. The chemical shifts of the sugar moieties signal ($\delta_C$ 98.1 (C-1'), 81.2 (C-2'), 78.5 (C-3'), 76.6 (C-5'), 75.5 (C-4'), 62.1 (C-6')) suggested the presence of a glucopyranoside. The coupling constant of the anomeric proton signal ($\delta_H$ 5.04, H-1') was 8.0 Hz, confirming β-D-glucopyranoside. Another sugar moiety ($\delta_C$ 103.0 (C-1''), 75.2 (C-3''), 74.6 (C-2''), 74.4 (C-5''), 71.9 (C-4''), 62.8 (C-6'')) suggested the presence of glucopyranoside; the coupling constant of the anomeric proton signal ($\delta_H$ 5.81, H-1'') was 3.6 Hz, confirming that the glucopyranose had a α-glucosidic linkage. The connection between the β-D-glucopyranosyl unit (C-1') and the C-20 of the aglycone and that of another α-D-glucopyranosyl unit (C-1'') with C-2' of the inner glucose was verified by the cross-peaks observed between the anomer proton signal at $\delta_H$ 5.04 (H-1') and the oxygenated quaternary carbon signal at $\delta_C$ 83.5 (C-20) and between the anomer proton signal at $\delta_H$ 5.81 (H-1'') and the oxygenated methine carbon signal at $\delta_C$ 81.2 (C-2') in the HMBC spectrum, respectively (Figure S5c,d). This was confirmed by the downfield shifts of the carbon ($\delta_C$ 78.5 (C-3')) and proton signals ($\delta_H$ 4.53 (H-3')) due to the glycosylation effect. Ultimately, the structure of G1-F1 was determined to be (20S)-3β,6α,12β -trihydroxydammar-24-ene-(20-O-β-D-glucopyranosyl-(1→2)-α-D-glucopyranoside), which has not been reported previously (Figure 2).

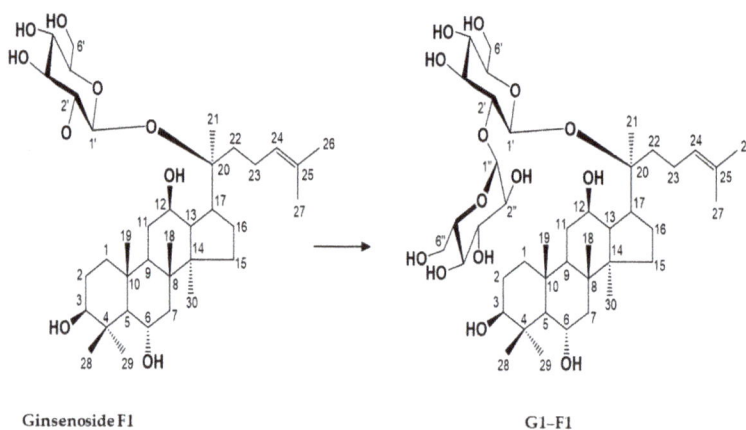

**Figure 2.** Chemical structures of ginsenoside F1 and its α-glycosylated F1 (G1–F1).

*3.4. Characterization of Novel α-Glycosylated Ginsenoside F1*

Water Solubility of Ginsenoside F1 and Novel α-Glycosylated Ginsenoside F1

Transglycosylation reactions catalyzed by CGTase are an efficient method to enhance the water solubility of various compounds [16,18,28]. Accordingly, the water solubility of α-glycosylated ginsenoside F1 was higher than that of F1 alone (data not shown). The soluble α-glycosylated ginsenoside F1 should not only facilitate investigation of the pharmacological activities of ginsenoside F1, but also may be useful as a cosmetics ingredient.

*3.5. Cell Cytotoxicity*

3.5.1. Comparison of Cell Viability of Ginsenoside F1 and Novel α-Glycosylated Ginsenoside F1 in Human Dermal Fibroblast Cells

To evaluate the effects of α-glycosylated ginsenoside F1 and ginsenoside F1 on the cell viability of HDFs, the cells were treated with different concentrations. Ginsenoside F1 reduced the cell viability of HDFs to a greater extent than α-glycosylated ginsenoside F1 (G1–F1) in a dose-dependent manner

(Figure 3). The α-glycosylated ginsenoside F1 showed lower toxicity toward HDFs than ginsenoside F1 up to a concentration of 5 mg/mL. The cell viability was greater than 90% of that of the control cells up to 2 mg/mL. These results showed that ginsenoside F1 and α-glycosylated ginsenoside F1 have no significant cytotoxicity against skin cells. Thus, the inhibitory effect of these compounds on collagenase expression was not due to cytotoxicity of these compounds at concentrations up to 2 mg/mL.

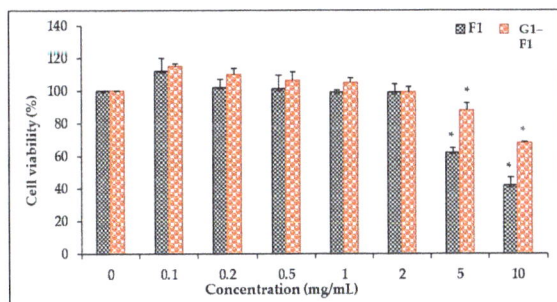

**Figure 3.** Cytotoxicity of ginsenoside F1 and α-glycosylated ginsenoside F1 in human dermal fibroblast cells. Cells were preincubated with or without compounds for 24 h, and cell viability was evaluated by 3-(4,5-dimethylthiazol-2-yl)-2,5-diphenyltetrazolium bromide (MTT) assay. Data represent the mean ± SD (standard deviation) of triplicate experiments. * $p < 0.05$ compared with the control. F1: ginsenoside F1; G1–F1: α-glycosylated ginsenoside F1.

3.5.2. Inhibition of Tyrosinase Activity by Ginsenoside F1 and G1–F1

To investigate the tyrosinase inhibitory activity of G1–F1, the half maximal inhibitory concentration (IC50) values against mushroom tyrosinase were measured. The tyrosinase inhibitory activity of α-glycosylated ginsenoside F1 was higher than that of ginsenoside F1 but weaker than that of arbutin (Figure 4).

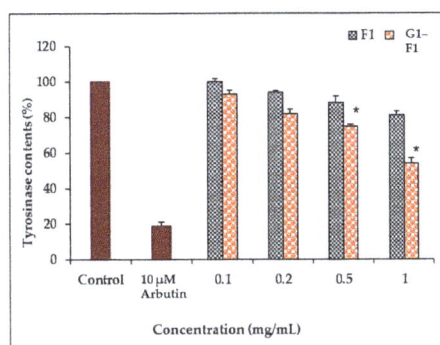

**Figure 4.** Inhibitory effects of ginsenoside F1 and α-glycosylated ginsenoside F1 on Mushroon tyrosinase activity. Tyrosinase activity was measured using 3.3 mM L-DOPA as a substrate. Results are expressed as the percentage of inhibition by ginsenoside F1 and α-glycosylated compound. Arbutin was used as a positive control. Data represent the mean ± SD of triplicate experiments. * $p < 0.05$ compared with the control. F1: ginsenoside F1; G1–F1: α-glycosylated ginsenoside F1.

It was previously reported that F1 can function as an anti-aging and antioxidant agent [11] and as a drug against skin cancer with antiproliferation and whitening functions [10]. Comparison of the inhibition of tyrosinase activity showed that α-glycosylated ginsenoside F1 had a greater inhibitory effect on tyrosinase activity than ginsenoside F1, indicating that α-glycosylated ginsenoside F1 might be an efficacious anti-tyrosinase agent for use in cosmetics.

### 3.5.3. Inhibition of Ultraviolet A (UVA)-Induced Matrix Metalloproteinase- (MMP-1) Expression of Ginsenoside F1 and G1–F1

Skin aging occurs as a result of collagen degradation through induction of MMPs by UV irradiation [29]. The α-glycosylated ginsenoside F1 exhibited a greater inhibitory effect against collagenase (MMP-1) than the ginsenoside F1 after UVA irradiation of HDF cell lines (Figure 5), indicating that the C-3-hydroxyl group in the compounds is important for inhibitory activity. (−)-*cis*-3,3′,4′,5,5′,7-Hexahydroxy-flavane-3-gallate (EGCG) was used as a positive control.

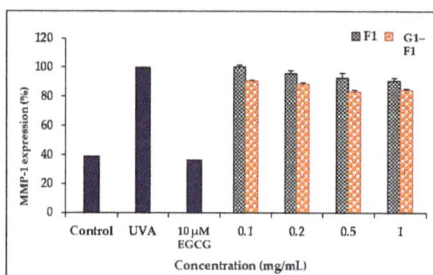

**Figure 5.** Inhibitory effects of ginsenoside F1 and α-glycosylated ginsenoside F1 on the expression of MMP-1 in UVA-irradiated human dermal fibroblasts. The cells were cultured in the presence of ginsenoside F1 and α-glycosylated ginsenoside F1 (0–1 mg/mL) for 24 h and subjected to ELISA. The results were expressed as the average ± SD of triplicate determinations. * $p < 0.05$ compared with UVA irradiation. F1: ginsenoside F1; G1–F1: α-glycosylated ginsenoside F1.

In addition to the number of sugars, their linkage positions and alpha vs. beta linkages affect pharmacological activities. For example, ginsenoside F1 and Rh1 have the same number of sugar moieties and the same molecular weight but different glucose attachment positions at C-20 and C-6, respectively. F1 showed significantly greater inhibition of viability than Rh1 in prostate cancer cell lines [30]. The glycosylation and nano formulations of ginseng saponins [13,25,26,31–33] and other steroidal saponins [19,27] has recently attracted increased interest.

The alpha isomers of glucose also exhibited significant activity, especially stronger inhibitory activity of α-arbutin on tyrosinase compared with β-arbutin [22]. Similarly, in comparison with the common beta isomers of glucose in ginsenosides, α-glycosyl ginsenoside was reported to have a reduced bitter taste [26], suggesting its potential as an additive in food products.

### 4. Conclusions

This study describes for the first time the glycosylation of ginsenoside F1 by CGTase and identification of a novel α-glucosylated F1 with an unusual α-D-glcp-(1→2)-β-D-glcp sugar chain (G1–F1). The novel compound G1–F1 showed lower cytotoxicity and stronger inhibitory activity against tyrosinase and collagenase (MMP-1) than ginsenoside F1. This novel G1–F1 may be a potential pharmacological active compound. A single α-glucosylated F1 was purified in this study, and other new glycosylated spots remain to be characterized.

**Supplementary Materials:** The following are available online at http://www.mdpi.com/2218-273X/8/4/142/s1. Figure S1: TLC analysis of transglycosylation of minor ginsenosides (Rh2, CK, PPD, Rh1, F1, PPT). S, standard; (i) Each ginsenoside with CGTase only and (ii) Each ginsenoside with CGTase and dextrin, Figure S2. (a). Effect of dextrin on transglycosylation of ginsenoside F1. Toruzyme® (20 μL) was incubated with ginsenoside F1 (1 mg) in 1 mL of 20 mM sodium phosphate buffer at 60 ± 1 °C for 2 h, (b). Effect of Toruzyme® on transglycosylation of ginsenoside F1. Toruzyme® (5–30 μL) was incubated with ginsenoside F1 (1 mg) and dextrin (5 mg) in 1 mL of 20 mM sodium phosphate buffer at 60 ± 1°C for 2 h. The yield was calculated as the increase in product by HPLC, Figure S3: TLC analysis of transglycosylation of ginsenoside F1 with Toruzyme® and dextrin at different times (min). S, standard of higher molecular weight ginsenosides than F1 in the same protopanaxatriol type ginsenosides; F1+toru (Control 1). Ginsenoside F1 and CGTase Toruzyme enzyme alone; Dextrin+toru (Control 2): Dextrin (sugar donor) and CGTase Toruzyme enzyme alone, Figure S4. (a). Infrared spectrum (FTIR) of novel α-glycosylated ginsenoside F1 (G1–F1), Figure S5. (a). $^1$H-NMR spectrum of novel α-glycosylated ginsenoside F1 (G1–F1). (b). $^{13}$C-NMR spectrum of novel α-glycosylated ginsenoside F1 (G1–F1). (c). gHSQC spectrum of novel α-glycosylated ginsenoside F1 (G1–F1). (d). Key gHMBC spectrum of novel α-glycosylated ginsenoside F1 (G1–F1).

**Author Contributions:** Conceptualization—H.J.L. and R.M.; Methodology—S.S.M., H.J.L., and J.W.M.; Validation—D.Y.L., Resources—Y.J.K.; Writing—original draft preparation—S.S.M., and H.J.L.; Writing—review, and editing—R.M. and Z.J.; Funding Acquisition—D.U.Y. and D.C.Y.; Project Administration and Supervision—D.C.Y.

**Funding:** This research received no external funding.

**Acknowledgments:** This research was supported by a grant from the Korea Institute of Planning & Evaluation for Technology in Food, Agriculture, Forestry, & Fisheries (KIPET NO: 317007-3), Republic of Korea.

**Conflicts of Interest:** The authors declare no conflicts of interest. The funders had no role in the design of the study; in the collection, analyses, or interpretation of data; in the writing of the manuscript; or in the decision to publish the results.

## References

1. Wong, A.S.; Che, C.M.; Leung, K.W. Recent advances in ginseng as cancer therapeutics: A functional and mechanistic overview. *Nat. Prod. Rep.* **2015**, *32*, 256–272. [CrossRef] [PubMed]

2. Mathiyalagan, R.; Subramaniyam, S.; Kim, Y.J.; Kim, Y.C.; Yang, D.C. Ginsenoside compound K-bearing glycol chitosan conjugates: Synthesis, physicochemical characterization, and in vitro biological studies. *Carbohydr. Polym.* **2014**, *112*, 359–366. [CrossRef] [PubMed]

3. Ahn, S.; Siddiqi, M.H.; Noh, H.-Y.; Kim, Y.-J.; Kim, Y.-J.; Jin, C.-G.; Yang, D.-C. Anti-inflammatory activity of ginsenosides in LPS-stimulated RAW 264.7 cells. *Sci. Bull.* **2015**, *60*, 773–784. [CrossRef]

4. Wee, J.J.; Mee Park, K.; Chung, A.S. Biological activities of ginseng and its application to human health. In *Herbal Medicine: Biomolecular and Clinical Aspects*, 2nd ed.; Benzie, I.F.F., Wachtel-Galor, S., Eds.; CRC Press: Boca Raton, FL, USA, 2011.

5. Sathishkumar, N.; Sathiyamoorthy, S.; Ramya, M.; Yang, D.U.; Lee, H.N.; Yang, D.C. Molecular docking studies of anti-apoptotic BCL-2, BCL-XL, and MCL-1 proteins with ginsenosides from *Panax ginseng*. *J. Enzyme Inhib. Med. Chem.* **2012**, *27*, 685–692. [CrossRef] [PubMed]

6. Yang, W.Z.; Hu, Y.; Wu, W.Y.; Ye, M.; Guo, D.A. Saponins in the genus *Panax* L. (Araliaceae): A systematic review of their chemical diversity. *Phytochemistry* **2014**, *106*, 7–24. [CrossRef] [PubMed]

7. Wakabayashi, C.; Murakami, K.; Hasegawa, H.; Murata, J.; Saiki, I. An intestinal bacterial metabolite of ginseng protopanaxadiol saponins has the ability to induce apoptosis in tumor cells. *Biochem. Biophys. Res. Commun.* **1998**, *246*, 725–730. [CrossRef] [PubMed]

8. Tawab, M.A.; Bahr, U.; Karas, M.; Wurglics, M.; Schubert-Zsilavecz, M. Degradation of ginsenosides in humans after oral administration. *Drug Metab. Dispos.* **2003**, *31*, 1065–1071. [CrossRef] [PubMed]

9. Han, J.; Lee, E.; Kim, E.; Yeom, M.H.; Kwon, O.; Yoon, T.H.; Lee, T.R.; Kim, K. Role of epidermal γδ T-cell-derived interleukin 13 in the skin-whitening effect of Ginsenoside F1. *Exp. Dermatol.* **2014**, *23*, 860–862. [CrossRef] [PubMed]

10. Yoo, D.S.; Rho, H.S.; Lee, Y.G.; Yeom, M.H.; Kim, D.H.; Lee, S.-J.; Hong, S.; Lee, J.; Cho, J.Y. Ginsenoside F1 modulates cellular responses of skin melanoma cells. *J. Ginseng Res.* **2011**, *35*, 86–91. [CrossRef]

11. Lee, E.H.; Cho, S.Y.; Kim, S.J.; Shin, E.S.; Chang, H.K.; Kim, D.H.; Yeom, M.H.; Woe, K.S.; Lee, J.; Sim, Y.C.; et al. Ginsenoside F1 protects human HaCaT keratinocytes from ultraviolet-B-induced apoptosis by maintaining constant levels of Bcl-2. *J. Investig. Dermatol.* **2003**, *121*, 607–613. [CrossRef] [PubMed]

12. Shibuya, M.; Nishimura, K.; Yasuyama, N.; Ebizuka, Y. Identification and characterization of glycosyltransferases involved in the biosynthesis of soyasaponin I in *Glycine max*. *FEBS Lett.* **2010**, *584*, 2258–2264. [CrossRef] [PubMed]

13. Mathiyalagan, R.; Kim, Y.-H.; Kim, Y.; Kim, M.-K.; Kim, M.-J.; Yang, D. Enzymatic Formation of Novel Ginsenoside Rg1-α-Glucosides by Rat Intestinal Homogenates. *Appl. Biochem. Biotechnol.* **2015**, *177*, 1701–1715. [CrossRef] [PubMed]

14. Nakano, H.; Kiso, T.; Okamoto, K.; Tomita, T.; Manan, M.B.; Kitahata, S. Synthesis of glycosyl glycerol by cyclodextrin glucanotransferases. *J. Biosci. Bioeng.* **2003**, *95*, 583–588. [CrossRef]

15. Li, S.; Li, W.; Xiao, Q.Y.; Xia, Y. Transglycosylation of stevioside to improve the edulcorant quality by lower substitution using cornstarch hydrolyzate and CGTase. *Food Chem.* **2013**, *138*, 2064–2069. [CrossRef] [PubMed]

16. Kometani, T.; Terada, Y.; Nishimura, T.; Takii, H.; Okada, S. Transglycosylation to hesperidin by cyclodextrin glucanotransferase from an alkalophilic *Bacillus* species in alkaline pH and properties of hesperidin glycosides. *Biosci. Biotechnol. Biochem.* **1994**, *58*, 1990–1994. [CrossRef]

17. Kamaruddin, K.; Illias, R.M.; Aziz, S.A.; Said, M.; Hassan, O. Effects of buffer properties on cyclodextrin glucanotransferase reactions and cyclodextrin production from raw sago (*Cycas revoluta*) starch. *Biotechnol. Appl. Biochem.* **2005**, *41*, 117–125. [PubMed]

18. Suzuki, Y.; Suzuki, K. Enzymatic formation of 4G-α-D-glucopyranosyl-rutin. *Agric. Biol. Chem.* **1991**, *55*, 181–187. [CrossRef] [PubMed]

19. Wang, Y.Z.; Feng, B.; Huang, H.Z.; Kang, L.P.; Cong, Y.; Zhou, W.B.; Zou, P.; Cong, Y.W.; Song, X.B.; Ma, B.P. Glucosylation of steroidal saponins by cyclodextrin glucanotransferase. *Planta Med.* **2010**, *76*, 1724–1731. [CrossRef] [PubMed]

20. Uchida, K.; Suzuki, Y. Enzymatic synthesis of a new derivative of thiamin, O-α-glucosylthiamin. *Biosci. Biotechnol. Biochem.* **1998**, *62*, 221–224. [CrossRef] [PubMed]

21. Seo, D.H.; Jung, J.H.; Ha, S.J.; Cho, H.K.; Jung, D.H.; Kim, T.J.; Baek, N.I.; Yoo, S.H.; Park, C.S. High-yield enzymatic bioconversion of hydroquinone to α-arbutin, a powerful skin lightening agent, by amylosucrase. *Appl. Microbiol. Biotechnol.* **2012**, *94*, 1189–1197. [CrossRef] [PubMed]

22. Sugimoto, K.; Nishimura, T.; Nomura, K.; Sugimoto, K.; Kuriki, T. Syntheses of arbutin-α-glycosides and a comparison of their inhibitory effects with those of α-arbutin and arbutin on human tyrosinase. *Chem. Pharm. Bull.* **2003**, *51*, 798–801. [CrossRef] [PubMed]

23. Quan, L.H.; Min, J.W.; Sathiyamoorthy, S.; Yang, D.U.; Kim, Y.J.; Yang, D.C. Biotransformation of ginsenosides Re and Rg1 into ginsenosides Rg2 and Rh1 by recombinant β-glucosidase. *Biotechnol. Lett.* **2012**, *34*, 913–917. [CrossRef] [PubMed]

24. Sim, G.-S.; Lee, B.-C.; Cho, H.; Lee, J.; Kim, J.-H.; Lee, D.-H.; Kim, J.-H.; Pyo, H.-B.; Moon, D.; Oh, K.-W.; et al. Structure activity relationship of antioxidative property of flavonoids and inhibitory effect on matrix metalloproteinase activity in UVA-irradiated human dermal fibroblast. *Arch. Pharm. Res.* **2007**, *30*, 290–298. [CrossRef] [PubMed]

25. Kim, M.J.; Kim, Y.H.; Song, G.S.; Suzuki, Y.; Kim, M.K. Enzymatic transglycosylation of ginsenoside Rg1 by rice seed α-glucosidase. *Biosci. Biotechnol. Biochem.* **2016**, *80*, 318–328. [CrossRef] [PubMed]

26. Kim, Y.H.; Lee, Y.G.; Choi, K.J.; Uchida, K.; Suzuki, Y. Transglycosylation to ginseng saponins by cyclomaltodextrin glucanotransferases. *Biosci. Biotechnol. Biochem.* **2001**, *65*, 875–883. [CrossRef] [PubMed]

27. Zhou, W.B.; Feng, B.; Huang, H.Z.; Qin, Y.J.; Wang, Y.Z.; Kang, L.P.; Zhao, Y.; Wang, X.N.; Cai, Y.; Tan, D.W.; et al. Enzymatic synthesis of α-glucosyl-timosaponin BII catalyzed by the extremely thermophilic enzyme: *Toruzyme* 3.0L. *Carbohydr. Res.* **2010**, *345*, 1752–1759. [CrossRef] [PubMed]

28. Sato, T.; Nakagawa, H.; Kurosu, J.; Yoshida, K.; Tsugane, T.; Shimura, S.; Kirimura, K.; Kino, K.; Usami, S. α-anomer-selective glucosylation of (+)-catechin by the crude enzyme, showing glucosyl transfer activity, of *Xanthomonas campestris* WU-9701. *J. Biosci. Bioeng.* **2000**, *90*, 625–630. [CrossRef]

29. Kligman, A.M. Early destructive effect of sunlight on human skin. *JAMA* **1969**, *210*, 2377–2380. [CrossRef] [PubMed]

30. Li, W.; Liu, Y.; Zhang, J.W.; Ai, C.Z.; Xiang, N.; Liu, H.X.; Yang, L. Anti-androgen-independent prostate cancer effects of ginsenoside metabolites in vitro: Mechanism and possible structure-activity relationship investigation. *Arch. Pharm. Res.* **2009**, *32*, 49–57. [CrossRef] [PubMed]

31. Luo, S.L.; Dang, L.Z.; Zhang, K.Q.; Liang, L.M.; Li, G.H. Cloning and heterologous expression of UDP-glycosyltransferase genes from *Bacillus subtilis* and its application in the glycosylation of ginsenoside Rh1. *Lett. Appl. Microbiol.* **2015**, *60*, 72–78. [CrossRef] [PubMed]

32. Wang, D.D.; Jin, Y.; Wang, C.; Kim, Y.J.; Perez, Z.E.J.; Baek, N.I.; Mathiyalagan, R.; Markus, J.; Yang, D.C. Rare ginsenoside Ia synthesized from F1 by cloning and overexpression of the UDP-glycosyltransferase gene from *Bacillus subtilis*: Synthesis, characterization, and in vitro melanogenesis inhibition activity in BL6B16 cells. *J. Ginseng Res.* **2018**, *42*, 42–49. [CrossRef] [PubMed]

33. Mathiyalagan, R.; Yang, D.C. Ginseng nanoparticles: A budding tool for cancer treatment. *Nanomedicine* **2017**, *12*, 1091–1094. [CrossRef] [PubMed]

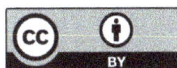

![biomolecules logo] *biomolecules*

MDPI

*Article*

# Squalene Found in Alpine Grassland Soils under a Harsh Environment in the Tibetan Plateau, China

**Xuyang Lu [1,2], Shuqin Ma [3,*], Youchao Chen [4], Degyi Yangzom [5] and Hongmao Jiang [1,6]**

1   Institute of Mountain Hazards and Environment, Chinese Academy of Sciences, Chengdu 610041, China;
    xylu@imde.ac.cn (X.L.); jianghongmao@163.com (H.J.)
2   Key Laboratory of Mountain Surface Processes and Ecological Regulation, Chinese Academy of Sciences,
    Chengdu 610041, China
3   College of Tourism, Henan Normal University, Xinxiang 453007, China
4   Wuhan Botanical Garden, Chinese Academy of Sciences, Wuhan 430074, China; chenyouchao@wbgcas.cn
5   Ecological Monitoring & Research Center, Tibetan Environment Monitoring Station, Lhasa 850000, China;
    dejiyangzong09@126.com
6   University of Chinese Academy of Sciences, Beijing 100049, China
*   Correspondence: mashuqin@htu.edu.cn; Tel.: +86-181-5309-5206

Received: 10 October 2018; Accepted: 14 November 2018; Published: 20 November 2018

**Abstract:** Squalene is found in a large number of plants, animals, and microorganisms, as well as other sources, playing an important role as an intermediate in sterol biosynthesis. It is used widely in the food, cosmetics, and medicine industries because of its antioxidant, antistatic, and anti-carcinogenic properties. A higher natural squalene component of lipids is usually reported as being isolated to organisms living in harsh environments. In the Tibetan Plateau, which is characterized by high altitude, strong solar radiation, drought, low temperatures, and thin air, the squalene component was identified in five alpine grasslands soils using the pyrolysis gas chromatography–mass spectrometry (Py-GC/MS) technique. The relative abundance of squalene ranged from 0.93% to 10.66% in soils from the five alpine grasslands, with the highest value found in alpine desert and the lowest in alpine meadow. Furthermore, the relative abundance of squalene in alpine grassland soils was significantly negatively associated with soil chemical/microbial characteristics. These results indicate that the extreme environmental conditions of the Tibetan Plateau may stimulate the microbial biosynthesis of squalene, and the harsher the environment, the higher the relative abundance of soil squalene.

**Keywords:** squalene; alpine grassland; Py-GC/MS; soil microorganism; Tibetan Plateau

## 1. Introduction

Squalene is named after the shark family Squalidae, and is a triterpene with the formula $C_{30}H_{50}$. It is an intermediate in the biosynthesis of sterols and hopanoids in the plant, animal, human, and microorganism worlds [1,2]. From the moment life appeared on Earth, squalene appeared in microorganisms. The cell membranes of higher organisms from the Precambrian contained great proportions of squalene, which was an essential substance for their survival in the hostile oxygen-free environment [2]. Squalene and its related compounds such as oxidosqualene and bis-oxidosqualene are precursors of thousands of bioactive triterpenoids and are also a carbon source which can be utilized by some microorganisms [3].

Squalene itself has several beneficial properties and values. For instance, it is a hydrophilic natural antioxidant which serves in health-promoting functions including skin hydration and tumor-suppression. It has cardio-protective, antibacterial/antifungal, immunity-boosting, and cholesterol-lowering effects. It can also be used as a drug delivery agent, and has been used as a feasible source of biofuels [4,5]. Thus, squalene has recently attracted a great deal of attention due to its industrial value as a lubricant, health-promoting agent, and/or as a form of biofuel.

The richest known source of squalene in the living world is the liver of certain species of fish, especially sharks living in the deep sea [1,6]. As the main organ for lipid storage, as an energy source, and for adjusting buoyancy, the liver of sharks comprises 50–80% unsaponifiable matter, with the great majority thereof being squalene. For example, *Centrophorus artomarginatus* deep-sea sharks can survive in waters with a depth of 600–1000 m, where with the environmental characteristics include lack of sunlight, consistently high pressure, and very poor oxygen supply. This survival is due to squalene from their liver, which accounts for 25–30% of their total body weight [2,7].

Squalene was also identified in many plant oils over broad ranges. The first vegetable oil in which it was found was olive oil, with a concentration of 5.64–5.99 g kg$^{1}$. In other vegetable oils, it is also quite prominent in soybean, grape seed, hazelnuts, peanuts, corn, pumpkin, rice bran, amaranth, and camellia oils [2,8]. Human serum also contains 10–13% squalene as one of its major constituents [3,9]. In addition, microbial squalene production has become a promising alternative in recent years due to the advantages of fast and massive growth, although microorganisms do not accumulate as much squalene as plants or shark livers [10–12].

The Tibetan Plateau, as the roof of the world, is considered to be the third "pole" of the world. The plateau is peculiarly cold due to its latitude, and is colder than anywhere else outside the polar regions. It has an average elevation of 4 km above sea level, and possesses one of the largest ice masses on Earth [13–15]. The plants, animals, and microorganisms living in the Tibetan Plateau endure extreme circumstances, characterized by high altitude, strong solar radiation, drought, low temperatures, thin air, and so on [16–18]. Low temperature and low oxygen pose key physiological challenges for those living in these harsh conditions on the plateau, a situation which is to some extent similar to that of sharks living within a deep-sea environment.

Squalene has been identified from some Tibetan plant components, including the lipophilic extracts from flowers (0.29–0.77%) and leaves (0.56–1.16%) of *Lamiophlomis rotate*, and the volatile oil from roots (1.73%) of *Rhodiola crenulata* [19,20]. The Tibetan yak can thrive well at altitudes of 2000–5000 m above sea level, and provides meat, milk, and other necessities for the local people. The highest squalene content in lipids was reported to exist in the longissimus muscle (20.99 mg/100 g), the biceps femoris muscle (59.82 mg/100 g), the liver (6.94 mg/100 g), the subcutaneous adipose tissue (7.06 mg/100 g), and the abdominal adipose tissue (7.06 mg/100 g) of the Tibetan yak [21]. Therefore, the chemical component of squalene has been found in some plants and animals on the Tibetan Plateau. Could this component also be identified from some microorganisms which likewise live in high-altitude, low-temperature, low-oxygen alpine conditions? As a variety of microorganisms were found to distributed in alpine soils of the Tibetan Plateau [22–24], in the present study alpine soils from five types of alpine grassland were analyzed by using pyrolysis gas chromatography–mass spectrometry (Py-GC/MS) to identify the squalene component. The aim of this study was to compare squalene content among different alpine grassland soils and further to explore the relationships between the squalene content and the soil environmental factors in the harsh conditions on the Tibetan Plateau.

## 2. Materials and Methods

### 2.1. Study Area

Tibet covers a total area of more than 1.2 million km$^2$ and represents is approximately one-eighth of the total area of China, with an average altitude higher than 4000 m. It regulates climate change and water resources in China and eastern Asia due to its geomorphological uniqueness in the world [25,26]. Because of its extensive territory and highly dissected topography, this region has a diverse range of climate and vegetation zones. Solar radiation is strong, with annual radiation varying between 140 and 190 kcal cm$^{-2}$. Due to the geographical conditions and atmospheric circulation, the average annual temperature is rather low, with the temperature varying from 18 to −4 °C, decreasing gradually from the southeast to the northwest. The average annual precipitation is less than 1000 mm in most areas of Tibet; annual precipitation rates can reach up to 2817 mm in the east and drop down to approximately 70 mm in the west [27].

Alpine grasslands are the most dominant ecosystems in Tibet, covering more than 70% of the whole plateau's area. It ranks first among all Chinese provinces and autonomous regions in the diversity of its grassland ecosystems, comprising 17 types of grassland based on the classification system used for the whole country [28,29]. Among all grassland types, alpine meadow (AM) is composed of perennial mesic and mesoxeric herbs under cold and wet climate conditions, occupying approximately 31.3% of the total grassland area of Tibet. Alpine steppe (AS) is composed of drought-tolerant perennial herbs or small shrubs under cold and arid/semiarid climate conditions, representing approximately 38.9% of the total Tibetan grassland area. Alpine desert (AD) is a grassland type developed and controlled by cold and extreme drought conditions, covering 6.71% of the total grassland area. Alpine meadow steppe (AMS) is a transitional type of alpine grassland from the meadow to the steppe, and alpine desert steppe (ADS) is a transitional type of alpine grassland from the steppe to the desert, covering 7.32% and 10.7% of the total grassland area in Tibet, respectively [27].

*2.2. Soil Sampling*

In this research, the study area was located at 30.75°–33.43° N, 79.75°–92.07° E, and the sampling sites were located in 10 counties from east to west in the Tibet Autonomous Region of China. Five sampling sites were selected at each of the three main natural grassland types, including AM, AS, and ADS. Three sampling sites were selected from the relatively small natural grassland area, including AMS and AD, in August 2016. At each sample site, three 1 m × 1 m quadrats were laid out at intervals of approximately 50 m. In total, 63 quadrats of alpine grassland in Tibet were sampled with 45 quadrats (15 sites × 3 quadrats) for AM, AS, and ADS and 18 quadrats (6 sites × 3 quadrats) for AMS and AD, respectively. At each quadrat, all aboveground plants and litter were removed from the soil surface before the sampling. Five soil samples were obtained for each quadrat at depths of 0–15 cm, and five soil samples were mixed as a soil sample for the soil chemical and microbial properties analysis. All soils were transported to the lab with cooler, and stored in sealed containers at 4 °C before the measurement. For the determination of soil bulk density, soil cores (5.4 cm in diameter) were also taken from each layer using a stainless-steel cylinder. In addition, the location and elevation of each site were measured using Global Positioning System (GPS) (Garmin MAP62CSX made in Garmin Ltd., Olathe, KS, USA).

*2.3. Soil Analyses*

In the lab, soil samples for soil chemical and microbial properties analyses were sieved to pass through a 2-mm-mesh sieve, and roots and stones were removed by hand. Then the samples were divided into three sub-samples. One sub-sample was air-dried and the squalene component was identified by pyrolysis gas chromatography–mass spectrometry (Py-GC/MS); the second was stored at 4 °C prior to determine soil microbial phospholipid fatty acids (PLFAs); and the third was sieved through 250-μm mesh for analysis of soil pH, soil organic carbon (SOC), dissolved organic carbon (DOC), total nitrogen (TN), and total inorganic nitrogen (TIN) contents.

Py-GC/MS tests were performed in a pyrolyzer (CDS5200). For this, 25 mg of soil was placed in quartz tubes (2 cm in length, 2 mm inside diameter) and quantified using a Mettler microbalance (Mettler–Toledo, Greifensee, Switzerland). The pyrolysis chamber was full of He. The soil samples were heated from ambient to 700 °C at a rate of 20 °C/ms and kept for 15 s. The pyrolyzer was coupled with PerkinElmer Clarus680GC-SQ8MS Systems (PerkinElmer, Santa Clara, CA, USA), and the carrier gas was He. For operation, the temperature program of the capillary column (HP-5, 0.25 mm) of GC was as follows: 3 min at 40 °C, then temperature was increased to 280 °C at a rate of 10 °C/min and kept at 280 °C for 5 min. The injector temperature was 280 °C. The MS indicator was operated in the electron impact mode at electron energy of 70 eV, and the ion source temperature was kept at 250 °C. The pyrolysis products were identified using identifications of the NIST 2014 library and the report by other researchers. Pyrolysis products were quantified by using the surface of two characteristics ion fragments of each product. The relative percentage of squalene compound was calculated according to peak height above baseline. For each sample, the relative peak height of squalene compound was calculated by normalizing results to the largest peak measured in the chromatogram. The percentage of squalene compound reported herein, therefore, is the relative percentage of that compound with respect to the largest peak compounds identified, not the absolute abundance of compounds of squalene in soils.

The soil microbial community was characterized by PLFA analysis. Lipids were extracted from soils by using one-phase chloroform, methanol, and water extractant, then fractionated into neutral lipids, glycolipids, and phospholipids on a silicic acid column. The quantification of PLFAs was performed by GC chromatography (GC Agilent 6890-Agilent Technology, Santa Clara, CA, USA) using a flame ionization detector (FID), split injector, and an HP7673 auto sampler. He as a carrier gas was operated with a flow rate at 0.8 mL min$^{-1}$ and a pressure of 35 psi. The injector and detector temperatures were 250 °C and 300 °C, respectively [30]. PLFAs were designated $X:Y\omega Z$. $X$: the total number of carbon atoms; $Y$: the number of unsaturated olefinic bond; $\omega$: the end of methyl; $Z$: the location of the keys or cyclopropane chain; a (anteriso) and i (iso): branching chain; 10Me: a methyl group tenth at the end of the pitch molecule carbon atoms; and cy: a cyclopropyl group on the carbon chain [31].

The absolute abundance of PLFAs is expressed as nmol/g dry soil, and the sum of absolute abundances of PLFAs was the microbial biomass [31]. The PLFAs, which were present in <3 samples at very low concentrations, were discarded from analysis. The bacterial PLFAs were estimated as the sum of general bacteria and non-specific bacteria. PLFA biomarkers included i13:0, 14:0, i14:0, i15:0, a15:0, i15:1 G, 16:0, i16:0, 16:1 2OH, 16:1G, 16:1ω5c, 16:1ω9c, i17:0, a17:0, cy17:0, 17:1ω8c, 18:1ω5c, 18:0, and cy19:0ω8c [32–36]. Actinomycete bacteria are represented by 10Me17:0 and 10Me18:0 [37]. Fungal groups included 18:1ω9c [37].

Soil pH was measured electrochemically (Model PHS-3E Meter, Leici Instruments Co. Ltd., Shanghai, China) in $H_2O$ at a soil: solution ratio of 1:2.5 [38]. Soil organic carbon content was detected by the potassium dichromate sulfuric acid oxidation technique [39]. Total nitrogen was detected by the Kjeldahl method [40]. Total inorganic nitrogen and dissolved organic carbon content were detected by extracting 5 g fresh-weight soil with 25 mL 0.5 mol $K_2SO_4$; then the soil extraction was passed through filter paper, with filtrates then analyzed by an Autosampler (SEAL XY-2 Sampler, Bran & Luebbe, Sydney, Australia) [41].

### 2.4. Data Analysis and Statistics

One-way ANOVA followed by Duncan's multiple comparisons was employed to test the differences in soil chemistries, including squalene relative abundance, SOC, DOC, TIN, and TN among soils collected from the AM, AS, AMS, ADS, and AD grassland types. The squalene relative abundance and soil chemical/microbial characteristics were subjected to principal component analysis (PCA), based on linear combinations of the original variables on independent orthogonal axes, while the squalene relative abundance and soil chemical/microbial traits were subjected to redundancy analysis (RDA), performed using Canoco 5 (Microcomputer Power, Ithaca, NY, USA, 2012). All statistical analyses were conducted using SPSS 20.0 (IBM, Chicago, IL, USA, 2011) with a significance level of $p < 0.05$. All figures were made by Sigmaplot® Version 10 software (Systat Software Inc., Chicago, IL, USA, 2007).

## 3. Results

### 3.1. Squalene Relative Abundance

The squalene component was identified from the soils in all five alpine grasslands, including AM, AS, AMS, ADS, and AD in the Tibetan Plateau using Py-GC/MS (Figure 1). There were significant differences in the squalene relative abundance of the soils among five alpine grassland types (Figure 2).

The relative abundance of squalene of the soils in AD was the highest, with a value of 10.66 ± 2.07%, and that of the soils in ADS was the second highest, with a value of 5.42 ± 1.38%. The squalene relative abundances of the soils in AM, AS, and AMS were significantly lower than those of the soils in AD, with values of 0.93 ± 0.22%, 3.12 ± 1.23%, 1.61 ± 0.52%, respectively.

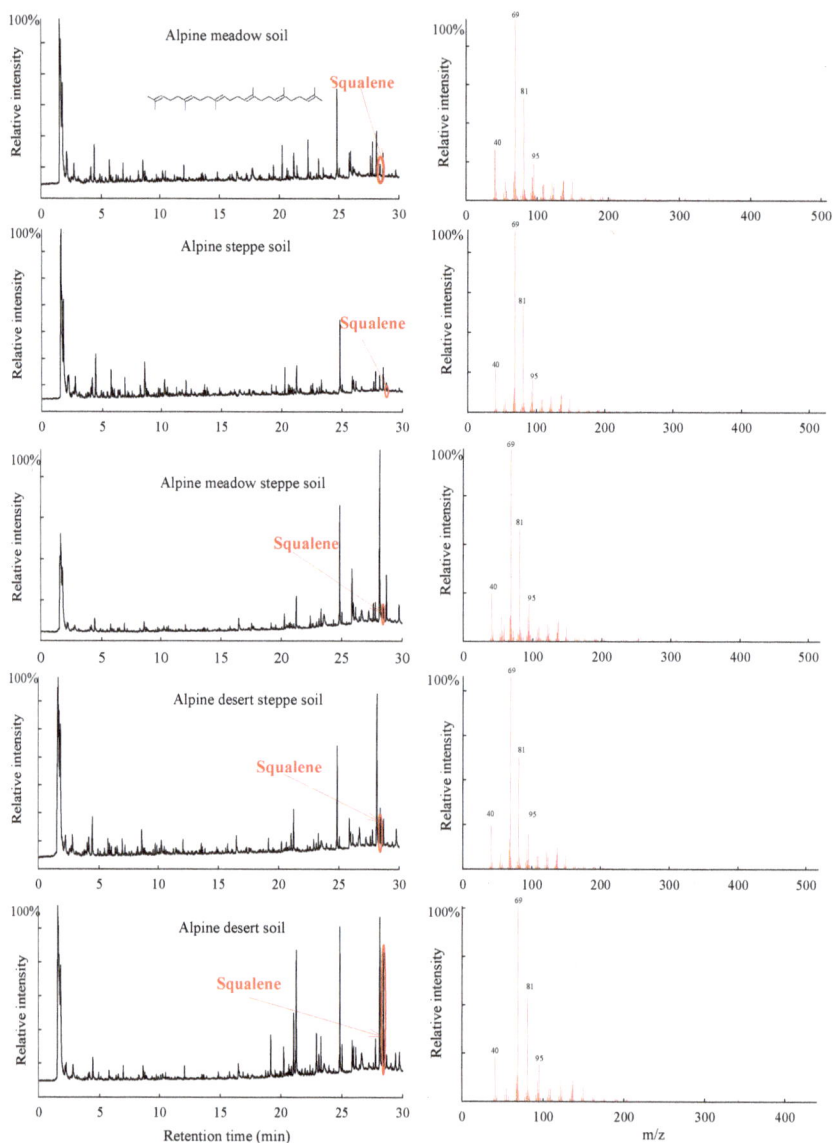

**Figure 1.** The squalene chromatograms (**left**) and mass spectrums (**right**) obtained from alpine grassland soils by pyrolysis gas chromatography–mass spectrometry (Py-GC/MS) in the Tibetan Plateau. m/z: mass-to-charge ratio.

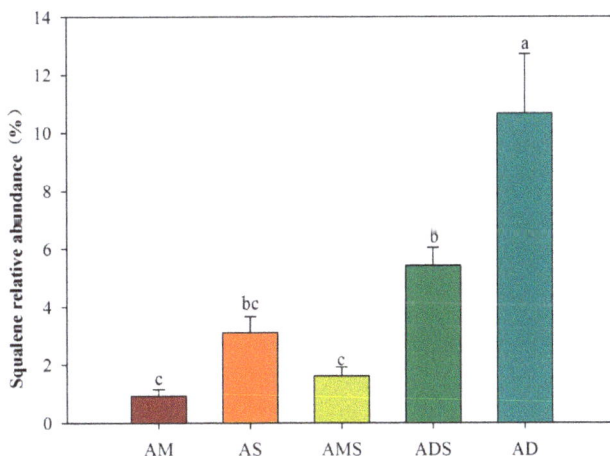

**Figure 2.** Squalene relative abundance in alpine grassland soils in the Tibetan Plateau. AM: alpine meadow, AS: alpine steppe, AMS: alpine meadow steppe, ADS: alpine desert steppe, AD: alpine desert.

*3.2. Soil Chemical/Microbial Characteristics*

Soil pH of the soils in five alpine grasslands was in the range of 7.57–9.52, with the highest value in the AMS soil and the lowest in the AS soil. Significant differences in the soil chemical characteristics were observed among the five types of alpine grassland in northern Tibet (Table 1). The SOC, DOC, TN, and TIN contents were the highest in the AM soil (34.97 ± 2.89 g kg$^{-1}$, 98.39 ± 27.30 mg kg$^{-1}$, 1.18 ± 0.24 g kg$^{-1}$, 39.65 ± 6.68 mg kg$^{-1}$, respectively); these values were 8.02, 4.63, 7.87, and 14.58 times those of the AD soil, respectively, which had the lowest indexes.

**Table 1.** The soil chemical characteristics of alpine grasslands in the Tibetan Plateau.

| Soil Chemical Indexes | pH | SOC (g kg$^{-1}$) | DOC (mg kg$^{-1}$) | TN (g kg$^{-1}$) | TIN (mg kg$^{-1}$) |
|---|---|---|---|---|---|
| AM | 8.00 ± 0.15 [c] | 34.97 ± 2.89 [a] | 98.39 ± 27.30 [a] | 1.19 ± 0.54 [a] | 39.65 ± 6.68 [a] |
| AS | 7.57 ± 0.03 [d] | 17.26 ± 2.48 [b] | 66.21 ± 9.03 [ab] | 0.75 ± 0.32 [ab] | 14.52 ± 2.39 [b] |
| AMS | 9.52 ± 0.21 [a] | 9.75 ± 5.58 [bc] | 41.91 ± 12.84 [b] | 0.42 ± 0.20 [bc] | 13.58 ± 1.16 [b] |
| ADS | 8.46 ± 0.29 [b] | 8.74 ± 1.99 [c] | 36.38 ± 6.28 [b] | 0.34 ± 0.12 [bc] | 5.72 ± 2.71 [b] |
| AD | 8.16 ± 0.11 [bc] | 4.36 ± 0.58 [c] | 21.24 ± 2.73 [b] | 0.15 ± 0.10 [c] | 2.72 ± 1.48 [b] |

AM: alpine meadow, AS: alpine steppe, AMS: alpine meadow steppe, ADS: alpine desert steppe, AD: alpine desert, SOC: soil organic carbon, DOC: dissolved organic carbon, TN: total nitrogen, TIN: total inorganic nitrogen. Values are mean values of soil chemical characteristics ± standard error (S.E.) in alpine grasslands. Values within the same row followed by the same letter are not significantly different at $p < 0.05$.

The absolute abundance of PLFAs in five grassland type soils showed that the richness order of soil samples was as follows: total PLFA, bacteria, fungi, and actinomycetes (Table 2). The total PLFA values were the highest in the AM soils (23.58 ± 2.76 nmol g soil$^{-1}$), at 2.00, 2.37, 5.30 and 6.45 times those of the AS, AMS, ADS and AD soils. The bacterial PLFAs showed a generally similar pattern to that of total PLFAs. The predominant bacteria were most prevalent in the AM soils (22.84 ± 2.95 nmol g soil$^{-1}$) of these five grassland types, and were least prevalent in AD soil (2.57 ± 0.69 nmol g soil$^{-1}$). The amounts of the fungi and actinomycetes were also the highest in the AM soil, at 3.70 ± 0.54 nmol g soil$^{-1}$, and 1.96 ± 0.27 nmol g soil$^{-1}$, respectively, but the lowest values were found in the ADS soils at 0.96 ± 0.15 nmol g soil$^{-1}$ and 0.37 ± 0.15 nmol g soil$^{-1}$, respectively.

**Table 2.** The soil microbial composition characteristics of alpine grasslands in the Tibetan Plateau.

| PLFAs (nmol g$^{-1}$) | Bacteria | Fungi | Actinomycetes | Total |
|---|---|---|---|---|
| AM | 22.84 ± 2.95 [a] | 3.70 ± 0.54 [a] | 1.96 ± 0.27 [a] | 23.58 ± 2.76 [a] |
| AS | 11.32 ± 1.43 [b] | 2.03 ± 0.31 [b] | 1.22 ± 0.15 [b] | 11.81 ± 1.41 [b] |
| AMS | 9.23 ± 1.22 [bc] | 1.86 ± 0.30 [b] | 0.84 ± 0.18 [bc] | 9.96 ± 1.27 [bc] |
| ADS | 3.72 ± 0.93 [cd] | 0.96 ± 0.15 [b] | 0.36 ± 0.15 [c] | 4.45 ± 0.98 [cd] |
| AD | 2.57 ± 0.69 [d] | 1.05 ± 0.25 [b] | 0.55 ± 0.11 [c] | 3.66 ± 0.93 [d] |

PLFAs: phospholipid fatty acids, AM: alpine meadow, AS: alpine steppe, AMS: alpine meadow steppe, ADS: alpine desert steppe, AD: alpine desert. Values are mean values of soil microbial PLFA characteristics ± standard error (S.E.) in alpine grasslands. Values within the same row followed by the same letter are not significantly different at $p < 0.05$.

### 3.3. Relationships between Squalene Relative Abundance and Soil Chemical/Microbial Characteristics

Two principal components were used as tools to distinguish the different grassland ecosystems (AM, AS, AMS, ADS, and AD), considering all properties together (SOC, DOC, TN, TIN, pH, PLFAs, and relative abundance of squalene). The cumulative variation in the distribution of the selected variable was 74.86% and 86.04% for the sum of the principal components PC1 and PC2 in the evaluation performed with soil chemical traits and PLFAs (Figure 3). The analysis of the interaction showed an integrated effect of the grassland ecosystem, soil chemical characteristics, and PLFAs on the relative abundance of soil squalene. For soil chemical characteristics, the relative abundance of squalene had a negative correlation with SOC ($r = -0.616$, $p < 0.01$), DOC ($r = -0.510$, $p < 0.05$), TN ($r = -0.612$, $p < 0.01$), and TIN ($r = -0.579$, $p < 0.01$). Nevertheless, the squalene relative abundance was not in correlation with soil pH. For soil microbial characteristics, the relative abundance of squalene was also significantly negatively correlated with soil PLFA quantity, including soil total PLFA ($r = -0.642$, $p < 0.01$), bacteria PLFAs ($r = -0.650$, $p < 0.01$), fungi PLFAs ($r = -0.576$, $p < 0.01$), and Actinomycete PLFAs ($r = -0.583$, $p < 0.01$).

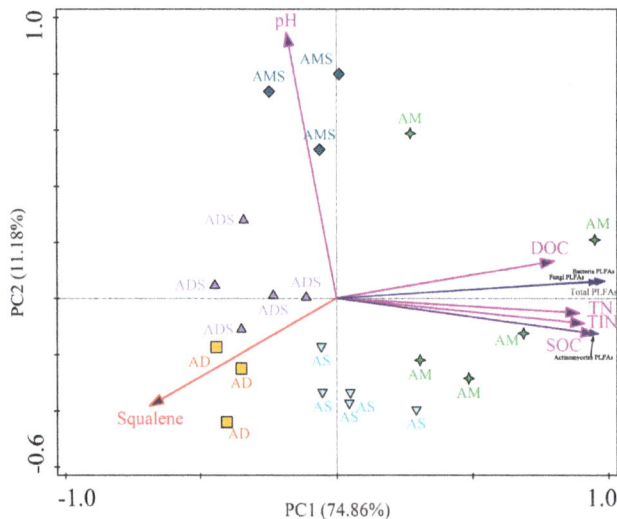

**Figure 3.** The relationships between squalene relative abundances and soil chemical/microbial characteristics in alpine grassland in the Tibetan Plateau. AM: alpine meadow, AS: alpine steppe, AMS: alpine meadow steppe, ADS: alpine desert steppe, AD: alpine desert, PLFAs: phospholipid fatty acids, SOC: soil organic carbon, DOC: dissolved organic carbon, TN: total nitrogen, TIN: total inorganic nitrogen.

## 4. Discussion

Squalene is a natural triterpene known to be an important intermediary of cholesterol/phytosterol biosynthesis in animals, plants, humans, and microorganisms. It is used widely in the food, cosmetic, and medicine industries due to its multiple functions [2,4]. Scientists have discovered that when squalene is found in great proportions in some animals and microorganisms, it is likely to be essential to their survival in extreme environments, especially hostile environments free of oxygen. Some animals include sharks, which live in the deep sea with dark, cold, high-pressure, and oxygen-poor conditions [6]. Other examples include moles, which inhabit a damp environment [12], and yaks, which thrive at altitudes of 2000–5000 m above sea level [21]. Squalene is absorbed and distributed to different organs from many biological sources, and is present in varying quantities [5]. In recent years, the bioavailability of squalene has been well established in cell cultures, animal models, and in humans, and further progress has been made concerning on the intracellular transport of this lipophilic molecule. Squalene accumulates in the animal liver and decreases levels of hepatic cholesterol and triglycerides, with these actions being exerted via a complex network of changes in gene expression at both transcriptional and post-transcriptional levels [5].

The Tibetan Plateau, the highest and most extensive highland in the world, is characterized by a harsh environment and fragile ecosystems at high altitude, with strong solar radiation, drought, low temperatures, and poor levels of oxygen [43]. In the present study, the squalene component was identified from five alpine grassland soils in the Tibetan Plateau by using the Py-GC/MS technique. Py-GC/MS served as a valuable analytical technique because pyrolysis products could be separated by gas chromatography and detected by mass spectrometry. The data by Py-GC/MS do not provide insight into the absolute abundance of compounds across samples, an approach that would require multiple internal standards. However, it is an efficient tool for revealing chemical characteristics in the organic matter of soils through semi-quantitative analyses with a comparison of abundance ratios of selected pyrolysis products [44–46]. A squalene component was found from all the soils in the five alpine grasslands, with relative abundance ranging from 0.93% to 10.66% in the Tibetan Platea, as shown using the Py-GC/MS technique (Figures 1 and 2). Nevertheless, at present the squalene component has only been found in very few soils in other regions, such as tropical rainforest soils in Indonesia [47], temperate broadleaved forest soils in Belgium [48], Mediterranean forest soil located in Spain [49], and agricultural soil in Canada [50]. For most of the soils, the squalene component was not obtained using the same technique [50–54].

In the Tibetan Plateau, squalene was identified in all the alpine grassland soils and some distribution characteristics are shown in Figure 3. The points were scattered among different alpine grassland types, while the points were concentrated in same grassland type. That is to say, the squalene relative abundances were different among different alpine grassland types, while they were similar in the same alpine grassland type (Figure 3). Comparing the five alpine grassland types, the squalene relative abundance was the highest in alpine desert soils, with a value of 10.66 ± 2.07%, and it was the lowest in alpine meadow soils, with the value 0.93 ± 0.22% (Figure 2). Thus, the relative abundance of squalene relative in alpine desert soils was 11.5 times that of alpine meadow soils. This could be attributed to the different environmental conditions in two alpine grassland types. Alpine deserts are distributed in harsher environments; they are the highest and driest grassland type in China and the world [55]. The average annual temperature ranges from $-10\,^{\circ}C$ to $-8\,^{\circ}C$, the average annual precipitation from 20.6 mm to 53.8 mm, and the vegetation total cover from 5% to 14% in the alpine desert area. In the alpine meadow area, the average annual temperature is around $0\,^{\circ}C$, the average annual precipitation ranges from 450 mm to 600 mm, and the total vegetation cover is from 50% to 90% [55–57].

In general, the squalene relative abundance was significantly negatively correlated with soil chemical/microbial characteristics in the Tibetan Plateau (Figure 3). This indicated that the relative abundance of squalene is higher in soils with low microbial quantities and confirmed that squalene is a product of biological adaptation to extreme environments. Soil microbial PLFA quantities in alpine grasslands were positively associated with mean annual temperature, mean annual precipitation, soil organic carbon, and aboveground biomass, and negatively associated with elevation, indicating that the harsh environmental conditions may not benefit the survival of soil microorganisms in the Tibetan Plateau [22,58,59]. Thus, microorganisms may adapt to harsh environmental conditions by increasing the levels of squalene in their bodies. It has been reported that each molecule of squalene could be formed by fusing two molecules of farnesyl diphosphate in microorganisms, and that some special mechanism exists to allow certain microorganisms to independently adapt to extreme environments [3,60]. For instance, prokaryotic hopanoid biosynthesis does not require molecular oxygen as a substrate, and the squalene is directly cyclized by the enzyme squalene-hopene cyclase in hypoxic environments [60]. Squalene has a role in facilitating tighter packing of archaeal lipid mixtures and also influences spatial organization in archaeal membranes of *Halobacterium salinarum*, an extremely halophilic archaeon [61]. Soil organic matter provides energy and the nitrogen elements constituting the nutrients required for the life activity process for microorganisms [62,63]. Therefore, the relationships between squalene abundance and soil chemical characteristics were consistent with its relationships to soil microbes in the Tibetan Plateau (Figure 3).

## 5. Conclusions

Squalene, which is attracting great biological interest due to its beneficial properties and is generally considered to be a product of biological adaptation to extreme environments, was found in all the soils in five alpine grasslands in the Tibetan Plateau using the Py-GC/MS technique. The relative abundance of squalene is higher in soil with low microbial quantities, which in the harsh environmental conditions may not benefit the survival of soil microorganisms in the Tibetan Plateau. This suggests that squalene is possibly a bioactive component for microorganisms in alpine grassland soils to adapt to harsh environmental conditions, especially in oxygen-poor environments. Furthermore, the relative abundance of squalene in alpine grassland soils had a significantly negative correlation with soil chemical/microbial characteristics. Therefore, the harsher the environment, the higher the relative abundance of squalene needed to adapt to this environment in the Tibetan Plateau.

In general, the present study represents preliminary research for squalene in alpine grassland soils; we still do not know which species or populations of microorganisms could biosynthesize squalene, what the mechanism of squalene biosynthesis is in the body of microorganisms, and why and how the extreme environmental conditions stimulate the production of squalene in the soils. In addition, Py-GC/MS is an analytic technique that uses semi-quantitative analyses with a comparison of abundance ratios of selected pyrolysis products. The absolute content of squalene in soils needs to be determined by using an authenticated external standard of squalene. Thus, further in-depth studies concerning squalene distribution, its biosynthesis mechanism, and its relationship with environmental factors are still needed in the Tibetan Plateau.

**Author Contributions:** Conceptualization, X.L. and S.M.; Methodology, X.L. and Y.C.; Software, Y.C. and H.J.; Validation, X.L., S.M., Y.C., D.Y. and H.J.; Formal Analysis, D.Y.; Investigation, S.M.; Resources, X.L.; Data Curation, X.L. and Y.C.; Writing—Original Draft Preparation, X.L.; Writing—Review and Editing, X.L. and S.M.; Funding Acquisition, X.L. and D.Y.

**Funding:** This research was funded by the Natural Science Foundation of China (Grant No. 41671262 and 41877338); the Natural Science Foundation of Tibet Autonomous Region, and the Key Laboratory of Mountain Processes and Ecological Regulation, Chinese Academy of Sciences.

**Conflicts of Interest:** The authors declare no conflict of interest.

## References

1. Amarowicz, P. Squalene: A natural antioxidant? *Eur. J. Lipid Sci. Technol.* **2009**, *111*, 411–412. [CrossRef]
2. Popa, O.; Bsbeanu, N.E.; Popa, I.; Nită, S.; Dinu-Pârvu, C.E. Methods for obtaining and determination of squalene from natural sources. *BioMed Res. Int.* **2015**, *2015*, 367202. [CrossRef] [PubMed]
3. Spanova, M.; Daum, G. Squalene—Biochemistry, molecular biology, process biotechnology, and applications. *Eur. J. Lipid Sci. Technol.* **2011**, *113*, 1299–1320. [CrossRef]

4.  Katabami, A.; Li, L.; Iwasaki, M.; Furubayashi, M.; Saito, K.; Umeno, D. Production of squalene by squalene synthases and their truncated mutants in *Escherichia coli*. *J. Biosci. Bioeng.* **2015**, *119*, 165–171. [CrossRef] [PubMed]

5.  Lou-Bonafonte, J.M.; Martínez-Beamonte, R.; Sanclemente, T.; Surra, J.C.; Herrera-Marcos, L.V.; Sanchez-Marco, J.; Arnal, C.; Osada, J. Current insights into the biological action of squalene. *Mol. Nutr. Food Res.* **2018**, *62*, e1800136. [CrossRef] [PubMed]

6.  Hall, D.W.; Marshall, S.N.; Gordon, K.C.; Killee, D.P. Rapid quantitative determination of squalene in shark liver oils by Raman and IR spectroscopy. *Lipids* **2016**, *51*, 139–147. [CrossRef] [PubMed]

7.  Vadalà, M.; Laurino, C.; Palmieri, L.; Palmieri, B. Shark derivatives (Alkylglycerols, Squalene, Cartilage) as putative nutraceuticals in oncology. *Eur. J. Oncol.* **2017**, *22*, 5–20.

8.  Yuan, C.; Xie, Y.; Jin, R.; Ren, L.; Zhou, L.; Zhu, M.; Ju, Y. Simultaneous analysis of tocopherols, phytosterols, and squalene in vegetable oils by high-performance liquid chromatography. *Food Anal. Methods* **2017**, *10*, 3716–3722. [CrossRef]

9.  Fooshee, D.R.; Aiona, P.K.; Laskin, A.; Laskin, J.; Nizkorodov, S.A.; Baldi, P.F. Atmospheric oxidation of squalene: Molecular study using COBRA modeling and high-resolution mass spectrometry. *Environ. Sci. Technol.* **2015**, *49*, 13304–13313. [CrossRef] [PubMed]

10. Ghimire, G.P.; Thuan, N.H.; Koirala, N.; Sohng, J.K. Advances in biochemistry and microbial production of squalene and its derivatives. *J. Microbiol. Biotechnol.* **2016**, *26*, 441–451. [CrossRef] [PubMed]

11. Xu, W.; Ma, X.; Wang, Y. Production of squalene by microbes: An update. *World J. Microbiol. Biotechnol.* **2016**, *32*, 195. [CrossRef] [PubMed]

12. Fagundes, M.B.; Vendruscolo, R.G.; Maroneze, M.M.; Barin, J.S.; de Menezes, C.R.; Zepka, L.Q.; Jacob-Lopes, E.; Wagner, R. Towards a sustainable route for the production of squalene using cyanobacteria. *Waste Biomass Valorization* **2018**, *3*, 1–8. [CrossRef]

13. Qiu, J. China: The third pole. *Nature* **2008**, *454*, 393–396. [CrossRef] [PubMed]

14. Yao, T.; Thompson, L.G.; Mosbrugger, V.; Zhang, F.; Ma, Y.; Luo, T.; Xu, B.; Yang, X.; Joswiak, D.R.; Wang, W.; et al. Third Pole Environment (TPE). *Environ. Dev.* **2012**, *3*, 52–64. [CrossRef]

15. Yang, Y.; Gao, Y.; Wang, S.; Xu, D.; Yu, H.; Wu, L.; Lin, Q.; Hu, Y.; Li, X.; He, Z.; et al. The microbial gene diversity along an elevation gradient of the Tibetan grassland. *ISME J.* **2014**, *8*, 430–440. [CrossRef] [PubMed]

16. Guo, G.; Kong, W.; Liu, J.; Zhao, J.; Du, H.; Zhang, X.; Xia, P. Diversity and distribution of autotrophic microbial community along environmental gradients in grassland soils on the Tibetan Plateau. *Appl. Microbiol. Biotechnol.* **2015**, *99*, 8765–8776. [CrossRef] [PubMed]

17. Pugnaire, F.I.; Zhang, L.; Li, R.; Luo, T. No evidence of facilitation collapse in the Tibetan plateau. *J. Veg. Sci.* **2015**, *26*, 233–242. [CrossRef]

18. Pan, S.; Zhang, T.; Rong, Z.; Hu, L.; Gu, Z.; Wu, Q.; Dong, S.; Liu, Q.; Lin, Z.; Deutschova, L.; et al. Population transcriptomes reveal synergistic responses of DNA polymorphism and RNA expression to extreme environments on the Qinghai-Tibetan Plateau in a predatory bird. *Mol. Ecol.* **2017**, *26*, 2993–3010. [CrossRef] [PubMed]

19. Liu, J.; Nan, P.; Wang, L.; Wang, Q.; Tsering, T.; Zhong, Y. Chemical variation in lipophilic composition of *Lamiophlomis rotata* from the Qinghai-Tibetan Plateau. *Chem. Nat. Compd.* **2006**, *42*, 525–528. [CrossRef]

20. Yuan, L.; Zhong, G.; Quan, H.; Tian, F.; Zhong, Z.; Lan, X. GC-MS study on chemical components of volatile oil from roots of *Rhodiola crenulata* growing in Tibet. *Chin. J. Exp. Tradit. Med. Formulae* **2012**, *18*, 67–70, (In Chinese with English Abstract).

21. Liu, C.; Jin, G.; Luo, Z.; Li, S.; Sun, S.; Li, Y.; Ma, M. Chinese yak and yellow cattle exhibit considerable differences in tissue content of squalene, tocopherol, and fatty acids. *Eur. J. Lipid Sci. Technol.* **2015**, *117*, 899–902. [CrossRef]

22. Chen, Y.L.; Ding, J.Z.; Peng, Y.F.; Li, F.; Yang, G.B.; Liu, L.; Qin, S.Q.; Fang, K.; Yang, Y.H. Patterns and drivers of soil microbial communities in Tibetan alpine and global terrestrial ecosystems. *J. Biogeogr.* **2016**, *43*, 2027–2039. [CrossRef]

23. Qi, Q.; Zhao, M.; Wang, S.; Ma, X.; Wang, Y.; Gao, Y.; Lin, Q.; Li, X.; Gu, B.; Li, G.; et al. The biogeographic pattern of microbial functional genes along an altitudinal gradient of the Tibetan pasture. *Front. Microbiol.* **2017**, *8*, 976. [CrossRef] [PubMed]

24. Yang, T.; Adams, J.M.; Shi, Y.; He, J.S.; Jing, X.; Chen, L.; Tedersoo, L.; Chu, H. Soil fungal diversity in natural grasslands of the Tibetan Plateau: Associations with plant diversity and productivity. *New Phytol.* **2017**, *215*, 756–765. [CrossRef] [PubMed]

25. Immerzeel, W.W.; Beek, L.P.H.; Bierkens, M.F.P. Climate change will affect the Asian water towers. *Science* **2010**, *328*, 1382–1385. [CrossRef] [PubMed]

26. Bibi, S.; Wang, L.; Li, X.; Zhou, J.; Chen, D.; Yao, T. Climatic and associated cryospheric, biospheric, and hydrological changes on the Tibetan Plateau: A review. *Int. J. Climatol.* **2018**, *38*, e1–e17. [CrossRef]

27. Lu, X.; Yan, Y.; Sun, J.; Zhang, X.; Chen, Y.; Wang, X.; Cheng, G. Carbon, nitrogen, and phosphorus storage in alpine grassland ecosystems of Tibet: Effects of grazing exclusion. *Ecol. Evol.* **2015**, *5*, 4492–4504. [CrossRef] [PubMed]

28. Gai, J.P.; Christie, P.; Cai, X.B.; Fan, J.Q.; Zhang, J.L.; Feng, G.; Li, X.L. Occurrence and distribution of arbuscular mycorrhizal fungal species in three types of grassland community of the Tibetan Plateau. *Ecol. Res.* **2009**, *24*, 1345–1350. [CrossRef]

29. Lu, X.; Yan, Y.; Sun, J.; Zhang, X.; Chen, Y.; Wang, X.; Cheng, G. Short-term grazing exclusion has no impact on soil properties and nutrients of degraded alpine grassland in Tibet, China. *Solid Earth* **2015**, *6*, 1195–1205. [CrossRef]

30. Prayogo, C.; Jones, J.E.; Baeyens, J.; Bending, G.D. Impact of biochar on mineralisation of C and N from soil and willow litter and its relationship with microbial community biomass and structure. *Biol. Fertil. Soils* **2014**, *50*, 695–702. [CrossRef]

31. Hannam, K.D.; Quideau, S.A.; Kishchuk, B.E. Forest floor microbial communities in relation to stand composition and timber harvesting in northern Alberta. *Soil Biol. Biochem.* **2006**, *38*, 2565–2575. [CrossRef]

32. Pankhurst, C.E.; Yu, S.; Hawke, B.G.; Harch, B.D. Capacity of fatty acid profiles and substrate utilization patterns to describe differences in soil microbial communities associated with increased salinity or alkalinity at three locations in South Australia. *Biol. Fertil. Soils* **2001**, *33*, 204–217. [CrossRef]

33. Arthur, M.A.; Bray, S.R.; Kuchle, C.R.; McEwan, R.W. The influence of the invasive shrub, *Lonicera maackii*, on leaf decomposition and microbial community dynamics. *Plant Ecol.* **2012**, *213*, 1571–1582. [CrossRef]

34. McMahon, S.; Schimel, J.P. Shifting patterns of microbial N-metabolism across seasons in upland Alaskan tundra soils. *Soil Biol. Biochem.* **2017**, *105*, 96–107. [CrossRef]

35. Sun, S.Q.; Liu, T.; Wu, Y.H.; Wang, G.X.; Zhu, B.; DeLuca, T.H.; Wang, Y.Q.; Luo, J. Ground bryophytes regulate net soil carbon efflux: Evidence from two subalpine ecosystems on the east edge of the Tibet Plateau. *Plant Soil* **2017**, *417*, 363–375. [CrossRef]

36. Jílková, V.; Cajthaml, T.; Frouz, J. Relative importance of honeydew and resin for the microbial activity in wood ant nest and forest floor substrate—A laboratory study. *Soil Biol. Biochem.* **2018**, *117*, 1–4. [CrossRef]

37. Yang, B.; Pang, X.Y.; Hu, B.; Bao, W.K.; Tian, G.L. Does thinning-induced gap size result in altered soil microbial community in pine plantaton in eastern Tibetan Plateau? *Ecol. Evol.* **2017**, *7*, 2986–2993. [CrossRef] [PubMed]

38. Jiao, F.; Shi, X.R.; Han, F.P.; Yuan, Z.Y. Increasing aridity, temperature and soil pH induce soil C-N-P imbalance in grasslands. *Sci. Rep.* **2016**, *6*, 1–9. [CrossRef] [PubMed]

39. Chen, Q.Q.; Sun, Y.M.; Shen, C.D.; Peng, S.L.; Yi, W.X.; Li, Z.A.; Jiang, M.T. Organic matter turnover rates and $CO_2$ flux from organic matter decomposition of mountain soil profiles in the subtropical area, south China. *Catena* **2002**, *49*, 217–229. [CrossRef]

40. Liang, B.; Yang, X.Y.; He, X.H.; Zhou, J.B. Effects of 17-year fertilization on soil microbial biomass C and N and soluble organic C and N in loessial soil during maize growth. *Biol. Fertil. Soils* **2011**, *47*, 121–128. [CrossRef]

41. Kalbitz, K.; Geyer, S. Different effects of peat degradation on dissolved organic carbon and nitrogen. *Org. Geochem.* **2002**, *33*, 319–326. [CrossRef]

42. Downing, D.T.; Stewart, M.E. Skin surface lipids of the mole *Scalopus aquaticus*. *Comp. Biochem. Physiol. Part B Comp. Biochem.* **1987**, *86*, 667–670. [CrossRef]

43. Sun, J.; Zhou, T.; Liu, M.; Chen, Y.; Shang, H.; Zhu, L.; Shedayi, A.A.; Yu, H.; Cheng, G.; Liu, G.; et al. Linkages of the dynamics of glaciers and lakes with the climate elements over the Tibetan Plateau. *Earth-Sci. Rev.* **2018**, *185*, 308–324. [CrossRef]

44. Dai, X.Y.; Ping, C.L.; Michaelson, G. J. Characterizing soil organic matter in Arctic tundra soil by different analytical approaches. *Org. Geochem.* **2002**, *33*, 407–419. [CrossRef]

45. Grandy, A.; Sinsabaugh, R.; Neff, J.; Stursova, M.; Zak, D. Nitrogen deposition effects on soil organic matter chemistry are linked to variation in enzymes, ecosystems and size fractions. *Biogeochemistry* **2008**, *91*, 37–49. [CrossRef]

46. Ma, S.Q.; Chen, Y.C.; Lu, X.Y.; Wang, X.D. Soil Organic Matter Chemistry: Based on Pyrolysis-Gas Chromatography- Mass Spectrometry (Py-GC/MS). *Mini-Rev. Org. Matter* **2018**, *15*, 389–403. [CrossRef]

47. Yassir, I.; Buurman, P. Soil organic matter chemistry changes upon secondary succession in Imperata Grasslands, Indonesia: A pyrolysis–GC/MS study. *Geoderma* **2012**, *173–174*, 94–103. [CrossRef]

48. Vancampenhout, K.; De Vos, B.; Wouters, K.; Swennen, R.; Buurman, P.; Deckers, J. Organic matter of subsoil horizons under broadleaved forest: Highly processed or labile and plant-derived? *Soil Biol. Biochem.* **2012**, *50*, 40–46. [CrossRef]

49. Campo, J.; Nierop, K.G.J.; Cammeraat, E.; Andreu, V.; Rubio, J.L. Application of pyrolysis-gas chromatography/mass spectrometry to study changes in the organic matter of macro- and microaggregates of a Mediterranean soil upon heating. *J. Chromatogr. A* **2011**, *1218*, 4817–4827. [CrossRef] [PubMed]

50. Jeannottea, R.; Hamela, C.; Jabaji, S.; Whalena, J.K. Pyrolysis-mass spectrometry and gas chromatography-flame ionization detection as complementary tools for soil lipid characterization. *J. Anal. Appl. Pyrolysis* **2011**, *90*, 232–237. [CrossRef]

51. Dai, X.Y.; White, D.; Ping, C.L. Comparing bioavailability in five Arctic soils by pyrolysis-gas chromatography/mass spectrometry. *J. Anal. Appl. Pyrolysis* **2002**, *62*, 249–258. [CrossRef]

52. Buurman, P.; Peterse, F.; Martin, G.A. Soil organic matter chemistry in allophanic soils: A pyrolysis-GC/MS study of a Costa Rican Andosol catena. *Eur. J. Soil Sci.* **2007**, *58*, 1330–1347. [CrossRef]

53. Grandy, A.S.; Strickland, M.S.; Lauber, C.L.; Bradford, M.A.; Fierer, N. The influence of microbial communities, management, and soil texture on soil organic matter chemistry. *Geoderma* **2009**, *150*, 278–286. [CrossRef]

54. Carr, A.S.; Boom, A.; Chase, B.M.; Meadows, M.E.; Roberts, Z.E.; Britton, M.N.; Cumming, A.M.J. Biome-scale characterisation and differentiation of semi-arid and arid zone soil organic matter compositions using pyrolysis–GC/MS analysis. *Geoderma* **2013**, *200–201*, 189–201. [CrossRef]

55. Land Management Bureau of Tibet. *Grassland Resources in Tibet Autonomous Region*; Sciences Press: Beijing, China, 1994. (In Chinese)

56. Yu, G.; Tang, L.; Yang, X.; Ke, X.; Harrison, S.P. Modern pollen samples from alpine vegetation on the Tibetan Plateau. *Glob. Ecol. Biogeogr.* **2001**, *10*, 503–520. [CrossRef]

57. Yan, Y.; Lu, X. Is grazing exclusion effective in restoring vegetation in degraded alpine grasslands in Tibet, China? *PeerJ* **2015**, *3*, e1020. [CrossRef] [PubMed]

58. Xu, M.; Li, X.; Cai, X.; Gai, J.; Li, X.; Christie, P.; Zhang, J. Soil microbial community structure and activity along a montane elevational gradient on the Tibetan Plateau. *Eur. J. Soil Biol.* **2014**, *64*, 6–14. [CrossRef]

59. Liu, X.; Cong, J.; Lu, H.; Xue, Y.; Wang, X.; Li, D.; Zhang, Y. Community structure and elevational distribution pattern of soil Actinobacteria in alpine grasslands. *Acta Ecol. Sin.* **2017**, *37*, 213–218. [CrossRef]

60. Takishita, K.; Chikaraishi, Y.; Leger, M.M.; Kim, E.; Yabuki, A.; Ohkouchi, N.; Roger, A.J. Lateral transfer of tetrahymanol-synthesizing genes has allowed multiple diverse eukaryote lineages to independently adapt to environments without oxygen. *Biol. Direct* **2012**, *7*, 5. [CrossRef] [PubMed]

61. Gilmore, S.F.; Yao, A.I.; Tietel, Z.; Kind, T.; Facciotti, M.T.; Parikh, A.N. Role of squalene in the organization of monolayers derived from lipid extracts of *Halobacterium salinarum*. *Langmuir* **2013**, *29*, 7922–7930. [CrossRef] [PubMed]

62. Yang, Y.; Zhang, N.; Xue, M.; Lu, S.T.; Tao, S. Effects of soil organic matter on the development of the microbial polycyclic aromatic hydrocarbons (PAHs) degradation potentials. *Environ. Pollut.* **2011**, *159*, 591–595. [CrossRef] [PubMed]

63. Kuzyakov, Y.; Xu, X. Competition between roots and microorganisms for nitrogen: Mechanisms and ecological relevance. *New Phytol.* **2013**, *198*, 656–669. [CrossRef] [PubMed]

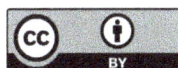

MDPI

St. Alban-Anlage 66

4052 Basel

Switzerland

Tel. +41 61 683 77 34

Fax +41 61 302 89 18

www.mdpi.com

*Education Sciences* Editorial Office

E-mail: education@mdpi.com

www.mdpi.com/journal/education

www.ingramcontent.com/pod-product-compliance
Lightning Source LLC
Chambersburg PA
CBHW041218220326
41597CB00033BA/6029